GEORGE HENRY LEWES

THE PHYSICAL BASIS OF MIND

BEING THE SECOND SERIES

OF

PROBLEMS OF LIFE AND MIND

Elibron Classics
www.elibron.com

Elibron Classics series.

ISBN 0-543-97580-0 (paperback)
ISBN 0-543-97579-7 (hardcover)

This Elibron Classics Replica Edition is an unabridged facsimile
of the edition published in 1877 by Trübner and Co., London.

THE

PHYSICAL BASIS OF MIND.

Works by the same Author.

PROBLEMS OF LIFE AND MIND. *The Foundations of a Creed.* Two Vols. Third Edition.

CONTENTS: The Method of Science and its Applications to Metaphysics—The Rules of Philosophizing—Psychological Principles—The Limitations of Knowledge—The Principles of Certitude—From the Known to the Unknown—Matter and Force—Force and Cause—The Absolute in the Correlations of Feeling and Motion.

HISTORY OF PHILOSOPHY FROM THALES TO COMTE. Two Vols. Fourth Edition.

THE LIFE OF GOETHE. Third Edition.

ARISTOTLE. A CHAPTER FROM THE HISTORY OF SCIENCE, INCLUDING ANALYSES OF ARISTOTLE'S SCIENTIFIC WRITINGS.

THE PHYSIOLOGY OF COMMON LIFE. Two Vols. With Illustrations.

SEASIDE STUDIES AT ILFRACOMBE, TENBY, THE SCILLY ISLES, AND JERSEY. With Illustrations. Second Edition.

STUDIES IN ANIMAL LIFE. With Illustrations.

THE PHYSICAL BASIS OF MIND.

With Illustrations.

BEING THE SECOND SERIES

OF

PROBLEMS OF LIFE AND MIND.

BY

GEORGE HENRY LEWES.

LONDON:
TRÜBNER & CO., LUDGATE HILL.
1877.

PRINTED BY BALLANTYNE, HANSON AND CO.
EDINBURGH AND LONDON

PREFACE.

THE title indicates that this volume is restricted to the group of material conditions which constitute the organism in relation to the physical world—a group which furnishes the data for one half of the psychologist's quest; the other half being furnished by historical and social conditions.

The Human Mind, so far as it is accessible to scientific inquiry, has a twofold root, man being not only an animal organism but an unit in the social organism; and hence the complete theory of its functions and faculties must be sought in this twofold direction. This conception (which has been declared "to amount to a revolution in Psychology"), although slowly prepared by the growing conviction that Man could not be isolated from Humanity, was first expounded in the opening volume of these *Problems of Life and Mind;* at least, I am not aware that any predecessor had seen *how* the specially human faculties of Intellect and Conscience were products of social factors co-operating with the animal factors.

In considering the Physical Basis a large place must be assigned to the mechanical and chemical relations which are involved in organic functions; yet we have to recognise that this procedure of Analysis is artificial and preparatory, that none of its results are final, none represent the synthetic reality of *vital* facts. Hence one leading object of the following pages has been everywhere to substitute the biological point of view for the metaphysical and mechanical points of view which too often obstruct research—the one finding its expression in spiritualist theories, the other in materialist theories; both disregarding the plain principle that the first requisite in a theory of biological phenomena must be to view them in the light of biological conditions: in other words, to fix our gaze upon what passes in the organism, and not on what may pass in the laboratory, where the conditions are different. Analysis is a potent instrument, but is too often relied on in forgetfulness of what constitutes its real aid, and thus leads to a disregard of all those conditions which it has artificially set aside. We see this in the tendency of anatomists and physiologists to assign to *one* element, in a complex cluster of co-operants, the significance which properly belongs to that cluster: as when the property of a tissue is placed exclusively in a single element of that tissue, the function of an organ assigned to its chief tissue, and a function of the organism to a single organ.

Another object has been to furnish the reader uninstructed in physiology with such a general outline of the structure and functions of the organism, and such details respecting the sentient mechanism, as may awaken an interest in the study, and enable him to understand the application of Physiology to Psychology. If he comes upon details which can only interest specially educated students, or perhaps only by them be really understood, he can pass over these details, for their omission will not seriously affect the bearing of the general principles. I have given the best I had to give; and must leave each reader to find in it whatever may interest him. The uses of books are first to stimulate inquiry by awakening an interest; secondly, to clarify and classify the knowledge already gained from direct contemplation of the phenomena. They are stimuli and aids to observation and thought. They should never be allowed to see for us, nor to think for us.

The volume contains four essays. The first, on the *Nature of Life*, deals with the speciality of organic phenomena, as distinguished from the inorganic. It sets forth the physiological principles which Psychology must incessantly invoke. In the course of the exposition I have incorporated several passages from four articles on Mr. Darwin's hypotheses, contributed to the *Fortnightly Review* during the year 1868. I have also suggested a modification of the hypothesis of Natural Selection, by extending to the *tissues and organs* that principle of competition which Mr. Darwin has so luminously applied to *organisms.* Should this generalisation of the "struggle for existence" be accepted, it will answer many of the hitherto unanswerable objections.

The second essay is on the *Nervous Mechanism,* setting forth what is known and what is inferred respecting the structure and properties of that all-important system. If the sceptical and revolutionary attitude, in presence of opinions currently held to be established truths, surprises or pains the reader unprepared for such doubts, I can only ask him to submit my statements to a similar scepticism, and confront them with the ascertained evidence. After many years of laborious investigation and meditation, the conclusion has slowly forced itself upon me, that on this subject there is a "false persuasion of knowledge" very fatal in its influence, because unhesitatingly adopted as the ground of speculation both in Pathology and Psychology. This persuasion is sustained because few are aware how much of what passes for observation is in reality sheer hypothesis. I have had to point out the great extent to which Imaginary Anatomy has been unsuspectingly accepted; and hope to have done something towards raising a rational misgiving in the student's mind respecting "the superstition of the nerve-cell"—a superstition which I freely confess to have shared in for many years.

The third essay treats of *Animal Automatism.* Here the constant insistance on the biological point of view, while it causes a rejection of the mechanical theory, admits the fullest recognition of all the mechanical relations involved in animal movements, and thus endeavours to reconcile the contending schools. In this essay I have also attempted a psychological solution of that much-debated question —the relation between Body and Mind. This solution explains why physical and mental phenomena must necessarily present to our apprehension such profoundly diverse characters; and shows that Materialism, in attempting to deduce the mental from the physical, puts into the conclusion what the very terms have excluded from the premisses; whereas, on the hypothesis of a physical process being only the objective aspect of a mental process, the attempt to interpret the one by the other is as legitimate as the solution of a geometrical problem by algebra.

In the final essay the *Reflex Theory* is discussed; and here once more the biological point of view rectifies the error of an analysis which has led to the denial of Sensibility in reflex actions, because that analysis has overlooked the necessary presence of the conditions which determine Sensibility. In these chapters are reproduced several passages from the *Physiology of Common Life.*

According to my original intention, this volume was to have included an exposition of the part I conceive the brain to play in physiological and psychological processes, but that must be postponed until it can be accompanied by a survey of psychological processes which would render the exposition more intelligible.

The Priory, *March* 1877.

CONTENTS.

PROBLEM I. THE NATURE OF LIFE.

CHAPTER I.

CHAPTER II.

CHAPTER III.

CHAPTER IV.

CHAPTER V.

PROBLEM II. THE NERVOUS MECHANISM.

CHAPTER I.

CHAPTER II.

CHAPTER III.

CHAPTER IV.

CHAPTER V.

CHAPTER VI.

CHAPTER VII.

CHAPTER VIII.

PROBLEM III. ANIMAL AUTOMATISM.

CHAPTER I.

CHAPTER II.

CHAPTER III.

CHAPTER IV.

CHAPTER V.

CHAPTER VI.

CHAPTER VII.

PROBLEM IV. THE REFLEX THEORY.

CHAPTER I.

CHAPTER II.

CHAPTER III.

CHAPTER IV.

PROBLEM I.

THE NATURE OF LIFE.

"La Physiologie a pour but d'exposer les phénomènes de la vie humaine et les conditions d'où ils dépendent. Pour y arriver d'une manière sûre, il faut nécessairement avant tout déterminer quels sont les phénomènes qu'on désigne sous le nom de *vie* en général. C'est pourquoi la première chose à faire est d'étudier les propriétés générales du corps qu'on appelle organiques ou vivans."

TIEDEMANN: *Traité de Physiologie de l'Homme*, i. 2.

"Some weak and inexperienced persons vainly seek by dialectics and far-fetched arguments either to upset or establish things that are only to be founded on anatomical demonstration and believed on the evidence of the senses. He who truly desires to be informed of the question in hand must be held bound either to look for himself, or to take on trust the conclusions to which they who have looked have come to."

HARVEY: *Second Dissertation to Riolan.*

THE NATURE OF LIFE.

CHAPTER I.

THE PROBLEM STATED.

1. ALTHOUGH for convenience we use the terms Life and Mind as representing distinct orders of phenomena, the one objective and the other subjective, and although for centuries they have designated distinct entities, or forces having different substrata, we may now consider it sufficiently acknowledged among scientific thinkers that every problem of Mind is necessarily a problem of Life, referring to one special group of vital activities. It is enough that Mind is never manifested except in a living organism to make us seek in an analysis of organic phenomena for the material conditions of every mental fact. Mental phenomena when observed in others, although interpretable by our consciousness of what is passing in ourselves, can only be objective phenomena of the vital organism.

2. On this ground, if on this alone, an acquaintance with the general principles of structure and function is indispensable to the psychologist; although only of late years has this been fully recognised, so that men profoundly ignorant of the organism have had no hesitation in theorising on its highest functions. In saying that such knowledge is indispensable, I do not mean that in the absence of such knowledge a man is debarred from understanding much of the results reached by investigators, nor that he may not himself

make useful observations and classifications of psychological facts. It is possible to read books on Natural History with intelligence and profit, and even to make good observations, without a scientific groundwork of biological instruction; and it is possible to arrive at empirical facts of hygiene and medical treatment without any physiological instruction. But in all three cases the absence of a scientific basis will render the knowledge fragmentary and incomplete; and this ought to deter every one from offering an opinion on debatable questions which pass beyond the limit of subjective observations. The psychologist who has not prepared himself by a study of the organism has no more right to be heard on the genesis of the psychical states, or of the relations between body and mind, than one of the laity has a right to be heard on a question of medical treatment.

THE POSITION OF BIOLOGY.

3. Science is the systematic classification of Experience. It postulates unity of Existence, with great varieties in the Modes of Existence; assuming that there is one Matter everywhere the same, under great diversities in the complications of its elements. The distinction of Modes is not less indispensable than the identification of the elements. These Modes range themselves under three supreme heads: Force, Life, Mind. Under the first, range the general properties exhibited by *all* substances; under the second, the general properties exhibited by *organised* substances; under the third, the general properties exhibited by organised *animal* substances. The first class is subdivided into *Physics*, celestial and terrestrial, and *Chemistry*. Physics treats of substances which move as masses, or which vibrate and rotate as molecules, without undergoing any appreciable change of structural integrity: they show changes of *position* and *state*, without corresponding changes in their elements. Chemistry treats of substances which undergo molecular changes of composition *destructive* of their integrity. Thus the blow which simply moves one body, or makes it vibrate, explodes

another. The friction which alters the temperature and electrical state of a bit of glass, ignites a bit of phosphorus, and so destroys its integrity of structure, converting phosphorus into phosphoric acid.

4. The second class, while exhibiting both physical and chemical properties, is markedly distinguished by the addition of properties called vital. Their peculiarity consists in this: they undergo molecular changes of composition and decomposition which are simultaneous, and *by this simultaneity preserve their integrity of structure.* They change their state, and their elements, yet preserve their unity, and even when differentiating continue specific. Unlike all other bodies, the organised are born, grow, develop, and decay, through a prescribed series of graduated evolutions, each stage being the indispensable condition of its successor, no stage ever appearing except in its serial order.

5. The third class, while exhibiting all the characteristics of the two preceding classes, is specialised by the addition of a totally new property, called Sensibility, which subjectively is Feeling. Here organised substance has become animal substance, and Vegetality has been developed into Animality by the addition of new factors—new complexities of the elementary forces. Many, if not most, philosophers postulate an entirely new Existence, and not simply a new Mode, to account for the manifestations of Mind; they refuse to acknowledge it to be a vital manifestation, they demand that to Life be added a separate substratum, the Soul. This is not a point to be discussed here. We may be content with the assertion that however great the phenomenal difference between Humanity and Animality (a difference we shall hereafter see to be the expression of a new factor, namely, the social factor), nevertheless the distinctive attribute of Sensibility, out of which rise Emotion and Cognition, marks the inseparable *kinship* of mental with vital phenomena.

Thus all the various Modes of Existence may, at least in their objective aspect, be ranged under the two divisions of Inorganic and Organic—Non-living and Living—and these are respectively the objects of the cosmological and the biological sciences.

6. The various sciences in their serial development develop the whole art of Method. Mathematics develops abstraction, deduction, and definition; Astronomy abstraction, deduction, and observation; Physics adds experiment; Chemistry adds nomenclature; Biology adds classification, and for the first time brings into prominence the important notion of *conditions of existence*, and the variation of phenomena under varying conditions: so that the relation of the organism to its medium is one never to be left out of sight. In Biology also clearly emerges for the first time what I regard as the true notion of causality, namely, the *procession* of causes,—the combination of factors in the product, and not an *ab extra* determination of the product. In Vitality and Sensibility we are made aware that the causes are *in* and not *outside* the organism; that the organic effect is the organic cause in operation; that there is autonomy but no autocracy; the effect issues as a resultant of the co-operating conditions. In Sociology, finally, we see brought into prominence the *historical conditions of existence*. From the due appreciation of the conditions of existence, material and historical, we seize the true significance of the principle of Relativity.

7. Having thus indicated the series of the abstract sciences we have now to consider more closely the character of Biology. The term was proposed independently yet simultaneously in Germany and France, in the year 1802, by Treviranus and Lamarck, to express "the study of the forms and phenomena of Life, the conditions and laws by which these exist, and the causes which produce them." Yet only of late years has it gained general acceptance in France and England. The term Cosmology, for what are usually called the Physical Sciences, has not yet come into general use, although its appropriateness must eventually secure its recognition.

Biology—the abstract science of Life—embracing the whole organic world, includes Vegetality, Animality, and Humanity;

the biological sciences are Phytology, Zoology, and Anthropology. Each of the sciences has its cardinal divisions, statical and dynamical, namely, Morphology—the science of form,—and Physiology—the science of function.

Morphology embraces—1°, *Anatomy, i.e.,* the description of the parts then and there present in the organism; and these parts, or organs, are further described by the enumeration of their constituent tissues and elements; and of these again the proximate principles, so far as they can be isolated without chemical decomposition. 2°, *Organogeny, i.e.,* the history of the evolution of organs and tissues.

Physiology embraces the properties and functions of the tissues and organs—the primary conditions of Growth and Development out of which rise the higher functions bringing the organism into active relation with the surrounding medium. The first group of properties and functions are called those of vegetal, or organic life; the second those of animal, or relative life.

ORGANISMS.

8. It will be needful to fix with precision the terms, Organism, Life, Property, and Function.

An organism, although usually signifying a more or less complex unity of organs, because the structures which first attracted scientific attention were all thus markedly distinguished from inorganic bodies, has by the gradual extensions of research been necessarily generalised, till it now stands for any organised substance capable of independent vitality: in other words, any substance having the specific combination of elements which manifests the serial phenomena of growth, development, and decay. There are organisms that have no differentiated organs. Thus a microscopic formless lump of semifluid jelly-like substance (Protoplasm) is called an organism, because it feeds itself, and reproduces itself. There are advantages and disadvantages in such extensions of terms. These are notable in the parallel extension of the term Life, which originally expressing only the complex activities of complex organisms, has come to express the simplest activities of protoplasm. Thus a Monad is an organism; a Cell is an organism; a Plant is an organism; a Man is an organism. And each of these organisms is said to have its Life, because

> "Through all the mighty commonwealth of things
> Up from the creeping worm to sovereign man" *

there is one fundamental group of conditions, one organised substance, one vitality.

Obviously this unity is an abstraction. In reality, the life manifested in the Man is *not* the life manifested in the Monad: he has Functions and Faculties which the Monad has no trace of; and if the two organisms have certain vital characteristics in common, this unity is only recognised in an *ideal construction* which lets drop all concrete differences. The Life is different when the organism is different. Hence any definition of Life would be manifestly insufficient which while it expressed the activities of the Monad left unexpressed the conspicuous and important activities of higher organisms. A sundial and a repeater will each record the successive positions of the sun in the heavens; but although both are instruments for marking time, the sundial will not do the work of the repeater; the complexity and delicacy of the watch mechanism are necessary for its more varied and delicate uses. A semifluid bit of protoplasm will feed itself; but it will not feed and sustain a complex animal; nor will it feel and think.

9. Neglect of this point has caused frequent confusion in the attempts to give satisfactory definitions. Biologists ought to have been warned by the fact that some of the most widely-accepted definitions exclude the most conspicuous phenomena of Life, and are only applicable to the vegetable world, or to the vegetal processes in the animal world. A definition, however abstract, should not exclude essential characters. The general consent of mankind has made Life synonymous with Mode of Existence. By the life of an

* WORDSWORTH.

animal is meant the existence of that animal; when dead the *animal* no longer exists; the substances of which the organism was composed exist, but under another mode; their connexus is altered, and the organism vanishes in the alteration. It is a serious mistake to call the corpse an organism; for that *special* combination which constituted the organism is not present in the corpse. This misconception misleads some speculative minds into assigning life to the universe. The universe assuredly exists, but it does not live; its existence can only be identified with life, such as we observe in organisms, by a complete obliteration of the speciality which the term Life is meant to designate. Yet many have not only pleased themselves with such a conception, but have conceived the universe to be an organism fashioned, directed, and sustained by a soul like that of man —the *anima mundi.* This is to violate all scientific canons. The life of a plant-organism is not the same as the life of an animal-organism; the life of an animal-organism is not the same as the life of a human-organism; nor can the life of a human-organism be the same as the life of the world-organism. The unity of Existences does not obliterate the variety of Modes; yet it is the speciality of each Mode which Science investigates; to some of these Modes the term Life is consistently applied, to others not; and if we merge them all in a common term, we must then invent a new term to designate the Modes now included under Life.

10. In resisting this unwarrantable extension of the term I am not only pointing to a speculative error, but also to a serious biological error common in both spiritualist and materialist schools, namely that of assigning Life to other than organic agencies. Instead of recognising the speciality of this Mode of Existence as dependent on a speciality of the organic conditions, the spiritualist assigns Life to some extra-organic Vital Principle, the materialist assigns it to some inorganic agent—physical or chemical. Waiving for the present all discussion of Vitalism, let us consider in what sense we must separate organic from all inorganic phenomena.

11. There is a distinction between inorganic and organic which may fitly be called radical: it lies at the root of the phenomena, and must be accepted as an ultimate fact, although the synthesis on which it depends is analytically reducible to a complication of more primitive conditions. It has been already indicated in § 5. All organisms above the very simplest are syntheses of three terms: Structure, Aliment, and Instrument. Crystals, like all other anorganisms, have structure, and in a certain sense they may be said to grow (*Mineralia crescunt*), though the growth is by *increase* and not by *modification:* * the motherlye, which is the food of the crystal, is never brought to the crystal, nor prepared for it, by any instrumental agency of the crystal. Organisms are exclusively instrumental; the organ is an instrument. The structural integrity of an organism is thus preserved through an alimentation which is effected through special instruments. Nothing like this is visible in anorganisms.

The increase of a crystal is further distinguishable from the growth of an organism, in the fact of its being simple accretion without development; and the structure of the crystal is distinguishable from that of an organism in the fact that its integrity is preserved by the *exclusion* of all molecular change, and not by the simultaneous changes of molecular decomposition and recomposition. Inorganic substances are sometimes as unstable as organic, sometimes even more unstable; but their instability is the source of their structural destruction—they change into other species; whereas the instability of *organised* substances (*not* of organic) is the source of their structural integrity: the tissue is renovated, and its renovation is a consequence of its waste.

12. But while the distinction is thus radical, when we

* Crystals not only grow by assimilation, but even repair injuries, with a certain superficial resemblance to the repair of animal tissues. Thus, according to the experiments of JORDAN cited by Sir JAMES PAGET (*Lectures on Surgical Pathology*, i. 153, and 2nd ed. p. 115), an octohedral crystal of alum, if fractured and replaced in a motherlye will in a few days exhibit a complete restoration of the original form. The whole crystal increases, but the increase is greatest on the broken edge, and the octohedral form is completely renewed. (Comp. § 113.)

view the organism from the *real*—that is, from the synthetic point of view—we must also urge the validity of the analytical point of view, which seizes on the conditions here complicated in a special group, and declares these conditions to be severally recognisable equally in anorganisms and in organisms. All the fundamental properties of Matter are recognisable in organised Matter. The elementary substances and forces familiar to physicists and chemists are the materials of the biologist; nor has there been found a single organic substance, however special, that is not reducible to inorganic elements. We see, then, that organised Matter is only a special combination of that which in *other* combinations presents chemical and physical phenomena; and we are prepared to find Chemistry and Physics indispensable aids in our analysis of organic phenomena. Aids, but only aids; indispensable, but insufficient.

13. There is therefore an ambiguity in the common statement that organised matter is not *ordinary* matter. Indisputable in one sense, this is eminently disputable when it is interpreted as evidence of a peculiar Vital Force "wholly unallied with the primary energy of Motion." If by "ordinary matter" be meant earths, crystals, gases, vapours, then assuredly organised matter is not ordinary. "Between the *living* state of matter and its *non-living* state," says Dr. Beale, "there is an absolute and irreconcilable difference; so far from our being able to demonstrate that the non-living passes by gradations into or gradually assumes the scale or condition of the *living*, the transition is sudden and abrupt, and matter already in the living state may pass into the non-living condition in the same sudden and complete manner."* The ambiguity here is sensible in the parallel case of the difference between crystallisable and coagulable matter, or between one crystal and another. If we can decompose the organic into the inorganic, this shows that the elements of the one are elements of the other; and if we are not yet able to recompose the inorganic elements into organic matter (not

* Cited by DRYSDALE: *Life and the Equivalence of Force;* part ii. p. 149.

at least in its more complex forms), may this not be due to the fact that we are ignorant of the proximate synthesis, ignorant of the precise way in which the elements are combined? I may have every individual part of a machine before me, but unless I know the proper position of each, I cannot with the parts reconstruct the machine. Indeed the very common argument on which so much stress is laid in favour of some mysterious Principle as the source of organic phenomena, namely, that human skill is hopelessly baffled in the attempt to make organic substances, still more a living cell, is futile. Men can make machines, it is said, but not organisms, *ergo* organisms must have a spiritual origin. But the fact is that no man can make a machine, *unless* he take advantage of the immense traditions of our race, and apply the skill of millions who have worked and thought before him, slowly and tentatively discovering the necessary means of mechanical effect. The greatest thinker, or the deepest scholar, who did not place himself in the line of the tradition, and learn the principles of mechanism, and the properties of the materials, would be as incapable of making a watch, as the physiologist now is of making a cell. But the skill of man has already succeeded in making many organic substances, and will perhaps eventually succeed in making a cell, certainly will, if ever the special synthesis which binds the elements together should be discovered. Not that such a discovery would alter the position of Biology in relation to Chemistry. The making of albumen, nay, the construction of an organism in the laboratory, would not in the least affect the foundation of Biology, would not obliterate the radical difference between organisms and anorganisms. It is the speciality of organic phenomena which gives them a special place, although the speciality may only be due to a complication of general agencies.

VITAL FORCE.

14. A similar ambiguity to that of the phrase "ordinary matter" lies in the equally common phrase "Vital Force," which is used to designate a special group of agencies, and is

then made to designate an agent which has no kinship with the general group; that is to say, instead of being employed in its real signification—that which alone represents our knowledge—as the abstract statical expression of the complex conditions necessary to the manifestation of vital phenomena, or as the abstract dynamical expression of the phenomena themselves, it is employed as an expression of their unknown Cause, which, because unknown, is dissociated from the known conditions, and erected into a mysterious Principle, having no kinship with Matter. In the first sense the term is a shorthand symbol of what is known and inferred. The known conditions are the relations of an organism and its medium, the organism being the union of various substances all of which have their peculiar properties when isolated; properties that disappear in the union, and are replaced by others, which result from the combination—as the properties of chlorine and sodium all disappear in the sea-salt which results from their union; or as the properties of oxygen and the properties of hydrogen disappear and are replaced by the properties of water. When therefore Vital Force is said to be exalted or depressed, the phrase has rational interpretation in the alteration which has taken place in one or more of the conditions, internal and external: a change in the tissues, the plasma, or the environment, exalts or depresses the energy of the vital manifestations; and to suppose that this is effected through the agency of some extra-organic Principle is a purely gratuitous fiction.

15. That we are ignorant of one or more of the indispensable conditions symbolised in the abstract term Vitality or Vital Force, is no reason for quitting the secure though difficult path of Observation, and rushing into the facile but delusive path of Fiction, which proposes metempirical Agents (in the shape of Vital and Psychical Principles) to solve the problems of Life and Mind. We may employ the term Vital Force to label our observations, together with all that still remains unobserved; and we are bound to recognise the line which separates observation from inference, what is proved from what is inferred; but while marking the limits of the known,

we are not to displace the known in favour of the unknown. It is said that because of our ignorance we must assume these causes of Life and Mind to be *unallied* with known material causes, and belonging to a different order of existences. This is to convert ignorance into a proof; and not only so, but to allow what we do not know to displace what we do know. The organicist is ready to admit that much has still to be discovered; the vitalist, taking his stand upon this unknown, denies that what has been discovered is really important, and declares that the real agent is wholly unallied to it. How *can* he know this?

He does not know it; he assumes it; and the chief evidence he adduces is that the ordinary laws of inorganic matter are incapable of explaining the phenomena of organised matter; and that physical and chemical forces are controlled by vital force. I accept both these positions, stripping them, however, of their ambiguities. The laws of ordinary matter are clearly incompetent in the case of matter which is not ordinary, but *specialised* in organisms; and when we come to treat of Materialism we shall see how unscientific have been the hypotheses which disregard the distinction. The question of control is too interesting and important to be passed over here.

VITAL FORCE CONTROLLING PHYSICAL AND CHEMICAL FORCES.

16. The facts relied on by the vitalists are facts which every organicist will emphasise, though he will interpret them differently. When, for example, it is said that "Life resists the effect of mechanical friction," and the proof adduced is the fact that the friction which will thin and wear away a dead body is actually the cause of the thickening of a living—the skin of a labourer's hand being thickened by his labour; the explanation is not that Life, an extra-organic agent, "resists mechanical friction"—for the mechanical effect is *not* resisted (the skin is rubbed off the rower's hand sooner than the wood is rubbed off the oar)—but that Life, *i.e.*, organic activity, repairs the waste of tissue.

17. Again, although many of the physical and chemical

processes which invariably take place under the influences to which the substances are subjected out of the organism, will not take place at all, or will take place in different degrees, when the substances are in the organism, this is important as an argument against the notion of vital *phenomena* being deducible from physical and chemical *laws*, but is valueless as evidence in favour of an extra-organic agent. Let us glance at one or two striking examples.

18. No experimental inquirer can have failed to observe the often contradictory results which seemingly unimportant variations in the conditions bring about; no one can have failed to observe what are called chemical affinities wholly frustrated by vital conditions. Even the ordinary laws of Diffusion are not always followed in the organism. The Amœba, though semifluid, resists diffusion when alive; but when it dies it swells and bursts by osmosis. The exchange of gases does not take place in the tissues, precisely as in our retorts. The *living* muscle respires, that is, takes up oxygen and gives out carbonic acid, not on the principle of simple diffusion, but by two separable physiological processes. The carbonic acid is given out, even when there is no oxygen whatever present in the atmosphere, and its place may then be supplied by hydrogen; and this physiological process is so different from the physical process which goes on in the dead muscle (the result of putrefaction), that it has been proved by Ranke to go on when the temperature is so low that all putrefaction is arrested. The same experimenter finds * that whereas living nerve will take up, by imbibition, 10 per cent. of potash salts, it will not take up 1 per cent. of soda salts, presented in equal concentration; and he points to the general fact that the absorption of inorganic substances does *not* take place according to the simple laws of diffusion, but that living tissues have special laws, the nerve, for instance, having a greater affinity for neutral potash salts than for neutral soda salts. Let me add, by way of anticipating the probable argument that may urge this in favour of Vital Principle which is lightly credited with the prescience of final causes, that so far

* RANKE: *Die Lebensbedingungen der Nerven*, 1868, p. 80.

from this "elective affinity" of the tissues being intelligent and always favourable, Ranke's experiments unequivocally show that it is more active towards destructive, poisonous substances, than towards the reparative, alimentary substances. Which is indeed consistent with the familiar experience that poisons are more readily absorbed than foods, when both are brought to the tissues. Thus it is well known that of all the salts the sulphate of copper is that which plants most readily absorb—and it kills them. The special affinities disappear as the vitality disappears, and dying plants absorb all salts equally.

19. The more the organism is studied, the more evident it will become that the simple laws of diffusion, as presented in anorganisms rarely if ever take effect in tissues; in other words, what is called Imbibition in Physics is the somewhat different process of Absorption in Physiology. The difference is notable in this capital fact that whereas the physical diffusion of liquids and gases is determined by differences of density, the physiological absorption of liquids and gases is determined by the molecular organisation of the tissue, which is perfectly indifferent to, and resists the entrance of, all substances incapable of entering into organic combination either as aliment or poison. A curious example of the indifference of organised substances to some external influences and their reaction upon others is the impossibility of provoking ciliary movement in an epithelial cell, during repose, by any electrical, mechanical, or chemical stimuli except potash and soda. Virchow discovered that a minute quantity of either of these, added to the water in which the cell floated, at once called forth the ciliary movements.

20. The true meaning of the resistance of Vitality to ordinary chemical affinity is that the conditions involved in the phenomena of Vitality are not the conditions involved in the phenomena of Chemistry, in other words, that in the living

* "Il n'y a peut être pas un seul phénomène chimique dans l'organisme qui se fasse par les procédés de la chimie de laboratoire; en particulier il n'y a peut être pas une oxydation qui s'accomplisse par fixation directe d'oxygène."—CLAUDE BERNARD.

organism the substances are placed under conditions different from those in which we observe these substances when their chemical affinities are displayed in anorganisms. But we need not go beyond the laboratory to see abundant examples of this so-called resistance to chemical affinity, when the conditions are altered. The decomposition of carbonates by tartaric acid is a chemical process which is wholly resisted if alcohol instead of water be the solvent employed. The union of sulphur with lead is said to be due to the affinity of the one for the other; but no one supposes this affinity to be irrespective of conditions, or that the union will take place when any one of these conditions is absent. If we fuse a compound of lead and iron in a crucible containing sulphur, we find it is the iron, and not the lead, which unites with the sulphur; yet we do not conclude that there is a Crucible Principle which frustrates chemical affinity, and resists the union of sulphur and lead; we simply conclude that the presence of the iron is a condition which prevents the combination of the sulphur with the lead: not until all the iron has taken up its definite proportion of sulphur will the affinity of the lead come into play. This is but another illustration of the law that *effects are processions of their causes*, summations of the conditions of their existence. If the fire burns no hole in the tea-kettle so long as there is water to conduct the heat away, this is not due to any principle more mysterious than the presence of a readily-conducting water.*

* Dr. MADDEN, in his essay *On the Relation of Therapeutics to Medicine*, 1871, p. 5, gives a remarkable illustration of what may be called the frustration of chemical affinity effected by mechanical conditions. "Before calico can be printed every loose particle of cotton must be removed from the surface in order that the coloured inks may not run. This removal is effected by passing the calico over and in contact with a red-hot iron cylinder, and, by regulating the rapidity with which the cylinder revolves, the intense heat burns off the loose fibres, yet does no injury to the woven cloth. In other words, the changes in the relation of the high temperature and the cotton are too rapid to admit of the fibre combining with the oxygen. Let the rate of revolution be reduced but very little and the calico would burst into flames." Any one who has snuffed a candle with his fingers will understand this. Dr. Madden further instances certain fulminates which can be detonated in

21. In accordance with the law of Causation just mentioned, which has been expounded in detail in our First Series (vol. ii. p. 388), the special combinations of Matter in organisms must present special phenomena. Therefore since the province of Biology is that of explaining organic phenomena by means of their organic conditions, it must be radically distinguished from the provinces of Physics and Chemistry, which treat not of organised but of inorganic matter. It is idle, it is worse, for it is misleading, to personify the organic conditions, known and inferred, in a Vital Principle; idle, because we might with equal propriety personify the conditions of crystallisation in a Crystal Principle; misleading, because the artifice is quickly dropped out of sight, and the abstract term then becomes accepted as an entity, supposed to create or rule the phenomena it was invented to express.

22. Inquirers are but too apt to misconceive the value of Analysis, which is an artifice of Method indispensable to research, though needing the complementary rectification by Synthesis before a real explanation can be reached. Analysis decomposes the actual fact into ideal factors, separates the group into its components, and considers each of these not as it exists in the group, in the reality, but as it exists when theoretically detached from the others. The oxygen and hydrogen into which water is decomposed did not exist as these gases in the water; the albumen and phosphate we extract from a nerve did not exist *as* isolated albumen and phosphate in the nerve, they were molecularly combined. In like manner the physical and chemical processes which may analytically be inferred in vital processes do not really take place in the same way as out of the organism. The real process is always a vital process, and must be explained by the synthesis of all the co-operant conditions. The laws of Physics

contact with gun-cotton without causing it to explode—the extreme rapidity with which the fulminates expand is too great to enable the gun-cotton to adjust its movements to this new motion. Precisely the same kind of thing occurs in organised matter. If the rate of its changes be reduced below a certain point the ordinary chemical affinities will assert themselves.

and Chemistry formulate abstract expressions of phenomena, wherever and whenever these appear, without reference to the *modes of production;* and in *this* sense the movement of a limb is no less a case of Dynamics than the movement of a pulley—the decomposition of a tissue is a case of Chemistry no less than the decomposition of a carbonate; the electro-motor phenomena observed in muscle are as purely physical as those observed in a telegraph. But when a biologist has to explain the movements of the limbs, or the decompositions of tissues, he has to deal with the phenomena and their modes of production, he has a particular group before him, and must leave out nothing that is characteristic of it. The movements of the pulley do not depend on Contractility and Sensibility, which in turn depend on Nutrition. The decomposition of the carbonate does not depend on conditions resembling those of a living tissue. Vaucanson's duck was surprisingly like a living duck in many of its movements; but in none of its actions was there any real similarity to the actions of a bird, because the machine was unlike an organism in action. The antithesis of mechanism and organism will be treated of in § 78.

23. We conclude, then, that defining physical phenomena as the movements which take place *without* change of structure, and chemical phenomena as the movements *with* change of structure, although both classes may be said to take place in the organism, and to be the primary conditions on which organic phenomena depend, they do not embrace the whole of the conditions, nor are the sciences which formulate them capable of formulating either the special phenomena characteristic of organisms or their special modes of production. The biologist will employ chemical and physical analysis as an essential part of his method; but he will always rectify what is artificial in this procedure, by subordinating the laws of Physics and Chemistry to the laws of Biology revealed in the synthetic observation of the organism as a whole. The rectification, here insisted on, will be recognised as peculiarly urgent in Psychology, which has greatly suffered from the misdirection of Analysis.

24. No one will misunderstand this specialisation of Biology to mean a separation of Life from the series of objective phenomena, and the introduction of a new entity; the specialisation points to a Mode of Existence. All classifications are artifices, but they have their objective grounds; the ground of difference on which Biology is separated from Chemistry and Physics, though all three may be merged in a common identity, is such as to justify the term radical. A vital process is no more to be considered physico-chemical, because physico-chemical conditions are presupposed in it, than a feeling is to be considered a nutritive process, because Nutrition is presupposed in all Feeling. Organic substances have been made by chemists, and inorganic "cells" have also been made; but these substances were not organised, these "cells" would not live. The germ-cell is the workshop of generation, the secreting-cell the workshop of secretion, the muscle-cell the workshop of contraction. What is required over and above organic substances and cell-forms, is that special state called *organisation*. See § 49.

Those who contemplate the manifestations without also taking into account their modes of production may see nothing but physico-chemical facts in vital facts. It is by a similar limitation of the point of view that Vitality is often confounded with Movement, and portions of organic matter are said to live, simply on the evidence of their movements.*

* I am often reminded of the surprising movements of particles of carbonate of lime in water which my friend Professor PREYER showed me during a visit to Bonn. He had removed one of the concretions, usually found in connection with nerves along the spine of old frogs, and crushed it in water; under the microscope the seeming spontaneity and variety of the movements of the particles was such that had we not known their origin we should certainly have attributed them to vitality: no infusoria could have moved with more seeming spontaneity. It is hardly physiological to conclude that because fragments of tissue manifest amœbiform movements therefore they are alive (STRICKER: art. *Die Zelle* in his *Handbuch der Lehre von den Geweben*, 1868, p. 7), or that the heart removed from the body is *alive* because it still beats. LIEBERKÜHN: *Ueber Bewegungserscheinungen der Zellen*, 1870, pp. 357–359, cites examples of such movements in undeniably dead substances. For Life, we demand not only Movement, but Functional Activity.

CHAPTER II.

DEFINITIONS OF LIFE.

25. BIOLOGY, the science of Life, being thus assigned its place in the hierarchy of objective laws, we now proceed to consider what the term Life symbolises.

By a large preliminary simplification, Life may be defined as *the mode of existence of an organism in relation to its medium.* To render this of any value, however, a clear conception of the organism is first indispensable; and this must be preceded by an examination of the various attempts to define life in anticipation of such a clear conception.

26. Every phenomenon, or group of phenomena, may be viewed under two aspects—the *statical*, which considers the conditions of existence; and the *dynamical*, which considers these conditions in their resultant,—in their *action.* The statical definition of Life will express the connexus of the properties of organised substance, all those conditions, of matter, form, and texture, and of relation to external forces, on which the organism depends. These various conditions, condensed into a single symbol, constitute Vitality or Vital Force, and are hence taken as the Cause of vital phenomena. The dynamical definition will express the connexus of Functions and Faculties of the organism, which are the statical properties of organised substance in action, under definite relations.

It is obvious that the term Life must vary with the varying significates it condenses—every variation in the complexity of the organism will bring a corresponding fulness in the signification of the term. The life of a plant is less significant than the life of an animal; and the life of a mollusc less than that of a fish. But not only is the term one of varying significance, it is always an abstract term which drops out of sight particular concrete differences registering only the universal resemblances.

27. It would be a profitless labour to search out, and a wearisome infliction to set down, the various definitions which have been proposed and accepted; but certain characteristic examples may be selected. All that I am acquainted with belong to two classes: 1°, the *meta*physiological hypothesis of an *extra*-organic agent, animating lifeless matter by unknown powers; 2°, the physiological hypothesis which seeks the cause of the phenomena (*i.e.*, the conditions) *within* the organism itself—a group of conditions akin to those manifested elsewhere, but differently combined. The first hypotheses are known under the names of Animism and Vitalism—more commonly the latter. The second are known as Organicism and Materialism—but the latter term only applies to some of the definitions.

28. Under Vitalism are included all the hypotheses of a soul, a spirit, an archæus, a vital principle, a vital force, a *nisus formativus*, a plan or divine idea, which have from time to time represented the metaphysical stage of Biology. The characteristic of that stage is the personification of a mystery, accompanied by the persuasion that to name a mystery is to explain it. In all sciences when processes are imperfectly observed, the *theory* of the processes (which is a systematic survey of the available evidence marshalled in the order of causal dependence) is supplemented by *hypothesis*, which fills up with a guess the gap left by observation. The difference between the metaphysical and the positive stages of a science lies in the kind of guess thus introduced to supplement theory, and the degree of reliance accorded to it. I have more than once insisted on the scientific canon that "to be valid, an explanation must be expressed in terms of phenomena already observed;" now it is quite clear that most of the extra-organic hypotheses do not fulfil this condition; no one having ever *observed* a spirit, an archæus, or a vital principle; but only *imagined* these agents to explain the facts observed. As an

example of the difference, and a proof that the value of an hypothesis does not rest on the facility with which it connects observations, and seems to explain them, take the three hypotheses of animal spirits, nervous fluid, and electricity, by which neural processes have been explained. The animal spirits are imaginary; the nervous fluid is without a basis in observation, no evidence of such a fluid having been detected; but electricity (or, speaking rigorously, the movements classed as electrical), although not proved to be *the* agent in nerve-action, is proved to exist in nerves as elsewhere, and its modes of operation are verifiable. It, therefore, and it alone of the three hypotheses, is in conformity with the scientific canon. It may not, on full investigation, meet all requirements; it may be rejected as imperfect; but it is the kind of guess which scientific theory demands.

The second difference noticeable between the metaphysical and the positive stages, is the degree of reliance accorded to hypothesis; which is very much the same as that noticeable in the uncritical and critical attitudes of untrained and trained intellects. The one accepts a guess as if it were a proof; is fascinated by the facility of linking together isolated observations, and, relying on the guess as truth, proceeds to deduce conclusions from it; the other accepts a guess as an aid in research, trying by its aid to come upon some observation which will reveal the hidden process; but careful never to allow the guess to *supersede observation,* or to form a basis of deductions not immediately verified.

29. A glance at the metaphysiological definitions will detect both the kind of guess and the kind of reliance which prevailed. The mystery was not simply recognised, it was personified as an entity: Will and Intelligence were liberally accorded to it, for it was supposed to shape matter, and direct force into predestined paths by prescience of a distant end. The observed facts of the egg passing through successive changes into a complex organism, were so marvellous, so unlike any facts observable in the inorganic world, that they seemed to demand a cause drawn from higher sources. The mystery of life obtruded itself at every turn. It was named,

and men fancied it explained. But in truth no mystery is got rid of by explanation, however valid; it is only shifted farther back. Explanation is the resolution of a complex phenomenon into its conditions of existence—the product is reduced to its factors; the explanation is final when this resolution has been so complete that a reconstruction of the product is possible from the factors. The vast majority of explanations—especially in the organic region—are no more than what mathematicians call "a first approximation." It is through successive approximations that science advances; but even when the final stage is reached a mystery remains. We may know that certain elements combine in certain proportions to produce certain substances; but why they produce these, and not different substances, is no clearer than why muscles contract or organisms die. This Why is, however, an idle question. That alone which truly concerns us is the How, and not the Why.

30. Biology is still a long way off the How. But it can boast of many approximations; and its theories are to be tested by the degree of approximation they effect. In this light the physiological, *intra*-organic, hypotheses manifestly have the advantage. Many of them are indeed very unacceptable; they are guided by a mistaken conception of the truths reached by Analysis. For when men first began to discard the extra-organic hypotheses, and to look into the organism itself, they were so much impressed by the mechanical facts observed, that they endeavoured to reduce all the phenomena to Mechanics. The circulation became simply a question of hydraulics. Digestion was explained as trituration. The chemists then appeared, and their shibboleths were "affinities" and "oxidations." With Bichat arose the anatomical school, which decomposing the organism into organs, the organs into tissues, and these tissues into their elements, sought the analytical conditions of existence of the organism in the properties of these tissues, and the functions of these organs. The extra-organic agent was thus finally shown to be not only a fiction, but a needless fiction.

Every student of the history of the science will note how

from the very necessities of the case the metaphysiologists, without relinquishing their Vital Principle, have been led more and more to enter on the track of the physiologists, pursuing their researches more and more into the processes going on in the organism, and assigning more and more causal efficiency to these, with a corresponding restriction of the province of their extra-organic cause. Hence in the ranks of the vitalists have been found some of the very best observers and theorists; but they were such in despite of, and not in consequence of, their hypothesis, which was only invoked by them when evidence was at fault. Nor, unscientific as vitalism is, can we deny that it has been so far serviceable to the science, that it has corrected the materialist error of endeavouring to explain organic phenomena by physico-chemical laws; and has persistently kept in view the radical difference between organic and inorganic.

31. These remarks may justify a selection of definitions, classified under the two heads. The selection is fitly opened by the Aristotelian definition which prevailed for centuries.

Aristotle distinguishes Life, which he says means "the faculties of self-nourishment, self-development, and self-decay," from the Vital Principle. Every natural body manifesting life may be regarded as an essential existence (οὐσία); but *then it is an existence only as a synthesis* (ὡς συνθέτη); and since an organism is such a synthesis, being possessed of Life, it cannot be the Vital Principle (ψυχή). Therefore it follows that the Vital Principle must be an essence, as being the Form of a natural body holding life in *potentiality*. The Vital Principle is the primary reality of an organism. "It is therefore as idle to ask whether the Vital Principle and Organism are one, as whether the wax and the impress on it are one. . . . Thus if an eye were an animal, Vision would be its Vital Principle: for Vision is, abstractedly considered, the essence of the eye; but the eye is the body of Vision, and if Vision be wanting, then, save in name, it is no longer an eye."

Apart from certain metaphysical implications, inevitable at that period, there is profound insight in this passage. His adversary Telesio quite misconceives the meaning here assigned to the Vital Principle.*

32. Let us pass over all the intermediate forms of the hypothesis, and descend to Kant, who defines Life "an internal principle of action" (this does not distinguish it from fermentation); an organism he says is "that in which every part is at once means and end." "Each part of the living body has its cause of existence in the whole organism; whereas in non-living bodies each part has its cause in itself." Johannes Müller adopts a similar view: "The harmonious action of the essential parts of the individual subsist only by the influence of a force, the operation of which is extended to all parts of the body, and does not depend on any single parts; this *force must exist before the parts*, which are in fact formed by it during the development of the embryo. . . . The vital force inherent in them generates from the organic matter the essential organs which constitute the whole being. This *rational creative force* is exerted in every animal strictly in accordance with what the nature of each requires."

33. This is decidedly inferior to Aristotle, who did not confound the vegetative with the rational principle. It rests on the old metaphysical error of a *vis medicatrix*, an error which cannot sustain itself against the striking facts which constantly point to a *vis destructrix*, a destructive tendency quite as inexorable as the curative tendency. And the experimental biologist soon becomes impressed with the fact that the tissues have indeed a *selective* action, by which from out the nutrient material only these substances are assimilated which will enter into combination with them; but this selective action is fatal, no less than reparative: substances which poison the tissue are taken up as readily as those which nourish it. The idea of prescience, therefore, cannot be sustained; it is indeed seldom met with now in the writings of any but the Montpellier school, who continue the

* TELESIUS: *De Natura Rerum*, 1586, v. 184. TELESIO might have been saved from the mistake had he attended to what NIPHUS had said on the point in his *Expositio subtilissima*, 1559, p. 245. Comp. also PHILELPHUS: *Epist. Familiarum*, 1502, p. 253, *verso*.

traditions of Stahl's teaching. It has been so long exploded elsewhere that one is surprised to find an English physiologist clinging to a modification of it—I mean Dr. Lionel Beale, who repeatedly insists on Life as "a peculiar Force, *temporarily associated* with matter," a "power capable of controlling and directing both matter and force," an "*undiscovered* form of force *having no connection with primary energy or motion.*" "The higher phenomena of the nervous system are probably due primarily to the movements of the germinal matter due to vital power, which vital power of this the highest form of germinal matter is in fact the living *I.*"

34. Apart from the primary objection to all these definitions, namely, that they seek to express organic phenomena in terms of an extra-organic principle, to formulate the facts *observed* in terms of a cause *inferred*, there is the fatal objection that they speak confidently on what is avowedly unknown. If the force be, as Dr. Beale says, "undiscovered," on what grounds can he assert that it has *no* connection with the forces which are known? All that the observed facts warrant is the assertion that organic phenomena are special (which no one denies), and must therefore depend on special combinations of matter and force. But on this ground we might assume a crystallising Force, and a coagulating Force, having no connection with the molecular forces manifested elsewhere: these also are special phenomena, not to be confounded with each other.

35. Schelling defines Life as "a principle of individuation" and a "cycle of successive changes determined and fixed by this internal principle." Which is so vague that it may be applied in very different senses. Bichat's celebrated definition (which is only a paraphrase of a sentence in Stahl), "the sum of the functions which resist Death," although an endeavour to express the facts from the Intra-organic point of view, is not only vague, but misrepresents one of the cardinal conditions, by treating the External Medium as antagonistic to Life, whereas Life is only possible in the relation to a Medium.

36. Were it not so vague, the definition proposed by

Dugès and Béclard would be unexceptionable: the former says it is "the special activity of organised beings;" the latter, "the sum of the phenomena proper to organised bodies." When supplemented by a description of organised bodies, these formulæ are compendious and exact. The same remark applies to the definition of Lamarck: "that state of things which permits organic movements; and these movements, which constitute active life, result from a stimulus which excites them."

37. De Blainville, and after him Comte and Charles Robin, define it thus: "Life is the twofold internal movement of composition and decomposition at once general and continuous." This, excellent as regards what is called vegetal life, is very properly objected to by Mr. Herbert Spencer in that it excludes those nervous and muscular functions which are the most conspicuous and distinctive of vital phenomena. The same objection must be urged against Professor Owen's definition: "Life is a centre of intussusceptive assimilative force capable of reproduction by spontaneous fission."

38. In 1853, after reviewing the various attempts to express in a sentence what a volume could only approximately expound, I proposed the following: "Life is a series of definite and successive changes, both of structure and composition, which take place within an individual without destroying its identity." This has been criticised by Mr. Herbert Spencer and by Dr. Lionel Beale, and if I had not withdrawn it before their criticisms appeared, I should certainly have modified and enlarged it afterwards. I mention it, however, because it is an approach to a more satisfactory formula in so far as it specifies two cardinal characteristics distinguishing organisms from all anorganisms, namely, the incessant evolution through definite stages, and the preservation of specific integrity throughout the changes; not only the organism as a whole is preserved amidst incessant molecular change, but each tissue lives only so long as the reciprocal molecular composition and decomposition persist. On both of these points I shall have to speak hereafter. The

definition, however, is not only defective in its restriction to the molecular changes of Nutrition, taking no account of the Properties and Functions of the organism; but defective also in giving no expression to equally important relations of the organism to the medium.

39. This last point is distinctly expressed in Mr. Spencer's definition: "Life is the continuous adjustment of internal relations to external relations." Considered as a formula of the most general significance, embracing therefore what is common to all orders of vital phenomena, this is the best yet proposed.* If I propose another it will not be to displace but to run alongside with Mr. Spencer's; and this only for more ready convenience. Before doing so I must say a few words by way of clearing the ground.

40. What does the term Life stand for? What are the concrete significates of this abstract symbol? As before stated, it is sometimes a compendious shorthand for the special phenomena distinguishing living from non-living bodies; and sometimes it expresses not these observed phenomena, but their conditions of existence, which are by one school personified in an abstract and extra-organic cause. Thus the life of an animal, a man, or a nation, means—1°, the special manifestations of these organisms, and groups of organisms; or 2°, the causes which produce these manifestations. We are often misunderstood by others, and sometimes vague to ourselves, when we do not bear these two different meanings in view. It was probably some sense of this which made Aristotle distinguish Vitality from Life, as that of the one uniform cause separated from its multiple effects; it was certainly the motive of Fletcher, who thus expressly limits the meanings: "*Vitality* or *Irritability*, the property which

* The authorities just cited are ARISTOTLE: *De Anima*, lib. ii. c. i. KANT: *Kritik der Urtheilskraft.* MÜLLER: *Physiology.* BEALE: *Bioplasm*, and *Introduction to Todd and Bowman's Anatomy.* SCHELLING: *Erster Entwurf*, and *Transcendent. Idealismus.* BICHAT: *Recherches sur la Vie et la Mort.* STAHL: *Theoria Vera Medica.* DUGÈS: *Physiologie Comparée.* BÉCLARD: *Anatomie Générale.* LAMARCK: *Philosophie Zoologique.* COMTE: *Cours de Philosophie Positive.* OWEN'S *Hunterian Lectures*, 1854. HERBERT SPENCER: *Principles of Biology.*

characterises organised beings of being acted on by certain powers otherwise than either strictly mechanically or strictly chemically; *Life*, the sum of the actions of organised beings resulting directly from their vitality so acted on." *

Vitality and Life being thus discriminated as the statical and the dynamical aspects of the organism, we find in relation to the former two radically opposed conceptions: the metaphysiological or extra-organic, and the physiological or intra-organic. The first conceives Vitality to be a Vital Principle, or extra-organic agent, sometimes a soul, spirit, archæus, idea, and sometimes a force, which easily becomes translated into a property.

The conception of an entity must be rejected, because it is metempirical and unverifiable, § 34. The conception of a force must be rejected, because it is irreconcilable with any definite idea we have of force. What the term Force signifies in Physics and Chemistry, namely, mass animated by velocity, or *directed pressure*, which is the activity of the agent,—is precisely that which these vitalists pertinaciously exclude. They assume a force which has nothing in common with mass and velocity; which is *not a resultant, but a principle;* which instead of being a *directed quantity*, is itself autonomous and *directive*, shaping matter into organisation, and endowing it with powers not assignable to matter. If this vital force has any mass at its back, it is a spiritual mass; if it is directed, the direction issues from a "Mind somewhere." Now this conception is purely metempirical. Not only is it inexact to speak of Vitality as a force, it is almost equally inexact to speak of it as a property; since it is a term which includes a variety of properties; and when Fletcher assigns the synonym of Irritability, this at once reveals the inexactness; for beside this property, we must place Assimilation, Evolution, Disintegration, Reproduction, Contractility, and Sensibility,—all characteristic properties included in Vitality.

41. Having thus rejected the conceptions of entity, force,

* FLETCHER, as quoted by DRYSDALE: *Life and the Equivalence of Force*, part ii. p. 120.

and property, we are left in presence of—1°, the organic conditions as the elements, and 2°, of their synthesis (in the state called organisation) as the personified principle. Vital forces, or the vital force, if we adopt the term for brevity's sake, is a *symbol of the conditions of existence of organised matter;* and since organisms are specially distinguishable from anorganisms by this speciality of their synthesis, and not by any difference in the nature of the elements combined, this state of organisation is the "force" or "principle" of which we are in quest. To determine what Life means, we must observe and classify the phenomena presented by living beings. To determine what Vitality—or organisation—means, we must observe and classify the processes which go on in organised substances. These will occupy us in the succeeding chapters; here I may so far anticipate as to propose the following definitions:—

42. Life is the functional activity of an organism in relation to its medium, as a synthesis of three terms: Structure, Aliment, and Instrument; it is the sum of functions which are the resultants of Vitality; Vitality being the sum of the properties of matter in the state of organisation.

Vital phenomena are the phenomena manifested *in* organisms when external agencies disturb their molecular equilibrium; and *by* organisms when they react on external objects. Thus everything done in an organism, or by an organism, is a vital act, although physical and chemical agencies may form essential components of the act. If I shrink when struck, or if I whip a horse, the blow is in each case physical, but the shrinking and the striking are vital.

Every part of a living organism is therefore vital, as *pertaining* to Life; but no part has this Life when isolated; for Life is the synthesis of all the parts:—a federation of the organs when the organism is complex, a federation of the organic substances when the organism is a simple cell.

43. All definitions, although didactically placed at the introduction of a treatise, are properly the final expression of the facts which the treatise has established, and they cannot therefore be fully apprehended until the mind is familiarised with the details they express. Much, therefore, which to the reader may seem unintelligible or questionable in the foregoing definition, must be allowed to pass until he has gone through the chapters which follow.

CHAPTER III.

ORGANISM, ORGANISATION, AND ORGANIC SUBSTANCE.

45. THERE is a marked difference between organ*ic* and organ*ised* substances. The organic are non-living, though capable of living when incorporated in organised tissue (albumen is such a substance); or they may be incapable of living because they have lived, and are products of waste, *e.g.*, urea. The organised substance is a specific combination of organic substances of various kinds, a combination which is organisation. Any organised substance is therefore either an independent organism, or part of a more complex organism. Protoplasm, either as a separate organism or as a constituent of a tissue, is organised substance.

Organic substances are numerous and specific. They are various combinations of proximate principles familiar to the chemist, which may conveniently be ranged under three classes: The first class of organic substances comprises those composed of principles having what is called a mineral origin; these generally quit the organism unchanged as they entered it. The second class comprises those which are crystallisable, and are formed *in* the organism, and generally quit it in this state as excretions. The third class comprises the colloids, *i.e.*, substances which are coagulable and not crystallisable, and are formed in and decomposed in the organism, thus furnishing the principles of the second class. All the principles are in a state of solution. Water is the chief vehicle of the materials which enter and the materials which quit the organism; and bodies in solution are solvents of others, so that the water thus acquires new solvent properties.

45*a*. Two points must be noted respecting organic substances: they are mostly combinations of *higher multiples* of the elements; and their combinations are not *definite* in quantity. Albumen, for example, has (according to one of the many formulas which have been given) an elementary composition of 216 atoms of Carbon, 169 of Hydrogen, 27 of Nitrogen, 3 of Sulphur, and 68 of Oxygen; whereas in its final state, in which it quits the organism as Urea, it is composed of 2 atoms of Carbon, 4 of Hydrogen, 2 of Nitrogen, and 2 of Oxygen, all the Sulphur having disappeared in other combinations. In like manner in the organism Stearin falls from C_{114}, H_{110}, O_{12}, to Oxalic Acid, which is C_4, H_2, O_8. It is obvious that the necessary modifiability of organic substance is due to this multiplicity of its elementary parts and the variety of its molecular structure.

45*b*. Nor is the indefiniteness of the quantitative composition less important, though seldom adequately appreciated, or even suspected. Robin and Verdeil * are the only writers I can remember who have distinctly brought the fact into prominence. That all inorganic substances are definite in composition, every one knows. Quicklime, for example, may be got from marble, limestone, oyster-shells, or chalk; but however produced, it always contains exactly 250 ounces of calcium to 100 ounces of oxygen; just as water is always OH_2. Not so the pre-eminently vital substances, those which are coagulable and not crystallisable: no precise formula will express one of these; for the same specific substance is found to vary from time to time, and elementary analyses do not give uniform results. Thus, if after causing an acid to combine with one of these substances, we remove the acid, we are not certain of finding the substance as it was before—as we are, for example, after urea is combined with nitric acid and then decomposed. The same want of definiteness is of course even more apparent in the *combinations* of these proximate principles into organised substance. Protoplasm differs greatly in different places. Epithelial cells differ. Muscular and nervous fibres are never absolutely the same in different regions. A striped and unstriped

* Robin et Verdeil : *Traité de Chimie Anatomique*, 1853.

muscular fibre, the muscular fibre of a sphincter or of a limb, a nerve-fibre in a centre, in a trunk, or in a gland, will present variations of composition. The elastic fibres of the ligaments are larger in the horse than in man; and in other animals they are smaller. These differences are sometimes due to the constituents, and sometimes to the arrangement of the constituents; the conversion of Albumen into Fibrine without elementary loss or addition, is a good example of the latter. That the tissues of one man are not absolutely the same as the tissues of another, in the sense in which it is true to say that the chalk of one hill is the same as that of another, or as gold in Australia is the same as gold in Mexico, is apparent in their very different reactions under similar external conditions: the substance which poisons the one leaves the other unaffected. The man who has once had the smallpox, or scarlet fever, is never the same afterwards, since his organism has now become insusceptible of these poisons. And Sir James Paget has called attention to the striking fact revealed in disease, namely, that in the same tissue—say the bone or the skin—a morbid substance fastens only on certain small portions leaving all the rest unaltered, but fastens on exactly corresponding spots of the opposite sides of the body; so that on both arms, or both legs, only the corresponding bits of tissue will be diseased. "Manifestly when two substances display different relations to a third their composition cannot be identical; so that though we may speak of all bone or of all skin as if it were all alike, yet there are differences of intimate composition. No power of artificial chemistry can detect the difference; but a morbid material can." * It is to this variability of composition that we must refer individual peculiarities, and those striking forms of variety known as idiosyncrasies, which cause some organisms to be affected by what seem inexplicable influences—physical and moral.

In spite of all these variations, however, there are certain specific resemblances dependent of course on similarity of

* Paget: *Lectures on Surgical Pathology*, p. 14.

composition and structure, so that the muscle of a crustacean is classed beside the muscle of a vertebrate, although the elementary analysis of the two yields different results. Nerve-tissue, according to my experience, is the most variable of all, except the blood; variable not only from individual to individual, and from genus to genus, but even in the same individual it never contains the same quantities of water, phosphates, &c. Hence it is that different nerves manifest different degrees of excitability, and the same nerve differs at different times. Thus the fifth pair, in a poisoned animal, retains its excitability long after the others are paralysed; and the patient under chloroform feels a prick on the brow or at the temples, when insensible at any other spot. The pneumogastric which is excitable during digestion is—in dogs at least—inexcitable when the animal is fasting.

46. The organic substances are what analysis discovers in organised substances, but none of them, not even the highest, is living, except as organised. Albumen alone, or Stearin alone, is as incapable of Vitality, as Plumbago, or Soda; but all organic substances are capable of playing a part in vital actions; and this part is the more important in proportion to their greater molecular variety. Organisation is a special synthesis of substances belonging to all three classes; and the organised substance, thus formed, alone merits the epithet living. We see how organised substances being constituted by principles derived from the inorganic world, and principles derived from the organic world, have at once a dependence on the external Medium, and an independence of it, which is peculiar to living beings. An analogous dependence and independence is noticeable with respect to the parts; and this is a character not found in inorganic compounds. The organism even in its simplest forms is a structure of different substances each of which is complex. While one part of a crystal is atomically and morphologically identical with every other, and is the whole crystal "writ small," one part of an organism is unlike another, and *no part* is like the whole. Hence the dependence of one organ, and one tissue on another, and each on all. Yet, while

every part is, so to speak, a condition of existence of every other, and the unity of the organism is but the expression of this solidarity,—wherever organised substance has been differentiated into morphological elements (cells, &c.), each of these has its own course of evolution independently of the others,—is born, nourished, developed, and dies.

47. The interdependence of nerve and muscle is seen in this, that the more the muscle is excited the feebler its contractions become; this decrease in contractility is compensated by an increased excitability in its nerve, so that while the muscle demands a more powerful stimulus, the nerve acquires a more energetic activity. Ranke's curious and careful experiments seem to prove that this depends on the wearied muscle absorbing more water, owing to the acids developed by its activity, and on the nerve losing this water—a nerve being always more irritable when its quantity of water diminishes.

48. Herein we see illustrated the great law of organised activity that it is a simultaneity of opposite tendencies, as organised matter is a synthesis of compositions and decompositions, always tending towards equilibrium and disturbance, storing up energy and liberating it. Unlike what is observed in unorganised matter, the conditions of waste bring with them conditions of repair, and thus—within certain limits—every loss in one direction is compensated by gain in another. There is a greater flow of nutrient material, or more properly speaking, a greater assimilation of it by the tissue, where there has been made a greater opening for it by previous disintegration. The alkaline state of the nutrient material, and the acid state of the material that has been used,—the alkaline state which characterises repose and assimilation, and the acid state which characterises activity and deassimilation, are but cases of this general law: on the synthesis of these opposite tendencies depends the restless change, together with the continued specific integrity, of organised matter.

49. The state of organisation may therefore be defined as the *molecular union of the proximate principles of the three classes in reciprocal dissolution.* An organism is formed of

matter thus organised, which exists in two states—the *amorphous,* and the *figured.* The amorphous substances are liquid, semiliquid, and solid; the figured, are the cells, fibres, and tubes, called "anatomical elements." For these I prefer the term suggested, I believe, by Milne Edwards, namely, *organites,* because they are the individual elements which mainly constitute the organs, and are indeed by many biologists considered as elementary organisms. These organites, which go to form the tissues, and by the tissues the organs, have their specific form, volume, structure, and chemical reactions. They exist in textures or tissues, or separately (*e.g.*, blood - corpuscles), and are in many respects like the simplest organisms known, such as monads, vibrios, amœbæ, &c.

50. The simplest form of life is not—as commonly stated—a cell, but a microscopic lump of jelly-like substance, or protoplasm, which has been named *sarcode* by Dujardin, *cytode* by Haeckel, and *germinal matter* by Lionel Beale. This protoplasm, although entirely destitute of texture, and consequently destitute of organs, is nevertheless considered to be living, because it manifests the cardinal phenomena of Life: Assimilation, Evolution, Reproduction, Mobility, and Decay. Examples of this simplest organism are Monads, Protamœbæ, and Polythalamia.* Few things are more surprising than the vital activity of these organites, which puzzle naturalists as to whether they should be called plants or animals. All microscopists are familiar with the spectacle of a formless lump of albuminous matter (a Rhizopod) putting forth a process of its body as a temporary arm or leg, or else slowly wrapping itself round a microscopic plant, or morsel of animal substance, thus converting its whole body into a mouth and a stomach; but these phenomena are surpassed by those described by Cienkowski,† who narrates how one Monad fastens on to a plant and sucks the chlorophyll first from one cell and then from another; another Monad,

* Comp. HAECKEL, in *Siebold und Kölliker's Zeitschrift,* 1865, p. 342, and his *Generelle Morphologie,* 1866, I. 135, 336.

† In the *Archiv für mikros. Anatomie,* 1865, p. 211.

unable to make a hole in the cell-wall, thrusts long processes of its body into the opening already made, and drags out the remains of the chlorophyll left there by its predecessor; while a third Monad leads a predatory life, falling upon other Monads that have filled themselves with food. Here, as he says, we stand on the threshold of that dark region where Animal Will begins; and yet there is here only the simplest form of organisation.*

51. Now let our glance pass on to the second stage—the Cell. Here we have a recognised differentiation in the appearance of a nucleus amid the protoplasm. The nucleus is chemically different from the substance which surrounds it; and although perhaps exaggerated importance has been attributed to this nucleus, and mysterious powers have been ascribed to it, yet as an essential constituent of the cell it commands attention. Indeed, according to the most recent investigations, the definition of a cell is "a nucleus with surrounding protoplasm." The cell-wall, or delicate investing membrane—that which makes the cell a closed sac—is no longer to be regarded as a necessary constituent, but only as an accessory.†

* Here organisation is the simplest form of all—molecular organised structure, which in the higher forms becomes tissue structure, and organ structure. The word *structure* properly means orderly arrangement of different materials; and molecular structure refers to the different proximate principles which constitute the organised substance. Usually, however, the word *structureless* indicates the absence of *visible* arrangement of the parts: a cell has structure since it has nucleus and protoplasm.

† In the cell-theory established by SCHLEIDEN and SCHWANN, in 1838, and which has formed the basis of modern histology, the cell-wall was endowed with an importance which can no longer be upheld now that the existence of independent organisms, and of cells, without a trace of enveloping membrane has been abundantly observed. Cells without walls were first described by COSTE in the *Comptes Rendus*, 1845, p. 1372. They were also described by CHARLES ROBIN in 1855, *Dict. de la Médicine*, art. *Cellule*. But little notice was taken until MAX SCHULTZE, in his famous essay, *Ueber Muskelkörperchen und was man eine Zelle zu nennen habe*, which appeared in *Reichert und Du Bois Reymond's Archiv*, 1861,—BRUECKE, in his memoir, *Die Elementarorganismen*, 1861,—and LIONEL BEALE, in his *Structure of the Simple Tissues*, 1861,—

52. The cell may be either an organism or an organite. It may lead an isolated life as plant or animal, or it may be united with others and lead a more or less corporate existence; but always, even as an element of a higher organism, it preserves its own individuality. At first we see that the corporate union is very slight, merely the contact of one cell with another of its own kind, as in the filament of a Conferva. Rising higher, we see the cell united with others different from it: plants and animals appear, having structures composed of masses of various cells. Rising still higher, we see animal forms of which the web is woven out of myriads upon myriads of cells, with various cell-products, processes, fibres, tubes.

ORGANISM AND MEDIUM.

53. But we have only one half of the great problem of life, when we have the organism; and it is to this half that the chief researches have been devoted, the other falling into neglect. What is that other? The Medium in which the organism lives. Every individual object, organic or inorganic, is the product of two factors:—first, the relation of its constituent molecules to each other; secondly, the relation of its substance to all surrounding objects. Its properties, as an object or an organism, are the results of its constituent molecules, and of its relation to external conditions. Organisms are the results of a peculiar group

all about the same time began the reform in the cell-theory which has effected a decisive change in the classical teaching. LEYDIG claims, and with justice, to have furnished important data in this direction (*Vom Bau des thierischen Körpers*, 1864, I. p. 11). The student interested in this discussion should consult MAX SCHULTZE: *Das Protoplasma der Rhizopoden und der Pflanzenzellen*, 1863; HAECKEL: *Die Radiolarien*, 1862; the controversial papers by REICHERT, in his *Archiv* (beginning with the Report of 1863), and MAX SCHULTZE, in his *Archiv für mikros. Anat.*, with HENLE's judgment in his *Jahresberichte*, and KÖLLIKER's summing-up in the last edition of his *Gewebelehre*. For a full yet brief history of the cell-theory see DRYSDALE: *The Protoplasmic Theory of Life*, 1874, pp. 95–106.

of forces, exhibiting a peculiar group of phenomena. Viewing these in the abstract, we may say that there are three regulative laws of life:—(1) The *Lex Formationis*—the so-called *nisus formativus*, or "organising force;" (2) the *Lex Adaptationis*, or adaptive tendency; (3) the *Lex Hereditatis*, or tendency to reproduce both the original form and its acquired modifications. We have always to consider the organising force in relation to all surrounding forces—a relation succinctly expressed in the word Adaptation. Just as water is water only under a certain relation of its constituent molecules to the temperature and atmospheric pressure—just as it passes into other forms (ice or steam) in adapting itself to other conditions; so, likewise, the organism only preserves its individuality by the adjustment of its forces with the forces which environ it.

54. This relation of Organism and Medium, the most fundamental of biological data, has had a peculiar fortune: never wholly unrecognised, for it obtrudes itself incessantly in the facts of daily experience, it was very late in gaining recognition as a principle of supreme importance; and is even now often so imperfectly apprehended that one school of philosophers indignantly rejects the idea of the Organism and Medium being the two factors of which Life is the product. Not only is there a school of vitalists maintaining the doctrine of Life as an entity independent both of Organism and Medium, and using these as its instruments; but there is also a majority among other biologists, who betray by their arguments that they fail to keep steadily before them the fundamental nature of the relation. Something of this is doubtless due to the imperfect conception they have formed of what constitutes the Medium: instead of recognising in it the sum of external conditions affecting the organism—*i.e.*, the sum of the relations which the organism maintains with external agencies,—they restrict, or enlarge it, so as to misapprehend its significance—restrict it to only a few of the conditions, such as climate, soil, temperature, &c., or enlarge it to embrace a vast array of conditions which stand in no directly appreciable relation to the organism. Every one understands that an organism is dependent on proper food, on oxygen, &c., and will perish if these are withheld, or be affected by every variation in such conditions. Every one understands that an animal which can devour or be devoured by another, will flourish or perish according to the presence of its prey or its enemy. But it is often forgotten that among external existences, all those which stand in no appreciable relation to the organism are not properly to be included in its Medium. In consequence of this oversight we frequently hear it urged as an objection to the Evolution Hypothesis, that manifold organisms exist under the *same* external conditions, and that organisms persist unchanged amid a great variety of conditions. The objection is beside the question. In the general sum of external forces there are certain items which are nearly related to particular organisms, and constitute their Medium; those items which are so distantly related to these organisms as to cause no reactions in them, are, for them, as if non-existent.* Of the manifold vibrations which the ether is supposed to be incessantly undergoing, only certain vibrations affect the eye as light; these constitute the Medium of Sight; the others are as if they were not. Only certain vibrations of the air affect the ear as Sound; to all other vibrations we

* At the time this was written, I had some fish ova in the course of development. Out of the same mass, and in the same vessel, all those which were supported by weed at a depth of half an inch from the surface, lived and developed; all those, without exception, that were at a depth of two to four inches, perished. In ordinary parlance, surely, nothing would be objected to in the phrase, "these ova were all in the *same* Medium;" the water was the same, the weed the same, the vessel the same; yet some difference of temperature and carbonic acid made all the difference between life and death. Another curious fact was observed: I removed eight of these ova with active embryos, and placed them in a large watch-glass containing a solution (one-half per cent.) of bichromate of ammonia. In this acid the embryos lived and were active fifty-seven hours, although other embryos placed in a similar watch-glass containing pond-water, survived only forty hours. The non-effect of the acid was probably due to the non-absorption which nullifies the effect of certain virulent poisons when they are swallowed; but why the fish should live longer in the acid than in the simple water, I do not at all comprehend.

are deaf; though ears of finer sensibility may detect them and be deaf to those which affect us.

55. "The external conditions of existence" is therefore the correct definition of the Medium. An animal may be surrounded with various foods and poisons, but if its organism is not directly affected by them they cannot be food or poison to it. An animal may be surrounded with carnivorous rivals, but if it is not adapted to serve them as food, or is too powerful to be attacked by them, they only indirectly enter into its Medium, by eating the food it would eat. The analogy is similar with anorganisms and their relation to their media. Every physical or chemical phenomenon depends on the concurrence of definite conditions: namely, the substance which manifests the change, and the medium in which the change is manifested. Alter the medium, solid, liquid, or gaseous, change its thermal or electrical state, and the phenomenon is altered. But although similar alterations in the medium notoriously influence the organism, yet, because a great many variations in external conditions are unaccompanied by appreciable changes in the organism, there are biologists who regard this as a proof of Life being independent of physical and chemical laws; an error arising from their not recognising the precise nature of organic conditions.

56. To give greater precision to the conception of a Medium it will be desirable to adopt the distinction much insisted on by Claude Bernard, namely, 1°, an External or Cosmical Medium, embracing the whole of the circumstances outside the organism, capable of directly affecting it, and 2°, an Internal or Physiological Medium, embracing the conditions inside the organism, and in direct relation with it—that is to say, the plasma in which its tissues are bathed, by which they are nourished. To these add its temperature and electrical conditions. Bernard only includes the nutritive fluid; but inasmuch as each organism possesses a temperature and electrical state of its own, and these are only indirectly dependent on the external temperature and electricity, and as it is with these internal conditions that

the organism is in direct relation, I include them with the plasma among the constituents of the Physiological Medium. Any change in the External Medium, whether of temperature or electricity, of food or light, which does not disturb the Internal Medium, will of course leave the organism undisturbed; and for the most part all the changes in the External Medium which do affect the organism, affect it by first changing the Internal Medium. External heat or cold raises or depresses the internal temperature *indirectly* by affecting the organic processes on which the internal temperature depends. We see here the rationale of acclimatisation. Unless the organism can adapt itself to the new External Medium by the readjustment of its Internal Medium, it perishes.

57. We are now enabled to furnish an answer to the very common objection respecting the apparent absence of any direct influence of external conditions. Let the objection first be stated in the words of a celebrated naturalist, Agassiz: "It is a fact which seems to be entirely overlooked by those who assume an extensive influence of physical causes upon the very existence of organised beings, that the most diversified types of animals and plants are everywhere found under identical circumstances. The smallest sheet of fresh water, every point of the sea-shore, every acre of dry land, teems with a variety of animals and plants. The narrower the boundaries which are assigned as the primitive home of all these beings, the more uniform must be the conditions under which they must be assumed to have originated; so uniform indeed that in the end the inference would be that the same physical causes can produce the most diversified effects."

Obviously there is a complete misstatement of the argument here; and the excess of the misstatement appears in the following passage: "The action of physical agents upon organised beings presupposes the very existence of those beings." Who ever doubted it? "The simple fact that there has been a period in the history of our earth when none of these organised beings as yet existed, and when, nevertheless, the material constitution of our globe and the physical forces acting upon it were essentially the same as they are now, shows that these influences are insufficient to call into existence any living being."* Although most readers will demur to the statement that because the material constitution of our globe was "essentially the same" before and after animal life appeared, therefore there could have been no special conditions determining the appearance of Life, the hypothesis of Evolution entirely rejects the notion of organic forms having been diversified by diversities in the few physical conditions commonly understood as representing the Medium. Mr. Darwin has the incomparable merit of having enlarged our conception of the conditions of existence so as to embrace *all* the factors which conduce to the result. In his luminous principle of the Struggle for Existence, and the Natural Selection which such a struggle determines, we have the key to most of the problems presented by the diversities of organisms; and the Law of Adaptation, rightly conceived, furnishes the key to all organic change.

58. In consequence of the defective precision with which the phrase "Medium," or its usual equivalent "physical conditions," is employed, several biological errors pass undetected. Haeckel † calls attention to the common mistake of supposing the organism to be passive under the influence of external conditions, whereas every action, be it of light or heat, of water or food, necessarily calls forth a corresponding reaction, which manifests itself in a modification of the nutritive process. He points out the obverse of this error in the current notion that Habit is solely due to the spontaneous action of the organism, in opposition to the influence of external agency,—as if every action were not the response to a stimulus. Corresponding with the fluctuations in the Medium there must necessarily be fluctuations of Adaptation, and I think we may safely assume that it is only when these fluctuations cease that the Adaptation becomes Habit. This is the interpretation of the phrase "Habit is *second* Nature," and is very different from the common interpretation which

* AGASSIZ: *Essay on Classification*, 1859, p. 15.
† HAECKEL: *Generelle Morphologie*, ii. 211.

attributes it to the use or disuse of organs; as if use or disuse were a spontaneous uncaused activity.

59. The organism, simple or complex, is, we have already seen, built up from materials originally derived from the External Medium, but proximately from the Internal Medium. This statement, however, requires some qualification, especially in view of the hypothesis that organised substance was originally created such as we now find it, and not evolved from inorganic materials. Whether this hypothesis be adopted, or rejected, we have the fact that the immense majority of organisms *now* existing—if not all—are products of pre-existing organisms; and therefore organised matter is now mainly, if not solely, formed by organised matter.

We take, therefore, as our point of departure, the protoplasm; this is the first of the three terms of the vital synthesis: Structure, Aliment, and Instrument. The evolution of this is proximately dependent on the *pabulum* afforded it in the Internal Medium, which is the true nutrient material, and to which what is usually called *food* stands in an external relation: for between the reception of food and its assimilation by the organite, there is an indispensable intermediary stage, through which matter passes from the unorganised to the organised state. This intermediate is now recognised in plants as in animals. The old belief that plants were nourished *directly* from the soil and atmosphere can no longer be sustained. The process of Nutrition is alike in both: in both the materials drawn from the External Medium are formed into proximate principles and organic substances. It is daily becoming more and more probable that the inorganic materials, water and oxygen, so freely entering into the organism, never pass directly from the External Medium to the tissues, but have to pass through the Internal Medium where they are changed, so that the water is no longer free, but exists in a fixed state which has no analogue out of the living substance. Only a part of the water can be pressed out mechanically; the rest—that which is already incorporated with the other elements—can only be got rid of in a vacuum and at a high temperature.

Oxygen, also, comports itself differently in the tissue; as is proved by the fact that its physiological absorption is markedly different from any chemical oxidation in a dead or decomposing tissue.* Be this as it may, we know that organic substances have to be unbuilt and rebuilt in the organism; that the albumen of our food never passes directly into the albumen of our tissues; any more than the milk drunk by a nursing mother will pass into her breasts, and increase her supply, except by nourishing her.

60. In the First Series of these Problems the term Bioplasm was employed to designate this organised part of the Internal Medium. I was led to adopt it as a corresponding term to that of Psychoplasm, by which I wished to designate the *sentient* material of the psychological medium. There can be little doubt that the term Bioplasm was an unconscious reproduction of the title of Dr. Beale's work, which I must have seen advertised. I withdraw it now that I have read Dr. Beale's work, and see that the signification he attaches to the term is almost identical with Protoplasm. In lieu thereof, the term Plasmode (from *plasma,* anything formed, and *odos,* a pathway) may be substituted: it represents the *nutrient* material on its way to form Protoplasm, which is *formative* material; while the materials *formed* may be termed Organites and Products: the organite being the cell or cell-derivative (fibre, tube); the products being the gaseous liquid and solid derivatives of vital processes, which are *secretions* when they form intercellular substance or return into the plasmode and re-enter the vital circle; *excretions* when they are rejected, as incapable of further assimilation. The liver-cell will furnish an example of each kind of product. The bile, though containing principles serviceable in the chemical transformations, is for the most part excreted; but besides bile, the liver-cell produces starchy and saccharine principles which are true secretions, and re-enter the plasmode.

61. The organite is thus composed of sap, substance, and

* See on this last point RANKE: *Die Lebensbedingungen der Nerven,* 1868, p. 34.

product; the organism, of plasmode, tissue, and product. A glance at the vegetable-cell shows it to be constituted by the primordial utricle, or protoplasm, the outermost layer of which is condensed into a membrance, or cell-wall, and the cavity thus enclosed is filled with sap. The cell-wall grows as the protoplasm grows, and the protoplasm draws its material from the plasmode. A glance at the blood, the great reservoir of the river of life, shows us plasmode in the serum, and organites in the corpuscles; the one distinguished by sodic salts, the other by potassic salts. The plasmode, or serum, is in a constant change of composition and decomposition, giving up to the various tissue-organites and intercellular plasmodes the requisite materials, and receiving from organites and plasmodes the products of their changes. The serum is fed from the food *and* the tissues; and it feeds the several plasmodes which bathe the several tissues. Passing into the capillaries, it becomes transformed as it passes through their walls into the intercellular spaces, saturating the acid products of the cell-activities with its alkalies, and furnishing the protoplasms with their needed materials.

62. It will be understood that, although in appearance these stages are sharply defined, in reality they are insensible. But from the analytical point of view we may regard Nutrition as the office of the plasmode, and Evolution as the office of the protoplasm. Although evolution or genesis of form depends on assimilation, it is not a necessary consequence: the plasmode or the protoplasm might preserve such perfect equality in the waste and repair, such complete equilibrium, as not to undergo any development. The ova, for example, which exist in the ovaries at birth are not all subsequently developed; and if with modern embryologists we conclude that there is no replacement of these by proliferation we shall in them have examples of organites remaining unchanged through a period of fifty years.* But such an equilibrium is perhaps only possible in complete inactivity.

* See WALDEYER: art. *Eierstock*, in STRICKER'S *Handbuch der Lehre von den Geweben*, 1870, p. 570. "I found in a fœtus, which, in a case of

63. Again, although the office of the plasmode is primarily that of forming protoplasm, I think there is evidence to suggest that it not only does this, but that some of it is used in the direct development of energy, especially heat and electricity. The various forms of starch and sugar taken in with the food or formed in the liver, certainly do not as such enter into protoplasm. The same with alcohol.

64. It is perhaps in forgetfulness of the artificial nature of analytical distinctions that controversies rage respecting what are called intercellular substances and cell-walls. Now that the wall is no longer regarded as an essential constituent of the cell, but as a secondary formation, two opinions are maintained: first, that it is merely a concentration of the external layer of protoplasm; secondly, that it is a product of secretion from the protoplasm. Both positions may be correct. Certainly in some cases there is no other appreciable difference between wall and protoplasm than that of a greater consistence; whereas in many other cases there exists a decided difference in their chemical reactions, showing a difference of composition. Taking both orders of fact, we may conclude that the cell-wall is sometimes part of the organite, and sometimes product: a blood-cell and a cartilage-cell may be cited as examples of each. And this argument applies to the intercellular substance also.

65. The terms plasmode and protoplasm are general, and include many species. There are different plasmodes for the different tissues, so that we find phosphates of soda in the blood-serum, phosphates of potash in the nerve-plasma, phosphates of magnesia in the muscle-plasma, and phosphates of lime in the bone-plasma; having severally to form the specifically different protoplasms of these tissues. Observe, moreover, the gradations of these in respect of their physical state: the blood being the most liquid, the nerve a degree more solid, the muscle still more solid, and the bone almost entirely solid; and since solubility of material is a necessary condition of the

extra-uterine pregnancy, had lain thirty years in the body of its mother, the structure of the muscles as intact as if it had been born at its full time."—VIRCHOW: *Cellular Pathologie,* lect. xiv.

chemical changes, we can understand how the blood, the nerve, the muscle, and the bone represent degrees of vital activity: the greater the instability of organised substance, the more active its molecular renovation. Many serious errors result from overlooking the specific differences of protoplasms; among them may be mentioned that very common one of asserting that the ovum of a man is not distinguishable from the ovum of any other mammal, nor the ovum of a mammal from that of a reptile; nay, we sometimes see it stated that the protoplasm from which a mammal may be developed is the same as that which is the germ of an oak. So long as this simply asserts that we have at present no means of distinguishing them by any chemical or physical tests, there can be no objection raised; but it is a serious misconception, which any embryological investigation ought to rectify, to suppose that the ovum is not specific from the first.

66. Between the organites and their plasmodes there is the necessary relation, which corresponds with the relation between organisms and their mediums. Once formed, the organites are arranged side by side, or end on end, into textures or tissues, and these are grouped into organs, every organ being constituted by a collection of tissues, as every apparatus is by a collection of organs, and the organism by the federation of all the parts. We have more than once insisted on the necessity of synthetic interpretation to complete the indications of analysis: which means that no account of vital phenomena is *real* unless it takes in all the co-operant factors, both those of the organism and the medium. Neglect of this canon vitiates Dr. Beale's otherwise remarkable labours.

THE HYPOTHESIS OF GERMINAL MATTER.

67. It may help to elucidate certain important points if I here examine the hypothesis which Dr. Beale has worked out with such patient skill, but with what seems to me such unphysiological results. He deserves, I think, more applause than has been awarded to him, not only for the admirable

patience with which he has pursued the idea, but also for the striking definiteness of the idea itself—always a great advantage in an hypothesis, since it gives precision to research. If biologists have paid but little attention to it, this is no doubt due to the theoretical, still more than to the observational contradictions it presents. Histologists dispute his facts, or his interpretations; while other biologists do not see their way in the application of his hypothesis. Respecting all disputed points of observation I shall be silent, for I have myself made no systematic researches in this direction, such as would entitle me to form an estimate of the evidence. But my dissent from the hypothesis is founded on biological principles so fundamental that I should be willing to take my stand entirely on the facts he himself puts forward.*

68. The hypothesis is that nothing in the organism has any claim to vitality except the minute masses of protoplasm (by him called bioplasm), which in the egg represent, he thinks, about the one-thousandth part of the whole mass, the rest being lifeless matter, namely, pabulum, and formed material. This bioplasm is the *germinal matter* out of which, by a *process of dying*, arise the tissues and humours constituting the *formed material*—these, with the pabulum which feeds the germinal matter, being all dead material. The germinal matter itself, though living, only lives because there is temporarily associated with it that Vital Force of which we have already spoken (§ 14). In virtue of this association, a particle of matter not exceeding the one hundred-thousandth of an inch in diameter is said to be alive; and, presumably, to contain within it all those manifold powers which the term Life condenses. The pabulum brought under the influence of this Vital Force is transformed into germinal matter which, escaping from this mysterious influence, *dies into tissue.* Muscle-fibres and nerve-fibres are thus not living parts, nor are their actions vital. So that to be consistent we must not speak of the organism as living, but as a dead structure *pro-*

* See BEALE: *The Structure of the Simple Tissues*, 1861; the Introd. to his edition of *Todd and Bowman's Physiological Anatomy*, 1866; and *How to Work with the Microscope*, 4th ed., 1868; also *Bioplasm*, 1872.

duced by the Vital Force, and *set in action* by the aid of scattered bits of germinal matter. He has not, I think, stated whether each of these bioplasms has its own Vital Force, so that the organism is the theatre of millions of Vital Forces; or whether it is one Vital Force which animates the whole organic world of plants and animals. But nothing can be less equivocal than his position respecting the lifelessness of every part of the organism except the germinal matter.

69. The germinal matter may be selected as the primary stage of the formed material, the initial point of growth, and thus stand for the pre-eminently distinctive centre of Nutrition; but were we to limit all Nutrition to the germinal matter, as defined by Dr. Beale, and deny the co-operation of all the formed material, we should still not be justified in restricting Life to simple Nutrition. We cannot exclude such phenomena as those of Sensation and Motion, nor can we assign these to the germinal matter.* To suppose this, would be equivalent to saying that the steam which issues from a tea-kettle is capable of the actions of a locomotive engine. The steam from the kettle is like the steam from the boiler, it has molecular energy, and by this will co-operate in the production of mechanical work, if the mechanism be adjusted to it. The molecular energy of the protoplasm in muscular fibre may be indispensable to the movements of the muscles, but these, and not the protoplasmic movements alone, are muscular contractions. An hypothesis, therefore, which is obliged to declare that muscle-fibre and nerve-fibre are not living, even when active in the organism, seems to me defective at its base. If we view these apart from the organism, they may, like all the other formed materials, be regarded as dead; and no one doubts that epidermis, nail, horn, hair, and bone are dead in this sense, that they cannot live independently, and do not reproduce themselves. But so long as even these form constituents of the living

* "The physical property of the tissue does not depend upon this matter, *nor is its function due to it.*"—BEALE: *Introduction to Todd and Bowman*, p. 11. That is to say, he regards even contractility and neurility as physical, not vital facts.

organism, they also are *living* (§ 42).* It is only by a misconception of the analytical artifice that so simple a truth could have been missed.

70. But this misconception meets us at many a turn. The Vitalist hypothesis of an extra-organic agent of course refuses to regard Life as the expression of all the co-operant conditions; and even opponents of that hypothesis often fall into the same error of principle, when they attempt to explain Life by localising it in the cells; which is simply a morphological substitution for the once popular doctrine that only the vascular parts were organised, and every part destitute of blood-vessels was dead. This idea seemed supported by the facts of the most highly vascular parts being the most vital, and of a parallelism existing between the vital activity of those organs which when injected seemed almost entirely composed of blood-vessels, as the liver and brain, and those which showed scarcely a trace of vessels, as cartilage and bone; it seemed supported also by the appearance of blood-vessels in all new formations, and by the idea of the blood as the nutrient fluid. Then came the cell-doctrine, and the belief that the cell was the really ultimate morphological element—which may be true—and that "here alone there is any manifestation of life to be found, so that we must not transfer the seat of vital action anywhere beyond the cell,"†—which is very questionable.

71. We have already seen that the cell is an anatomical element, or organite; the organism is but an aggregate of organites *and* their plasmodes. But Biology, which deals with the organism as a whole, and with functions which are

* In turning over the pages of a work which was celebrated some half-century ago—RUDOLPHI'S *Grundriss der Physiologie*—I was interested to find a clear recognition of this biological principle: "Alle Theile aller Organismen," he says, i. 233, "sie mögen noch so verschieden in ihrem Bau, in ihrer Mischung, und in ihrer Thätigkeit seyn, sind ohne Ausnahme *als organisch und mithin als lebend zu betrachten.*" In a note he adds that physiologists have considered certain solid parts—epidermis, nail, hair, and bones—to be dead; "but all these are organically developed, and are in direct connection with the other parts."

† VIRCHOW: *Die Cellular Pathologie*, 1860, lect. i.

the resultants of all the vital properties, must not be restricted to any single factor, however important. It would assuredly be deemed absurd to say that diamond rings and lead pencils were the same, because the diamond and the plumbago, which are the specific elements of each, are both the same chemical element,—carbon. The substance is really different in diamond and plumbago, is different in properties, and is, in rings and pencils, united with different substances into objects having very different properties. Whatever analysis may discover as to the identities of organic structures, we cannot explain a single vital phenomenon without taking into account the three terms Structure, Aliment, and Instrument; and whenever a cell is said to be the seat of vital action, these three terms must be implied. In Dr. Beale's hypothesis the restriction is carried to its extreme; not content with the cell, he withdraws vital action from the cell as a whole, assigning it to the protoplasm and nucleus—cell-contents and cell-wall being, in his view, dead. If it be true that the protoplasm is alone concerned in Nutrition, yet Nutrition is not Life. Occupied mainly with formative processes, it leaves other indispensable processes to other parts. He instances the removal of all the tissues during the metamorphoses of insects:—"new organs and textures are laid down afresh and developed *ab initio*, instead of being built up upon those first formed." But to show how he restricts the idea of Life, he adds: "Such complete change, however, necessitates a state of existence during which *action* or *function remains in complete abeyance.*"*

The muscles and nerves which are instrumental in this functional life are said to be dead. It is true that the muscle-fibre does not develop fresh fibres. But it is equally true that the protoplasm of muscle does not alone execute *muscular* contraction. Each has its special office. Hence I reject the idea that formed material is dead. He further says "formed material may *be* changed, it cannot *change* itself." The antithesis is doubly inexact: 1°, nothing changes itself, but only yields to pressure, or reacts on being stimulated;

* BEALE: *Bioplasm*, 104.

and 2°, all the evidence at hand is against the notion that the formed material is not the seat of incessant molecular change; it is wasted and repaired molecule by molecule. Kölliker properly protests against the growing tendency of histologists to deify protoplasm, and to make it the sole seat of vital changes, the cell-wall and cell-products having also, he says, their physiological importance. It is manifestly erroneous to deny vital changes to the red blood-corpuscles on the ground of their no longer containing germinal matter.*

72. The analytical view may separate certain parts as active, and other parts as passive, and thus regard the cells as the seats of vital activity, the intercellular substance as merely accessory and instrumental; but the real or synthetical view must recognise both parts as equally indispensable, equally vital. Take cartilage, for instance, with its enormous preponderance of intercellular substance (formed material), and consider how absolutely impossible any of its uses would be were it reduced to the germinal matter of its corpuscles! And so of all the tissues.

73. If formed material is not to be excluded from the living parts of the organism, neither is the plasmode, out of which the germinal matter arises, since here we have the nutritive changes in their highest activity; and because the property of Nutrition is here most active, the other property of Development is in abeyance. Dr. Beale holds that pabulum necessarily becomes germinal matter; but when we come to treat of Nutrition it will appear that this is not more true than that Food necessarily becomes Tissue: some of it does; but much of it is used up for heat and other purposes.

74. What is true, and important, in the distinction between germinal matter and formed material, is that from the former onwards there is a gradual process of devitalisation, the older parts of every organite and tissue approaching more and more to the state of inorganic matter. But to show how vain is the attempt to restrict Vitality to any one out of a complex of co-operant factors, we might set up a chemical hypothesis to the effect that Vitality depends on

* KÖLLIKER: *Gewebelehre*, 5th ed., 1867, p. 12.

phosphates; and with it explain the phenomena quite as well as with the hypothesis of germinal matter. For not only is it found that the productive quality of a soil depends on its richness in phosphates, but, as Lehmann has shown, wherever cells and fibres make their appearance phosphates are found, even in the lowest organisms, which however contain but little. Phosphates abound in seeds and ova; in muscles and ganglia; and are deficient in the woody parts of plants and the elastic fibres of animals. The infant absorbs phosphates in large quantities, and excretes them in small quantities. Nervous activity is accompanied by the consumption of a third more phosphorus than accompanies muscular activity. Phosphates are among the most energetic of organic stimulants. But who would endow the phosphates with Vitality, on the ground of their indispensable presence in all vital processes?

75. Life, as we saw, is the expression of the whole organism. Many of the parts are incapable of manifesting any vital phenomena except in connection with all the rest; and of those parts which may be separated from the organism and continue to manifest some vital phenomena, none are capable of manifesting all. When the connexus of the parts is destroyed the organism is dead. Long after that cessation which we call Death, there are still evidences of Vitality in some of the parts: the heart will continue to beat, the glands will secrete, the hair will grow, the temperature will still be above that of the surrounding medium, the muscles will be excitable; these vital properties are the activities of organised substances, and so long as the state of organisation is preserved they are preserved; but the Life, which is the synthesis of all the vital properties, vanishes with the destruction of that synthesis.

76. May we not generalise this, and say that every special form of existence, organic or inorganic, is determined by the synthesis of its elements? Atoms are grouped into molecules, molecules into masses, masses into systems. Out of the textureless germinal membrane and the yolk, with no additions from without except oxygen and heat, are developed all the textures and organs of the chick, and this chick weighs no more than the egg out of which it was evolved. The development has been a succession of syntheses—epigenesis upon epigenesis. We may, if we please, regard each organite, as it appears, living its separate life, and each tissue its separate life; but we must not confound under the same symbol modes of existence so widely different as the activities of an organite, and the activities of an organism constituted by millions of organites.

77. If therefore we cannot restrict Life to the processes of Nutrition, Dr. Beale's hypothesis, whatever value it may have as explaining histogenesis, is quite unacceptable. Neither Vital Force nor Bioplasm covers the whole ground. For the former there is no better evidence than our ignorance of the real synthesis; for the latter the evidence is positive in its nature, but its interpretation is questionable. Dr. Beale selects as the germinal matter those portions of tissue which are susceptible of being deeply stained by the carmine solution, the formed material being only stained in a faint degree; the nucleus and nucleolus are the portions of germinal matter which are most deeply stained; and hence he concludes that the older the matter the fainter will be its colouration. There is no dispute as to the value of the staining process, invented by Gerlach, for the discrimination of chemically different parts of a tissue; and Dr. Beale has made excellent use of it in his researches.* But I altogether dispute the conclusion that the staining process reveals the parts which are exclusively vital; and for this reason: it depends solely on the acid reaction of those parts; and we cannot divorce the acid from the alkaline agencies, both being indispensable. Nay, it has been proved that in the *living animal* no organised substance can be stained. Lord

* Nevertheless there are some facts directly contradicting his conclusions. For example, he considers the axis cylinder of the nerve to be formed material, and agrees with Max Schultze and others as to its fibrillated structure; yet according to Lister and Turner, Gerlach and Frey, the axis cylinder is deeply stained by carmine, and in this respect resembles the nucleus of protoplasm.

Godolphin Osborne first discovered in 1856 that the protoplasm of growing wheat was susceptible of colouration;* but Gerlach in 1858 found that this never took place in the *animal* during life. He kept tadpoles and intestinal worms for weeks in coloured fluids, without a single spot becoming stained; although no sooner did these animals die than the staining began. Nor even when he injected the coloured fluids under the skin, and into the stomach, was the slightest colouration produced.†

To Gerlach's testimony may be added that of Stein, who, in his magnificent work on *Infusoria*, says that not only has no foreign substance ever been found in the protoplasm of the *Opalina*, but in the *Acineta*, and all the embryos of the higher Infusoria known to him, he has been unable to colour the living substance.‡ This resistance of the living protoplasm is surely a serious objection to the hypothesis that only those parts of the dead organism which are stained were the truly vital parts. Ranke sums up the results of his experiments thus: "They all show that the living cell resists the imbibition of every substance which it cannot assimilate. It is precisely the impossibility of staining the cell that proves this conclusively, since every particle of carmine absorbed would have revealed its presence."

It is not to be supposed that Dr. Beale was unacquainted with Gerlach's experiments. He has at any rate so far qualified the statement of his hypothesis as to admit that it is only after death that the germinal matter is stained. "The living matter" (he says, *How to Work with the Microscope*, p. 107) "possesses an acid reaction, or to speak more correctly, an acid reaction is always developed immediately after its death." Now, since this acid reaction only presents itself after death, and it is this which is revealed

* From the quite recent experiments M. BAILLON has submitted to the *Académie des Sciences* (15th February 1875) it appears that although cut flowers absorb coloured fluids, the roots when intact only absorb the fluid, and reject the colouring matters, by a veritable dialysis.

† GERLACH cited by RANKE: *op. cit.*, p. 75.

‡ STEIN: *Der Organismus der Infusionsthierchen*, 1859, p. 76.

by the carmine, we have no right to conclude that the carmine singles out the vital parts. Every one knows that the living muscle and nerve, when in repose, present an alkaline or faintly neutral reaction, and after excitation this is changed into an acid reaction, which increases with the exhaustion of the tissue. In strict logic, therefore—if we could logically apply such a test—it is the unstained parts that ought to be called vital. But, in truth, alkalinity and acidity are equally indispensable.

78. The main object of my bringing this question forward was to illustrate the danger of being misled by analysis: a danger we shall see to be very serious in psychological inquiries. The aid derived from analysis need never be undervalued; all that we have to bear in mind is that it is only a logical artifice, and that our real explanation must always be synthetic. Because of the tendency to rely on analysis there has been an imperfect discrimination of the profound difference between

ORGANISMS AND MACHINES;

and while on the one hand the legitimate striving of the biologist to display the mechanism of organic actions has been denounced by a certain school as Materialism and a hateful attempt to "rob Life of its mystery," there has been on the other hand a misconception of this mechanism, as if its dependant actions were of the nature of machines, that is to say, as if organised mechanisms were strictly comparable with machines constructed of inorganic parts. No doubt the laws of Mechanics are the same in both, for these are abstract laws which take no account of concrete differences. But when elaborate parallels are drawn up between steam-engines and animal organisms, the coal consumed in the one likened to the food in the other, and the force evolved in the combustion in both being the same, there is a complete obliteration of all that specially distinguishes vital activity.

79. Between an organism and a machine there is the superficial resemblance that both have a complex structure,

and are constructed of different and dependant parts. But underneath this resemblance there is a radical diversity.* The arrangement of parts in the organism is more than a *juxtaposition*, it is a *solidarity*, arising from the fact of their being all differentiations from a common substance which is a special combination of the three classes of proximate principles. Thus they are not parts which have been *put together*, but which have been *evolved*, each out of a pre-existing part, and each co-operating in the very existence of the other. The machine is made of independent and primarily-unrelated parts; its integrity depends on the continued preservation of the substance of each part; waste is here destruction. The organism is constituted by interdependent and primarily-related parts; its integrity depends on the continued destruction and renovation of their substance; waste is a condition of vitality. The actions of the machine are *sub*ordinated; the actions of an organism are *co*-ordinated. The lever moves a wheel, and the wheel in moving liberates a spring, each transmitting a communicated impulse, but otherwise each acts independently—no slight modification in the structure or movement of the wheel will modify the structure or the movements of the lever, no alteration in the tension of the spring will affect the structure of the wheel. But in the organism all are parts of one sympathetic whole; each reacts on each; each is altered by the other. Not a nerve is stimulated, nor a muscle moved, but the entire organism is affected. A condensation here is the cause of a greater imbibition there. The injection of salt or sugar under the skin of the frog's leg will produce cataract in its eye. The activity of a secreting cell in the ovary, or liver, alters the condition of the brain; the activity of the brain will check the secretion of a gland, or relax the sphincters of the bladder. When we observe the growth of horns, or the appearance of the beard, concomitant with the secretion of spermatic cells—and especially when we observe with these a surprising change in the

* STAHL had a profound conviction of the radical difference, though he was not able to point out the conditions involved. See his *Disquisitio de mechanismi et organismi vera diversitate.*

physical and moral capabilities and tendencies of the organism —we understand how the remotest parts of this mechanism are bound together by one subtle yet all-powerful tie. Nothing of this is visible in a machine. In a machine the material is so far of secondary importance that it may be replaced by materials of various kinds: a pulley may be worked with a hempen cord, a silken cord, or an iron chain; a wheel may be wood, iron, copper, brass, or steel; the actions will in each case be similar. Not so the organic mechanism: the slightest variation, either in composition or intimate structure, will affect, and may frustrate the organic activity. It is only in the skeleton that the specific character of the materials may be changed; and here only in the substitution of one phosphate for another in the solid masonry.*

80. Another marked characteristic of the organism is that it has a connexus of actions, the simultaneous effect of a continuous evolution, appearing in stages and ages. And in the animal organism there is a *consensus* as well as a *connexus*, through which there is evolution of Mind; and in the Social Organism an evolution of Civilisation. This consensus forms an intermediate stage through which the animal actions are sensitive as well as nutritive, and the nutritive are regulated by the sensitive. It is obvious that nothing like this is to be found in a machine; and we conclude, therefore, that any view of the organism which regards its mechanism without taking in these cardinal characteristics must be radically defective. We no more deny the existence of mechanical phenomena in denying that the organism is like a machine, than we deny the existence of chemical phenomena in denying that Vitality is chemical.

* M. FERNAND PAPILLON has shown that animals may be fed with food deprived of phosphates of lime if its place is supplied with magnesia, strontia, or aluminia; they make their bones out of these as out of lime. But no such substitution is possible in muscle, nerve, or gland; we cannot replace the phosphate of magnesia in muscles by the phosphate of iron, lime, or potash, as we can replace the iron of a wheel by steel, copper, or brass.

CHAPTER IV.

THE PROPERTIES AND FUNCTIONS.

81. The terms Property and Function are not always used with desirable precision. There is, however, a marked distinction between the property which characterises a tissue in whatever organ the tissue may be found, and the function which is exhibited by an organ composed of several tissues. We ought never to speak of a function unless we imply the existence of a correlative organ; and it is therefore incorrect to speak of the function of Nutrition, since *all* the tissues nourish themselves; but we may speak of certain organs as special instruments in facilitating Nutrition. Thus also with Respiration, usually, but not accurately, spoken of as the function of the lungs; the lungs being simply the most effective of the instruments by which the interchange of gases (which also takes place in every tissue) is facilitated. If by Respiration we mean Breathing, then, indeed, Respiration is the function of the lungs; if we mean the absorption of oxygen and the exhalation of carbonic acid, Respiration is a general property of vital tissue. A fragment of muscle removed from the body respires, so long as its organisation is intact; but it does not *breathe*—it has no accessory instruments, nor does it need them. The co-operation of nerve centres, diaphragm, ribs, circulating system, &c., necessary in the complex organism to bring the due amount of oxygen to the tissues, and convey away the carbonic acid, is here needless. In the ascending animal series we find this necessity growing with the complexity of the organism. The whole skin respires in the amphibia, and to some extent in

man also: a frog will live for ten or fourteen days after extirpation of its lungs, the skin respiring sufficiently to keep up a feeble vitality. But the skin does not suffice; and, very early, certain portions are specialised into organs (at first in the shape of external gills, and finally as internal lungs), for the more energetic, because more specialised, performance of this office. In the simpler organisms the blood is easily reached by the air; therefore no instrument is needed. In primitive societies the transport of goods is effected by men and women carrying them; in civilised societies by the aid of horses and camels, and waggons drawn by oxen; till finally these are insufficient, and railways are created, whose power of transport transcends the earlier methods, as the breathing of a mammal transcends the respiration of a mollusc. Breathing is the special function of an organ—the lungs (or more strictly, the thoracic apparatus)—as Railway Transport is a special social function. Although each of the tissues forming this organ can, and does, exhale carbonic acid and absorb oxygen—and each of the railway servants can, and does, transport objects to and from the locomotive—yet the main work is thrown upon the special apparatus.

82. What is meant by properties of tissue and functions of organs may be thus illustrated. Let us suppose ourselves investigating the structure of a ship. We find it composed of various *materials* — wood, iron, copper, hemp, canvas, &c.; and these under various *configurations* are formed into particular parts serving particular purposes, such as deck, masts, anchor, windlass, chains, ropes, sails, &c. In all these parts the materials preserve their properties; and wherever wood or iron may be placed, whatever purpose the part may serve, the properties of wood and iron are unaffected; and it is through a combination of these properties that the part is effective; while through the connection of one part with another the purpose becomes realised. The purposes to which masts, ropes, or sails are subservient may be called their functions; and these of course only exist, *as such,* in the ship. It is the

same with the organism. We find it composed of various Tissues, and these are combined into various Organs or Instruments.* The properties of Tissues remain the same, no matter into what Organs they may be combined; they preserve and exert their physical, chemical, and vital properties, as wood and iron preserve their properties. Each Tissue has its characteristic quality; and the Organ which is constructed out of a combination of several Tissues, more or less modified, is effective solely in virtue of these properties,† while the Function of that organ comes into play through its combination with other organs. For example, muscular tissue has a vital property which is characteristic of it, Contractility; and muscles are organs constituted by this tissue and several others; ‡ such organs have the general function of Contraction, but whether this shall be specially manifested in the beating of the heart, the winking of the eyelid, the movement of the chest, or the varied movements of the limbs, will depend on the *anatomical connections.* The reader unfamiliar with Biology is requested to pay very particular attention to this point; he will find many obscurities dissipated if he once lays hold of the "principal connections."

82*a*. Although Bichat's conception was of great value, it was not sufficiently disengaged from the metaphysical mode of viewing biological phenomena. Both he and his disciples

* Anatomy resolves the Tissues into Organites (cells, fibres, tubes); here its province ends, and that of Chemistry begins by pointing out the molecular composition of the Organites.

† This luminous conception, though vaguely seized by PINEL, was first definitely wrought out by BICHAT. See his *Recherches sur la Vie et la Mort*—and especially his *Anatomie Générale*, 1812, i. p. lxx. It was one of the most germinal conceptions of modern times.

‡ Just as there go other materials besides canvas to make a sail, and others besides iron to make a windlass, so there go other tissues besides the muscular to form a muscle—there is the membranous envelope, the nerve, the blood-vessels, the lymphatics, the tendon, and the fat. Even in Contraction there is another property involved besides the Contractility of the muscular element, namely, the Elasticity of the fibrous wall of the muscular tube; but Contractility is the dominant property, and determines the speciality of the function.

will be found treating Properties as entities, and invoking them as *causes* of the phenomena instead of recognising them simply as abstract *expressions* of the phenomena. Readers of my First Series will remember how often I have had occasion to point out this common error: men having baptized observed facts with a comprehensive name, forget the process of baptism, and suppose the name to represent a mysterious agency. The fact that gases combine is expressed in the term affinity; and then Affinity is understood to be the cause of the combinations. The fact that bodies tend towards each other is called their gravitation, and Gravitation is then said to cause the tendency. The doctrine of vital properties has been thus misunderstood. While no one imagines that he can operate on affinity otherwise than by operating on the known conditions under which gases combine, many a biologist and physician speaks as if he could operate on the Irritability of a tissue, or the Co-ordination of muscles, by direct action on these abstractions.

Let it be therefore once for all expressly stated that by the property of a tissue is simply meant the *constant mode of reaction of that tissue under definite conditions.* The property is not a cause, otherwise than the conditions it expresses are a cause. And these conditions are first those of the organised structure itself, and secondly those of the medium in which it lives. Oxygen unites with Hydrogen to form water, but only under certain pressures; so likewise muscles manifest Contractility on being stimulated (that is their mode of reaction), but only under certain degrees of temperature, humidity, and a certain chemical composition of the plasmode. The property is so truly an expression of the co-operant conditions, that it is found to vary with those conditions, and to vanish when they vary beyond a certain limit.

An attempt has been made to restrict the notion of a property to an ultimate fact. Whatever is not reducible to known conditions is to be accepted as a property. Combustion, for example, is reducible to the molecular combination of oxygen and some other gas; but this combination itself is not reducible, and it is therefore christened affinity. I cannot accept this view. Admitting our inability to say *why* gases combine under certain conditions (and in this sense all facts are inexplicable and ultimate, unless we take the *how* as ample explanation of the *why*), I must still say that since affinity itself depends on the co-operation of known conditions, it is not less explicable than combustion. But the point is unimportant: what we have here to settle is the meaning of a property of tissue,—and that is the mode of reaction which that tissue manifests under constant conditions, internal and external.

83. The evolution of Life is the evolution of special properties and functions from general properties and functions. The organism rises in power as it ramifies into variety. Out of a seemingly structureless germinal membrane, by successive differentiations certain portions are set apart for the dominant, or exclusive, performance of certain processes; just as in the social organism there is a setting apart of certain classes of men for the dominant or exclusive performance of offices, which by their co-operation constitute Society. The soldier fights, but ceases to build or reap, weave or teach; the mason builds; the agriculturist sows and reaps; the priest and thinker teach; the statesman governs. In simple societies each does all, or nearly all; but the social life thus manifested is markedly inferior to the energetic life of a complex society. So with organisms. An amœba manifests the general properties of Nutrition, Reproduction, Sensibility, and Movement. But it has no special organs, consequently no special functions. The polype has a certain rudimentary specialisation of parts: it has a simple alimentary cavity, and prehensile tentacles; and although by these it can seize and digest its prey, it can only do so in a limited way—all the manifold varieties and power of prehension and digestion observed in more complex organisms are impossible with such organs as the polype possesses.

84. Differences of structure and connection necessarily bring about corresponding differences in Function, since

Function is the *directed energy* of the Properties of tissues. One organ will differ from another in structure, as the liver from the pancreas, or the kidney from the spleen; or one organ may closely resemble another but differ from it only in *connections,* as a sensory and a motor nerve, or an extensor and a flexor muscle. We must therefore always bear both points in mind. Every modification, structural or connectional, is translated by a corresponding modification in the office. The hand and the foot show this well. The tissues are the same in both, the properties are the same, and both have the same general function of Prehension; but their morphological differences carry corresponding differences in their uses.

Suppose we have a galvanic battery, we know that its electric force may be variously applied. Two pieces of charcoal fixed to the ends of its conducting wires give us the electric light; replacing the charcoal by a telegraphic apparatus we can transmit a message from one continent to the other; the wires dipped in a solution effect a chemical decomposition, dipped into a mixture of gases they effect a chemical composition. In these, and many other applications, the property of the battery is constant; but the functions it subserves have varied with the varying co-operants. So with the properties of tissue.* Not only have we to bear in mind the organic connections of the tissues, but also the relation of the organs to their media. Swimming and Walking, for example, are both functions of the locomotive apparatus, but they are specially differenced by the media in which the animal moves.

85. The properties of tissues are their peculiar modes of reaction, and each tissue has its dominant characteristic, such as the Contractility of the muscle, and the Neurility of the nerve. But there has of late years sprung up a misleading

* "L'élément musculaire peut être annexé à une foule de mécanismes divers ; tantôt à un os, tantôt à un intestin, tantôt à une vessie, tantôt à un vaisseau, tantôt à un conduit excréteur, tantôt enfin à des appareils tout à fait spéciaux à certaines espèces d'animaux."—CLAUDE BERNARD: *Rapport sur les Progrès de la Physiologie générale,* 1867, p. 38.

conception, partly a consequence of the cell-theory, and partly of the almost inevitable tendency of analysis to disregard whatever elements it provisionally sets aside; this conception is the removal of the property from its *tissue*, and the localisation of it in one of the *organites*—cell or fibre. This has been conspicuously mischievous in the case of the nerve-cell, which has been endowed with mysterious powers, and may be said to have usurped the place of nerve-tissue. I shall have to speak of this in the next problem. Here I only warn the student against the common error. The properties of a tissue depend on the structure and composition of that tissue, together with its plasmode and products; they vary as these vary. To select any one element in this complex, and ascribe the reaction of the tissue to that, is only permissible as a shorthand expression.

86. What has just been expounded may be condensed in the following biological law:—

Identity of tissue everywhere implies identity of property; and similarity of tissue corresponding similarity of property. Identity of organic connection everywhere implies identity of function; and similarity of organic connection similarity of function.

87. This law, first formulated by me in 1859, and then applied to the interpretation of nervous functions, was so little understood that for the most part it met with either decided denial or silent neglect; no doubt because of the general disinclination to admit that the properties and functions of the spinal cord could be *similar* to those of the brain, in correspondence with the similarity of their tissues and organic connections. Even Professor Vulpian, who adopted it, as well as my principal interpretations, hesitated, and relapsed into the orthodox view in assigning three different properties to one and the same tissue in cord, medulla oblongata, and cerebrum.* In the course of our inquiries we

* VULPIAN: *Leçons sur la Physiologie du Système Nerveux*, 1866, p. 581. In a work just published I find M. LUYS hesitating at the consistent application of this law. After pointing out the identity of the tissue

shall so frequently have to invoke this law that I earnestly beg the reader to meditate upon it, and ask himself upon what other grounds, save those of structure and connection, the properties and functions can possibly rest? If on no other, then similarity in structure and connection by logical necessity involves similarity in property and function.

DOES THE FUNCTION DETERMINE THE ORGAN?

88. Closely connected with this law, which simply formulates the self-evident principle that *every action is rigorously determined by the nature of the agent, and the conditions under which the act takes place*, is the surprising question whether functions are dependent upon organs, or organs dependent on functions?—a question which sometimes takes this shape: Is Life the result of organisation, or is organisation the result of Life?

The vitalist, who holds that Life is an extra-organic agent, is logical in declaring organisation to be the consequence of Life;* but there are many organicists who conclude from certain facts that organs are developed by functions, and that organisation is a result of Life. There seems, however, to be some equivoque here. I cannot otherwise understand how Mr. Spencer should have written:

in cerebrum and spinal cord, he is only prepared to say that we cannot deny that there is *no impossibility* in admitting physiological equivalence where there is morphological equivalence.—LUYS: *Actions Reflexes du Cerveau*, 1874, p. 14.

* It is because men converted the result into a principle, and supposed that Life preceded the Organism, that they were led to puzzle themselves over such facts as the continuance of vitality in divided organisms. ARISTOTLE felt the force of the objection: "Plants when divided are seen to live, and so are certain insects, as if still possessing the same Vital Principle (ψυχή) considered specifically (τῷ εἴδει) though not the same numerically (μὴ ἀριθμῷ). Each of these parts has sensation and locomotion for a time; and there is no room for surprise at their not continuing to manifest these properties, seeing that the organs necessary for their preservation are absent."—*De Anima*, lib. i. ch. iv. Compare BASSO: *Philos. Naturalis adversus Aristotelem*, Amsterdam, 1649, p. 260; and TAURELLUS: *Contra Cæsalpinum*, 1650, p. 850; neither of them grappling with the difficulty so firmly as ARISTOTLE.

"There is one fact implying that Function must be regarded as taking the precedence of Structure. Of the lowest rhizopods which present no distinctions of parts, and nevertheless feed and grow and move about, Professor Huxley has remarked that they exhibit Life without Organisation."* The equivoque here arises from the practice of calling all living bodies "organisms," even those destitute of the differentiations called organs; but if we substitute the term "living body" in lieu of "organism," the equivoque will disappear, and Function no longer seem to precede Structure. Neither Mr. Spencer nor Mr. Huxley would affirm that Life can be manifested without a living body; and every living body must have a structure of some sort—unless by structure be meant a special configuration of parts. The properties of a body, whether it be simple or complex in structure, result from the properties of its components; and the vital phenomena vary with these varying components. The substance of a Rhizopod is indeed simple as compared with that of higher organisms, but is complex as compared with anorganisms; and corresponding with this simplicity of structure there is simplicity of vital function.†

89. The *properties* of steam are exhibited by the kettle on the fire, no less than by the gigantic engine which animates a manufactory; but the *uses* of steam (the functions of the engine) vary with the varying structure, and the applications of that structure to other structures. Precisely analogous is the case of the organ and its function, in relation to the living substance of which it is a peculiar modification. Vital actions are manifested by a lump of protoplasm; but these actions are as sharply demarcated from the actions of more highly organised animals, as the phenomena of a steam-engine are from those of a tea-kettle.

90. Mr. Spencer has nowhere defined what he means by Structure, nor given a definition of Organ, and this neglect makes it difficult rightly to appreciate his view. But whether we take structure to signify the *substance* of the living body, or

* SPENCER: *Principles of Biology*, 1864, i. 153.

† Comp. LAMARCK: *Philos. Zool.*, ii. 114.

the *differentiations* of that substance into separate tissues and organs, in either case the actions (functions) of which this structure is the agent must be rigorously determined by it. Mr. Spencer has avowed this in declaring that the "general physiologist may consider functions in their widest sense as the correlatives of tissue." Is this true in the widest sense and not true in the narrowest? I am puzzled to find him insisting that "function from beginning to end is the determining cause of structure. Not only is this manifestly true where the modification of structure arises by reaction from modification of function; but it is also true where a modification of structure otherwise produced apparently initiates a modification of function." Such language would be consistent were he a vitalist who believed in a Principle independent of Matter which shapes matter into organic forms; but as a positive thinker he can scarcely escape the admission that since Function is the activity of the Agent (Function in the widest sense being the action of the whole Organism, and in its narrowest sense the action of the special Organ) there cannot be an *activity preceding the agent.* I suspect that he does not always bear in mind the distinction between Property and Function, and consequently is led into statements at variance with the principles he professes. As far as I understand the course of his thought, it runs somewhat thus: With the increased use of an organ its volume may be increased, its structure altered; this alteration will, by reaction, cause alterations in other organs, and thus the result of a change in the habitual activities of an animal will be an alteration in the arrangement of its parts.

91. We speak loosely of an organ being developed by increased activity; but this is loose speech, and investigation shows that the organ is not developed *by*, but accompanies the increased activity, every increment of activity being necessarily preceded by a corresponding increment of structure. This is evident *à priori:* the force manifested is inherent in the structure manifesting it. Thus we ought not to say "the vascular system furnishes good instances of the increased growth that *follows* increased function;" we ought

to say, "that *permits* increased function." The muscle having a contractile power represented by 10, expends, we will suppose, 7 units of force in its normal activity, and these are replaced by its normal nutrition. If from an extra demand upon it 9 units are expended, the muscle becomes fatigued, if 10, exhausted, and it will no longer contract, the whole disposable sum of its contractility being dissipated. During all these stages the structure of the muscle—or to prevent all equivoque, let us say the substance of the muscle—has been changing, not indeed in any degree appreciable to the eye, but appreciable by the more decisive tests of chemical and physiological reactions. Yet inasmuch as in the ordinary course of things the waste is quickly repaired, the muscle in repose once more regains its original state, once more represents 10 units of contractility. Now let us consider what takes place when extra labour is thrown upon the muscle, when exercise causes growth. At the outset of a walking tour we may not be able to compass more than twenty miles a day, at its close we manage thirty. Is it the increased activity of the function which has caused this increase of structure? In one sense, yes; but let us understand it. Had the increase of activity been temporary, there would have been only a temporary increase of structure. But when the ordinary expenditure of 7 units rises to 9, on several successive days, this extra expenditure of tissue has had to be met by an extra nutrition—*i.e.*, more plasmode has been formed and more protoplasm. It is a physiological law, easily explained, that, within due limits, extra waste brings about extra repair: as the channels are widened and multiplied, the *derived* currents become stronger, and the increased flow of nutrition which was temporary becomes permanent, because this increase is no longer dependent on an extra stimulus, but on an enlarged channel.* When the channels have not become multiplied or enlarged, which must be the case whenever the extra stimulus is fluctuating and temporary, the extra expenditure is not followed by increased

* Comp. SPENCER: *op. cit.*, ii. 362, 363, for good illustrations of this.

size of the muscle: the currents resume their old directions, no longer being diverted.

92. Let the social organism furnish us with an illustration. At the present moment there is a movement against the retail shopkeepers of London in favour of Co-operative Stores. The stimulus of getting better goods and cheaper, attracts the flow of custom from its old channels; and if this continue a certain time the new arrangements will be so thoroughly organised, and will work so easily, that Co-operative Stores will to a great extent supplant the retail shops. But if from any causes the stimulus slackens before this reorganisation has passed from the oscillating into the permanent stage—if the goods are not found to be superior, or the cheapness not worth the extra trouble—the old influences (aiding our indolence) which have been long and continuously at work, will cause the social organism to resume its old aspect, and the co-operative "varieties" will disappear, or exist beside the ancient "species."

In the one case as in the other a glance at the process is enough to detect that the increase in the activity has been preceded by a corresponding increase in the structure. The muscle has not been enlarged *by* extra activity, but *with* it. The co-operative action has grown with each additional co-operator. Looking at the cases from afar we may justly say that development has been due to function; but looking to the process we see that each increment of activity was necessarily dependent on an increment of substance. When changes of habit or adaptation are said to produce modifications in structures, this is true in as far as one modification of structure necessarily brings with it correlative modifications, the growth of one part affecting the growth of all more or less; but we must remember that to render the structure capable of new adaptations corresponding modifications must have been going on. The retail shopkeepers might securely laugh at the co-operative movement if the respectable families would not or could not become co-operant. When Mr. Spencer urges that "not only may leaf-stalks assume to a great degree the character of stems when they have to discharge the functions of stems by supporting many leaves, and very large leaves, but they may assume the characters of leaves when they have to undertake the functions of leaves," I would ask if he is not reversing the actual process? The stem cannot assume the functions of a leaf until it has first assumed the character of a leaf. The assumptions of both must be gradual, and *pari passu.*

93. The hand is an organ, its function is prehension. The performance of this function in any of its numerous applications is rigorously limited by the structure of the hand—the bones, muscles, nerves, circulating and absorbent vessels, connective tissue, fat, &c. Fatigue the nerve, and the function will be feebly performed; exhaust it, and the function ceases; diminish the action of the heart, tie an artery, or vitiate the structure of the blood, and the function will be correspondingly affected; stiffen the tendons, soften the bones, diminish the synovial fluid, or increase the fat—in short, make *any* alteration whatever in the structure of the hand, and an alteration is necessarily produced in its function. So rigorously is function dependent upon structure, that the hand of one man will execute actions which are impossible to another. The hand of a baby is said to be the same in structure as the hand of a man; and since the powers (functions) of the two are notoriously different, we might rashly conclude that here function was dissociated from structure. The case is illustrative. In baby and man the structure is similar, not the same; the resemblance is of kind, not of degree; and the function likewise varies with the degree. The penny cannon which delights the child is similar in structure to the ten-pounder which batters down walls; and though, speaking generally, we may say that the function of both is to fire gunpowder for human ends, no one expects the penny cannon to be employed in warfare. In physiology, as in mechanics, the effect varies with the forces involved.

There can be no doubt that an exaggerated activity will produce a modification in the active organ, for this is only the familiar case of increased growth with increased exercise, and this is the biological meaning in which Function can be said not, indeed, to *create*, but to *modify* an existing Organ. Preceding the activity there must be the agent. Every organ although having its special function has also the properties of all the tissues which constitute it. The function is only the synthesis of these properties to which a dominant tissue gives a special character. The eye, for example, though specially characterised by its retinal sensibility to light, is largely endowed with muscles, and its movements are essential to Vision. The intestinal canal, again, though specially characterised by its secretions for the decomposition of food, has muscles which are essential to Digestion. In many animals, especially vegetable-feeders, there is an exaggeration of the muscular activity in certain parts of the intestinal canal which is only possible through a corresponding development of the muscular tissue, so that in some birds, crustaceans, and molluscs we find a gizzard, which is wholly without a mucous membrane to secrete fluids, and which aids Digestion solely by trituration.

94. Mr. Spencer, as I have already suggested, seems to have been led into his view by not keeping distinctly present to his mind the differences between Properties of tissue and Function, the activity of an organ. "That function takes precedence of structure," he says, "seems implied in the definition of Life. If Life consist of inner actions so adjusted as to balance outer actions—if the actions are the *substance* of Life, while the adjustment constitutes its *form*; then may we not say that the actions formed must come before that which forms them—that the continuous change which is the basis of function must come before the structure which brings the function into shape?" The separation of "actions formed" from "that which forms them" is inadmissible. An action cannot come *before* the agent: it is the agent in act. The continuous change, which is the basis of Vitality, is a change of molecular arrangements; and the organ which gives a special *direction* to the vital activity, *e.g.*, which shapes the property of Contractility into the function of Prehension, this organ must itself be formed before it can manifest this function. It is true that in one sense the organs

are formed by, or are differentiated in, a pre-existent organism; true that the general activity of living substance must precede the special activity of any organ, as the expansions of steam must precede any steam-engine action; but the general activity depends on the general structure; and the special actions on the special structures. If by Organisation we are to understand not simply organised substance, but a more or less complex arrangement of that substance into separate organs, the question is tantamount to asking whether the simplest animals and plants have life? And to ask the question, whether Life precedes organic substance? is tantamount to asking whether the convex aspect of a curve precedes the concave? or whether the motions of a body precede the body? To disengage ourselves from the complicated suggestions of such a word as Life, let us consider one of the vital phenomena, Contraction. This is a phenomenon manifested by simple protoplasm, and by the highly differentiated form of protoplasm known as muscle. In one sense it would be correct to say that Contractility as a general property of tissue precedes Contraction, which is specialised in muscle. But it would be absurd to say that *muscular* contraction preceded the existence of muscle, and formed it. The contractions of the protoplasm are not the same as muscular contractions any more than the hand of a baby is the same as a man's; the general property which both have in common depends on the substance both have in common; the special property which belongs to the muscle depends on its special structure. An infinite activity of the contractile protoplasm would be incompetent to form a muscle, unless it were accompanied by that peculiar change in structure which constitutes muscle. The tea-kettle might boil for ever without producing a steam-engine or the actions of a steam-engine. That which is true of one function is true of all functions, and true of Life, which is the sum of vital activities.

95. It is this haziness which made Agassiz "regret to observe that it has almost become an axiom that identical functions presuppose identical organs. There never was a more incorrect principle leading to more injurious con-

sequences."* And elsewhere he argues that organs can exist without functions. But this is obviously to pervert the fundamental idea of an organ. "The teeth of the whale which never eat through the gums, and the breasts of the males of all classes of mammalia," are cited by him as examples of such organs without functions; but in the physiological significance of the term these are not organs at all. It is no more to be expected that the breasts of the male should act in lactation, than that the slackened string of a violin should yield musical tones; but the breasts of the male may be easily stimulated into yielding milk, and the slackened string of the violin may be tightened so as to yield tone. Even the breasts of the female do not yield milk except under certain conditions, and in the absence of these are on a par with those of the male.

96. Organised substance has the general properties of Assimilation, Evolution, Sensibility, and Contractility; each of the special tissues into which organised substance is differentiated manifests a predominance of one of these properties. Thus although the embryo-cells all manifest contractility, it is only the specialised muscle-cell which continues throughout its existence to manifest this property, and in a dominant form; the muscle-cell also assimilates and develops, but besides having these properties in common with all other cells, it has the special property of contracting with an energy not found in the others. All cells respire; but the blood-cells have this property of absorbing oxygen to a degree so far surpassing that of any other cell that physiologists have been led to speak of their containing a peculiar respiratory substance. In like manner all, or nearly all, the tissues contain *myeline*—which indeed is one of the chief constituents of the yolk of eggs—but only in the white sheath of the nerves is it detached and specialised as a tissue.

97. But while Sensibility and Contractility are general properties of organised substance, specialised in special tissues; Sensation and Contraction are functions of the

* AGASSIZ: *Essay on Classification*, p. 91.

organs formed by such tissues: and these organs are only found in animal organisms. It is a serious error, which we shall hereafter have to insist on, to suppose that Sensation can be the property of ganglionic cells, or, as it is more often stated, the property of the central grey matter. Sensation is the function of the organism; it varies with the varying organ: the sensation of Touch not being the same as the sensation of Sight, or of Sound.

98. We may consider the organism under two aspects —that of Structure, and that of Function. The latter has two broad divisions corresponding with the vegetal and animal lives; the one is Nutrient, the other Efficient. The one prepares and distributes Food, the other distributes Motion. Of course this separation is analytical. In reality the two are interblended; and although the neuro-muscular system is developed out of the nutritive system, it is no sooner developed than it plays its part as Instrument in the preparation and distribution of Aliment.

This not being a treatise on Physiology there can be no necessity for our here considering the properties and functions in detail. What is necessary to be said on Sensibility and Contractility will find its place in the course of future chapters; for the present we will confine ourselves to Evolution on account of its psychological, no less than its physiological, interest.

CHAPTER V.

EVOLUTION.

99. THAT organised substance has the property of nourishing itself by assimilating from its internal medium substances there present in an unorganised state, and that this is followed by a development or differentiation of structure, is familiar to every inquirer.

Every one who has pursued embryological researches, and in a lesser degree every one who has merely read about them, must have been impressed by this marvel of marvels: an exceedingly minute portion of living matter, so simple in aspect that a line will define it, passes by successive modifications into an organism so complex that a treatise is needed to describe it; not only do the cells in which the ovum and the spermatozoon originate, pass into a complex organism, reproducing the forms and features of the parents, and with these the constitutional peculiarities of the parents (their longevity, their diseases, their mental dispositions, nay, their very tricks and habits), but they may reproduce the form and features, the dispositions and diseases, of a grandfather or great-grandfather, which had lain dormant in the father or mother. Consider for an instant what this implies. A microscopic cell of albuminous compounds, wholly without trace of organs, not appreciably distinguishable from millions of other cells, does nevertheless contain within it the "possibilities" of an organism so complex and so special as that of a Newton or a Napoleon. If ever there was a case when the famous Aristotelian notion of a "potential existence" seemed justified, assuredly it is this. And although we can only by a fallacy maintain the oak to be *contained* in the acorn, or the animal contained in the ovum, the fallacy is so natural, and indeed so difficult of escape, that there is no ground for surprise when physiologists, on first learning something of development, were found maintaining that the perfect organism existed already in the ovum, having all its lineaments in miniature, and only growing into visible dimensions through the successive stages of evolution.* The preformation of the organism seemed an inevitable deduction from the opinions once universal. It led to many strange, and some absurd conclusions; among them, to the assertion that the original germ of every species contained within it all the countless individuals which in process of time might issue from it; and this in no metaphysical "potential" guise, but as actual boxed-up existences (*emboîtés*); so that Adam and Eve were in the most literal sense progenitors of the whole human race, and contained their progeny already shaped within them, awaiting the great accoucheur, Time.

100. This was the celebrated "emboîtement" theory. In spite of obvious objections it gained scientific acceptance, because physiologists could not bring themselves to believe that so marvellous a structure as that of a human organism arose by a series of successive modifications, or because they could not comprehend how it was built up, part by part, into forms so closely resembling the parent-forms. That many and plausible reasons pleaded in favour of this opinion is evident in the fact that illustrious men like Haller, Bonnet, Vallisneri, Swammerdamm, Réaumur, and Cuvier were its advocates; and if there is not a single physiologist of our day who accepts it, or who finds any peculiar difficulty in following the demonstrations of embryologists, how from the common starting-point of a self-multiplying epithelial cell parts so diverse as hairs, nails, hoofs, scales, feathers, crystalline lens, and secreting glands may be evolved, or how from the homogeneous germinal membrane the complex organism will arise, there are very few among the scorners of

* "Nulla in corpore animali pars ante aliam facta est, et omnes simul creatæ existunt."—HALLER, *Elementa Physiologiæ*, viii. 148.

the dead hypothesis who seem capable of generalising the principles which have destroyed it, or can conceive that the laws of Evolution apply as rigorously to the animal and vegetable *kingdoms* as to the individual *organisms.* The illustrious names of those who advocated the preformation hypothesis may serve to check our servile submission to the authorities so loudly proclaimed as advocates of the fixity of species. The more because the two doctrines have a common parentage. The one falls with the other; and no array of authorities can arrest the fall. That the manifold differentiations noticeable in a complex organism should have been evolved from a membrane wholly destitute of differences is a marvel, but a marvel which Science has made intelligible. Yet the majority of those to whom this has been made intelligible, still find an impossibility in admitting that the manifold forms of plant and animal were successively evolved from equally simple origins. They relinquish the hypothesis of preformation in the one case, and cling to it in the other. Evolution, demonstrable in the individual history, seems preposterous in the history of the class. And thus is presented the instructive spectacle of philosophers laughing at the absurdities of "preformation," and yet exerting all their logic and rhetoric in defence of "creative fiats"—which is simply the preformation hypothesis "writ large."

101. It would not be difficult to show that the doctrine of Epigenesis with which Wolff for ever displaced the doctrine of Preformation, leads by an inevitable logic to the doctrine of universal Evolution; and that we can no more understand the appearance of a new organism which is not the modification of some already existing organism, than we can understand the sudden appearance of a new organ which is not the modification of some existing structure. In the one case as in the other we may disguise the process under such terms as creative fiat and preformation; but these terms are no explanations; they re-state the results, they do not describe the process; whereas Epigenesis describes the process as it passes under the eye of science.

102. If any reader of these pages who, from theological or zoological suspicion of the Development Hypothesis, clings to the hypothesis of a creative Plan which once for all arranged the organic world in Types that could not change, will ask what rational interpretation can be given to the succession of phases each embryo is forced to pass through, it may help to give him pause. He will observe that *none* of these phases have any adaptation to the future state of the animal, but are in positive contradiction to it, or are simply purposeless; whereas all show stamped on them the unmistakable characters of *ancestral* adaptations and the progressions of Organic Evolution. What does the fact imply? There is not a single known example of a complex organism which is not developed out of simpler forms. Before it can attain the complex structure which distinguishes it, there must be an evolution of forms similar to those which distinguish the structures of organisms lower in the series. On the hypothesis of a Plan which pre-arranged the organic world, nothing could be more unworthy of a supreme intelligence than this inability to construct an organism at once, without previously making several tentative efforts, undoing to-day what was so carefully done yesterday, and *repeating for centuries the same tentatives, and the same corrections, in the same succession.* Do not let us blink this consideration. There is a traditional phrase much in vogue among the anthropomorphists, which arose naturally enough from the tendency to take human methods as an explanation of the divine—a phrase which becomes a sort of argument—"The Great Architect." But if we are to admit the human point of view, a glance at the facts of embryology must produce very uncomfortable reflections. For what should we say to an architect who was unable, or being able was obstinately unwilling, to erect a palace except by first using his materials in the shape of a hut, then pulling it down and rebuilding them as a cottage, then adding story to story and room to room, *not* with any reference to the ultimate purposes of the palace, but wholly with reference to the way in which houses were constructed in ancient times? What should we say to the architect who could not form a museum out of bricks and mortar, but was forced to begin as if going to build a mansion: and after proceeding some way in this direction, altered his plan into a palace, and that again into a museum? Yet this is the sort of succession on which organisms are constructed. The fact has long been familiar; how has it been reconciled with Infinite Wisdom? Let the following passage answer for a thousand:—"The embryo is nothing like the miniature of the adult. For a long while the body in its entirety and its details presents the strangest of spectacles. Day by day and hour by hour the aspect of the scene changes, and this instability is exhibited by the most essential parts no less than by the accessory parts. One would say that Nature feels her way, and only reaches the goal after many times missing the path—on dirait que la nature tâtonne et ne conduit son œuvre à bon fin qu'après s'être souvent trompée."* Writers have no compunction in speaking of Nature feeling her way and blundering; but if in lieu of Nature, which may mean anything, the Great Architect be substituted, it is probable that the repugnance to using such language of evasion may cause men to revise their conceptions altogether; they dare not attribute ignorance and incompetence to the Creator.

103. Obviously the architectural hypothesis is incompetent to explain the phenomena of organic development. Evolution is the universal process; not creation of a direct kind. Von Baer, who very properly corrected the exaggerations which had been put forth respecting the identity of the embryonic forms with adult forms lower in the scale, who showed that the mammalian embryo never was a bird, a reptile, or a fish, nevertheless emphasised the fact that the mammalian embryo passes through all the lower typical forms; so much so that, except by their size, it is impossible to distinguish the embryos of mammal, bird, lizard, or snake. "In my collection," he says, "there are two little embryos which I have omitted to label, so that I am now quite incompetent to say to what class they belong. They may be lizards, they may be

* QUATREFAGES: *Metamorphoses de l'Homme et des Animaux*, 1862, p. 42.

small birds, or very young mammals; so complete is the similarity in the mode of formation of the head and trunk. The extremities have not yet made their appearance. But even if they existed in the earliest stage we should learn nothing from them, for the feet of lizards, mammals, and the wings of birds, all arise from the same common form." He sums up with his formula: "The special type is always evolved from a more general type." *

Such reminiscences of earlier forms are intelligible on the supposition that originally the later form was a modification of the earlier form, and that this modification is repeated; or on the supposition that there was a similarity in the organic conditions, which similarity ceased at the point where the new form emerged. But on no hypothesis of creative Plan are they intelligible. They are useless structures, failing even to subserve a temporary purpose. Sometimes, as Mr. Darwin remarks, a trace of the embryonic resemblance lasts till a late age: "Thus birds of the same genus, and of closely allied genera, often resemble each other in their first and second plumage: as we see in the spotted feathers in the thrush group. In the cat tribe most of the species are striped and spotted in lines; and strips or spots can plainly be distinguished in the whelp of the lion and the puma. We occasionally, though rarely, see something of this kind in plants. . . . . . The points of structure in which the embryos of widely different animals of the same class resemble each other, often have no direct relation to their conditions of existence. We cannot, for instance, suppose that in the embryos of the vertebrata the peculiar loop-like courses of the arteries near the bronchial slits are related to similar conditions in the young mammal which is nourished in the womb of its mother, in the egg of a bird which is hatched in a nest, and in the spawn of a frog under water."

104. It would be easy to multiply examples, but I will content myself with three. The tadpole of the Salamander has gills, and passes his existence in the water; but the

* VON BAER: *Ueber Entwickelungsgeschichte*, 1828, i. 221.

Salamandra atra, which lives high up among the mountains, brings forth its young full-formed. This animal never lives in the water. Yet if we open a gravid female, we find tadpoles inside her with exquisitely feathered gills, and (as I have witnessed) these tadpoles "when from the mother's womb untimely ripped," if placed in water, swim about like the tadpoles of water newts. Obviously this aquatic organisation has no reference to the future life of the animal, nor has it any adaptation to its embryonic condition; it has solely reference to ancestral forms, it repeats a phase in the development of its progenitors. Again, in the embryo of the naked Nudibranch, we always observe a shell, although the animal is without a shell, and there can be no purpose served by the shell in embryonic life.* Finally, the human embryo has a tail, which is of course utterly purposeless, and which, although to be explained as a result of organic laws, is on the creative hypothesis only explained as an adherence to the general plan of structure—a specimen of pedantic trifling "worthy of no intellect above the pongo's." †

105. Humanly appreciated, not only is it difficult to justify the successive stages of development, the incessant building

* Curiously enough, while the Nudibranch, which is without a shell, possesses one during its embryonic life, there is another mollusc, *Neritina fluviatilis*, which possessing a shell in its subsequent life is without one during the early periods, and according to CLAPARÈDE begins an independent existence capable of feeding itself before it acquires one. See his admirable memoir on the *Neritina*, in *Müller's Archiv*, 1857.

† Has any advocate of the hypothesis that animals were created as we see them now, fully formed and wondrously adapted in all their parts to the conditions in which they live, ever considered the hind legs of the seal, which he may have watched in the Zoological Gardens? Here is an animal which habitually swims like a fish, and cannot use his hind limbs except as a rudder to propel him through the water; but instead of having a fish-like tail he has two legs flattened together, and nails on the toes—toes and nails being obvious superfluities. Now which is the more rational interpretation, that these limbs, in spite of their non-adaptation, were retained in rigid adherence to a Plan, or that the limbs were inherited from an ancestor who used them as legs, and that these legs have gradually become modified by the fish-like habits of the seal?

up of structures immediately to be taken down, but also to explain why development was necessary at all. Why are not plants and animals formed at once, as Eve was mythically affirmed to be taken from Adam's rib, and Minerva from Jupiter's head? The theory of Evolution answers this question very simply; the theory of Creation can only answer it by affirming that such was the ordained plan. But the theory of Evolution not only gives the simpler and more intelligible answer to this question, it gives an answer to the further question which leaves the theory of Creation no loophole except a sophism—namely, why the formation of organisms is constantly being frustrated or perverted? And, further, it gives an explanation of the law noticed by Milne Edwards, that Nature is as economical in her means as she is prodigal in her variation of them: "On dirait qu'avant de recourir à des ressources nouvelles elle a voulu épuiser, en quelque sorte, chacun des procédés qu'elle avait mis en jeu." * The applause bestowed on Nature for being economical, is a curious transference to Nature of human necessities. Why, with a whole universe at her disposal, should Nature be economical? Why must she always be working in the same groove, and using but a few out of the many substances at her command? Economy is a virtue only in the poor. If Nature, in organic evolutions, is restricted to a very few substances, and a very few modes of combination, always creating new forms by modification of the old, and apparently incapable of creating an organism at once, this must imply an inherent necessity which is very unlike the free choice that can render economy a merit.

106. There may indeed be raised an objection to the Development Hypothesis on the ground that if the complex forms were all developed from the simpler forms, we ought to trace the identities through all their stages. If the fish developed into the reptile, the reptile into the bird, and the bird into the mammal (which I, for one, think questionable), we ought to find, it is urged, evidence of this passage.

* MILNE EDWARDS, *Intro. à la Zoologie Générale*, 1851, p. 9.

And at one time it was asserted that the evidence existed; but this has been disproved, and on the disproof the opponents of Evolution take their stand. Although I cannot feel much confidence in the idea of such a passage from Type to Type, and although the passage, if ever it occurred, must have occurred at so remote a period as to leave no evidence more positive than inference, I cannot but think the teaching of Embryology far more favourable to it than to our opponents. Supposing, for the sake of argument, that the passage did take place, ought we to find the embryonic stages accurately reproducing the permanent forms of lower types? Von Baer thinks we ought; and lesser men may follow him without reproach. But it seems to me that he starts from an inadmissible assumption, namely, that the development must necessarily be in a straight line rather than in a multiplicity of divergent lines. "When we find the embryonic condition," he says, "differing from the adult, we ought to find a corresponding condition somewhere in the lower animals." * Not necessarily. We know that the mental development of a civilised man passes through the stages which the race passed through in the course of its long history, and the psychology of the child reproduces the psychology of the savage. But as this development takes place under conditions in many respects different, and as certain phases are hurried over, we do not expect to find a complete parallel. It is enough if we can trace general resemblances. Von Baer adds, "That certain correspondences should occur between the embryonic states of some animals and the adult states of others seems inevitable and of no significance (?). They could not fail, since the embyros lie within the animal sphere, and the variations of which the animal body is capable are determined for each type by the internal connection and mutual reaction of its organs, so that particular repetitions are inevitable." A profound remark, to which I shall hereafter have occasion to return, but its bearing on the present question is inconclusive. The fact that

* Von Baer, *op. cit.*, i. 203.

the embryonic stages of the higher animals resemble in general characters the permanent stages of the lower animals, and very closely resemble the embryonic stages of those animals, is all that the Development Hypothesis requires. Nor is its value lessened by the fact that many of the details and intermediate stages seem passed over in the development of the higher forms, for the recapitulation can only be of outlines, not of details; since there are differences in the forms, there must be differences in their histories.

107. In the preceding observations the object has simply been to show that the phenomena to be explained can be rationally conceived as resulting from gradual Evolution, whereas they cannot be so rationally interpreted on any other hypothesis. And here it may be needful to say a word respecting Epigenesis.

The Preformation hypothesis, which regarded every organism as a simple educt and not the product of a germ, was called by its advocates an evolution hypothesis—meaning that the adult form was an outgrowth of the germ, the miniature magnified. Wolff, who replaced that conception by a truer one, called his, by contrast, Epigenesis, meaning that there was not simply *out*-growth but *new* growth. "The various parts," he says, "arise one *after* the other, so that always one is secreted from (*excernirt*), or deposited (*deponirt*) on the other; and then it is either a free and independent part, or is only fixed to that which gave it existence, or else is contained within it. So that *every part is the effect of a pre-existing part, and in turn the cause of a succeeding part.*" * The last sentence expresses the conception of Epigenesis which embryologists now adopt; and having said this, we may admit that Wolff, in combating the error of preformation, replacing it with the truer notion of gradual and successive formation, was occasionally open to the criticism made by Von Baer, that he missed the true sense of Evolution, since the new parts are not *added on* to the old parts as new for-

* WOLFF: *Theorie der Generation*, 1764, § 67. The reader will find abundant and valuable corroboration of this biological principle in SIR JAMES PAGET'S *Lectures on Surgical Pathology*.

mations, but *evolved from* them as transformations. "The word Evolution, therefore, seems to me more descriptive of the process than Epigenesis. It is true that the organism is not preformed, but the course of its development is precisely the course which its parents formerly passed through. Thus it is the Invisible—the course of development—which is predetermined."* When the word Epigenesis is used, therefore, the reader will understand it to signify that necessary succession which determines the existence of new forms. Just as the formation of chalk is not the indifferent product of any combination of its elements, carbon, oxygen, and calcium, but is the product of only one series of combinations, an evolution through necessary successions, the carbon uniting with oxygen to form carbonic acid, and this combining with the oxide of calcium to form chalk, so likewise the formation of a muscle, a bone, a limb, or a joint has its successive stages, each of which is necessary, none of which can be transposed. The formation of bone is peculiarly instructive, because the large proportion of inorganic matter in its substance, and seemingly deposited in the organic tissue, would lead one to suppose that it was almost an accidental formation, which might take place anywhere; yet although what is called connective tissue will ossify under certain conditions, true bone is the product of a very peculiar modification, which almost always needs to be preceded by cartilage. That the formation of bone has its special history may be seen in the fact that it is the last to appear in the animal series, many highly organised fishes being without it, and all the other systems appearing before it in the development of the embryo. Thus although the mother's blood furnishes all the requisite material, the fœtus is incapable of assimilating this material and of forming bone, until its own development has reached a certain stage. Moreover, when ossification does begin, it generally begins in the skull (in man in the clavicle); and the only approach to an internal skeleton in the Invertebrates is the so-called skull of the Cephalopoda. Not only is bone a late

* VON BAER: *Selbstbiographie*, 1866, p. 319.

development, but cartilage is also; and although it is an error to maintain that the Invertebrates are wholly destitute of cartilage, its occasional presence having been fully proved by Claparède and Gegenbaur, the rarity of its presence is very significant. The animals which can form shells of chalk and chitine, are yet incapable of forming even an approach to bone.

108. Epigenesis depends on the laws of succession, which may be likened to the laws of crystallisation, if we bear in mind the essential differences between a crystal and an organism, the latter retaining its individuality through an incessant molecular change, the former only by the exclusion of all change. When a crystalline solution takes shape, it will always take a definite shape, which represents what may be called the *direction* of its forces, the polarity of its constituent molecules. In like manner, when an organic plasmode takes shape—crystallises, so to speak—it always assumes a specific shape dependent on the polarity of its molecules. Crystallographers have determined the several forms possible to crystals; histologists have recorded the several forms of Organites, Tissues, and Organs. Owing to the greater variety in elementary composition, there is in organic substance a more various polar distribution than in crystals; nevertheless there are sharply defined limits never overstepped, and these constitute what may be called the specific forms of Organites, Tissues, Organs, Organisms. An epithelial cell, for example, may be ciliated or columnar, a muscle-fibre striated or non-striated, a nerve-fibre naked or enveloped in a sheath, but the kind is always sharply defined. An intestinal tube may be a uniform canal, or a canal differentiated into several unlike compartments, with several unlike glandular appendages. A spinal column may be a uniform solid axis, or a highly diversified segmented axis. A limb may be an arm, or a leg, a wing, or a paddle. In every case the anatomist recognises a specific type. He assigns the uniformities to the uniformity of the substance thus variously shaped, under a history which has been similar; the diversities he assigns to the various conditions under which the processes of growth have been determined.

He never expects a muscular tissue to develop into a skeleton, a nervous tissue into a gland, an osseous tissue into a sensory organ. He never expects a tail to become a hand or a foot, though he sees it in monkeys and marsupials serving the offices of prehension and locomotion. He never expects to find fingers growing anywhere except from metacarpal bones, or an arm developed from a skull. The well-known generalisation of Geoffroy St. Hilaire that an organ is more easily annihilated than transposed, points to the fundamental law of Epigenesis. In the same direction point all the facts of growth. Out of a formless germinal membrane we see an immense variety of forms evolved; and out of a common nutritive fluid this variety of organs is sustained, repaired, replaced; and this not indifferently, not casually, but according to rigorous laws of succession: that which precedes determining that which succeeds as inevitably as youth precedes maturity, and maturity decay. The nourishment of various organs from plasmodes derived from a common fluid, each selecting from that fluid only those molecules that are like its own, rejecting all the rest, is very similar to the formation of various crystals in a solution of different salts, each salt separating from the solution only those molecules that are like itself. Reil long ago called attention to this analogy. He observed that if in a solution of nitre and sulphate of soda a crystal of nitre be dropped, all the dissolved nitre crystallises, the sulphate remaining in solution; whereas on reversing the experiment, a crystal of sulphate of soda is found to crystallise all the dissolved sulphate, leaving the nitre undisturbed. In like manner muscle selects from the blood its own materials which are there in solution, rejecting those which the nerve will select.

109. Nay, so definite is the course of growth, that when a limb or part of a limb is cut off from a crab or salamander, a new limb or new part is reproduced in the old spot, exactly like the one removed. Bonnet startled the world by the announcement that the *Naïs*, a worm common in ponds, spontaneously divided itself into two worms; and that when he cut it into several pieces, each piece reproduced head and

tail, and grew into a perfect worm. This had been accepted by all naturalists without demur, until Dr. Williams, in his "Report on British Annelida, 1851," declared it to be a fable. In 1858, under the impulse of Dr. Williams' very emphatic denial, I repeated experiments similar to those of Bonnet, with similar results. I cut two worms in half, and threw away the head-bearing segments, placing the others in two separate vessels, with nothing but water and a little mud, which was first carefully inspected to see that no worm lay concealed therein. In a few days the heads were completely reformed, and I had the pleasure of watching them during their reconstruction. When the worms were quite perfect, I again cut away their heads, and again saw these reformed. This was repeated, till I had seen four heads reproduced; after which the worms succumbed.

110. The question naturally arises, Why does the nutritive fluid furnish only material which is formed into a part like the old one, instead of reproducing another part, or one having a somewhat different structure? The answer to this question is the key to the chief problem of organic life. That a limb *in situ* should replace its molecular waste by molecules derived from the blood, seems intelligible enough (because we are familiar with it), and may be likened to the formation of crystals in a solution; but how is it that the limb *which is not in existence* can assimilate materials from the blood? how is it that the blood, which elsewhere in the organism will form other parts, here will only form this particular part? There is, probably, no one who has turned his attention to these subjects who has not paused to consider this mystery. The most accredited answer at present before the world is one so metaphysiological that I should pass it by, were it not intimately allied with that conception of Species, which it is the object of these pages to root out. It is this:

111. The organism is determined by its Type, or, as the Germans say, its Idea. All its parts take shape according to this ruling plan; consequently, when any part is removed, it is reproduced according to the Idea of the whole of which it forms a part. Milne Edwards, in a very interesting and suggestive work, concludes his survey of organic phenomena in these words: "Dans l'organisme tout semble calculé en vue d'un résultat déterminé, et l'harmonie des parties ne résulte pas de l'influence qu'elles peuvent exercer les unes sur les autres, mais de leur co-ordination sous l'empire d'une puissance commune, d'un plan préconçu, d'une force pré-existante." * This is eminently metaphysiological. It refuses to acknowledge the operation of immanent properties, refuses to admit that the harmony of a complex structure results from the mutual relations of its parts, and seeks *outside* the organism for some mysterious force, some plan, not otherwise specified, which regulates and shapes the parts. Von Baer, in his great work, has a section entitled, "The nature of the animal determines its development;" and he thus explains himself: "Although every stage in development is only made possible by the pre-existing condition [which is another mode of expressing Epigenesis], nevertheless the entire development is ruled and guided by the Nature of the animal which is about to be (von der gesammten Wesenheit des Thieres welches werden soll), and it is not the momentary condition which alone and absolutely determines the future, but more general and higher relations." † One must always be slow in rejecting the thoughts of a master, and feel sure that one sees the source of the error before regarding it as an error; but in the present case I think the positive biologist will be at no loss to assign Von Baer's error to its metaphysical origin. Without pausing here to accumulate examples both of anomalies and slighter deviations which are demonstrably due to the "momentary conditions" that preceded them, let us simply note the logical inconsistency of a position which, while assuming that *every separate stage* in development is the necessary sequence of its predecessor, declares the *whole of the stages* independent of such relations! Such a position is indeed reconcilable on the assumption that animal forms are moulded "like clay in the hands of the potter." But this

* MILNE EDWARDS: *Intro. à la Zoologie Générale*, 176.

† VON BAER: *Ueber Entwickelungsgeschichte*, i. 147.

is a theological dogma, which leads to very preposterous and impious conclusions; and whether it leads to these conclusions or to others, positive Biology declines theological explanations altogether. Von Baer, although he held the doctrine of Epigenesis, coupled it, as many others have done, with metaphysical doctrines to which it is radically opposed. He believed in Types as realities; he was therefore consistent in saying, "It is not the Matter and its arrangements which determine the product, but the nature of the parent form—the Idea, according to the new school." How are we to understand this Idea? If it mean an independent Entity, an agency external to the organism, we refuse to acknowledge its existence. If it mean only an *a posteriori* abstraction expressing the totality of the conditions, then, indeed, we acknowledge that it determines the animal form; but this is only an abbreviated way of expressing the law of Evolution, by which each stage determines its successor. The Type does not *dominate* the conditions, it *emerges* from them; the animal organism is not cast in a mould, but the imaginary mould is the form which the polarities of the organic substance assume. It would seem very absurd to suppose that crystals assumed their definite shapes (when the liquid which held their molecules in solution is evaporated) under the determining impulse of phantom-crystals, or Ideas; yet it has not been thought absurd to assume phantom forms of organisms.

112. The conception of Type as a determining influence arises from that fallacy of taking a resultant for a principle, which has played so conspicuous a part in the history of philosophy. Like many others of its class it exhibits an interesting evolution from the crude metaphysical to the subtle metaphysical point of view, which at last insensibly blends into the positive point of view. At first the Type or Idea was regarded as an objective reality, external to the organism it was supposed to rule. Then this notion was replaced by an approach to the more rational interpretation, the idea was made an internal not an external force, and was incorporated with the material elements of the organism, which were said to "endeavour" to arrange themselves according to the Type. Thus Treviranus declares that the seed "dreams of the future flower;" and "Henle, when he affirms that hair and nails grow in virtue of the Idea, is forced to add that the parts endeavour to arrange themselves according to this Idea." * Even Lotze, who has argued so victoriously against the vitalists, and has made it clear that an organism is a vital mechanism, cannot relinquish this conception of legislative Ideas, though he significantly adds, "these have no power in themselves, but only in as far as they are grounded in mechanical conditions." Why then superfluously add them to the conditions? If every part of a watch, in virtue of the properties inherent in its substance, and of the mutual reactions of these and other parts, has a mechanical value, and if the sum of all these parts is the time-indicating mechanism, do we add to our knowledge of the watch, and our means of repairing or improving it, by assuming that the parts have over and above their physical properties the metaphysical "tendency" or "desire" to arrange themselves into this specific form? When we see that an organism is constructed of various parts, each of which has its own properties inalienable from its structure, and its uses dependent on its relation to other parts, do we gain any larger insight by crediting these parts with desires or "dreams" of a future result which their union will effect? That which is true in this conception of legislative Ideas is that when the parts come together there is mutual reaction, and the resultant of the whole is something very unlike the mere addition of the items, just as water is very unlike oxygen or hydrogen; further, the connexus of the whole impresses a peculiar direction on the development of the parts, and the law of Epigenesis necessitates a serial development, which may easily be interpreted as due to a pre-ordained plan.

113. In a word, this conception of Type only adds a new name to the old difficulty, adding mist to darkness. The law

*LOTZE : Art. *Lebenskraft*, in *Wagner's Handwörterbuch der Physiologie*, p. xxvi.

of Epigenesis, which is simply the expression of the material process determined by the polarity of molecules, explains as much of the phenomena as is explicable. A lost limb is replaced by the very processes, and through the same progressive stages as those which originally produced it. We have a demonstration of its not being reformed according to any Idea or Type which exists apart from the immanent properties of the organic molecules, in the fact that it is not reformed at once, but by gradual evolution; the mass of cells at the stump are cells of embryonic character, cells such as those which originally "crystallised" into muscles, nerves, vessels, and integument, and each cell passes through all its ordinary stages of development. It is to be remembered that so intimately dependent is the result on the determining conditions, that any external influence which disturbs the normal course of development will either produce an anomaly, or frustrate the formation of a new limb altogether. One of my tritons bit off the leg of his female;* the leg which replaced it was much malformed, and curled over the back so as to be useless; was this according to the Idea? I cut it off, and examined it; all the bones were present, but the humerus was twisted, and of small size. In a few weeks a new leg was developed, and this leg was normal. If the Idea, as a ruling power, determined the growth of this third leg, what determined the second, which was malformed? Are we to suppose that in normal growth the Idea prevails, in abnormal the conditions? That it is the polarity of the molecules which at each moment determines the group those molecules will

* I had kept these tritons four years in the hope that they would breed; but in spite of their being subjected to great varieties of treatment—for months well supplied with food, and for months reduced almost to starvation—they never showed the slightest tendency to breed; another among the many illustrations of the readiness with which the generative system is affected even in very hardy and not very impressionable animals. CLAPARÈDE observed the still more surprising fact that the *Neritina fluviatilis* (a river snail) not only will not lay eggs, but will not even feed in captivity. He attributes it to the stillness of the water in the aquarium, so unlike that of the running streams in which the mollusc lives. See *Müller's Archiv*, 1857.

assume, is well seen in the experiment of Lavalle mentioned by Bronn.* He showed that if when an octohedral crystal is forming, an angle be cut away, so as to produce an artificial surface, a similar surface is produced spontaneously on the corresponding angle, whereas all the other angles are sharply defined. "Valentin," says Mr. Darwin, "injured the caudal extremity of an embryo, and three days afterwards it produced rudiments of a double pelvis, and of double hind limbs. Hunter and others have observed lizards with their tails reproduced and doubled. When Bonnet divided longitudinally the foot of the salamander, several additional digits were occasionally formed." † Where is the evidence of the Idea in these cases?

114. I repeat, the reproduction of lost limbs is due to a process which is in all essential respects the same as that which originally produced them; the genesis of one group of cells is the necessary condition for the genesis of its successor, nor can this order be transposed. But—and the point is very important—it is not every part that can be reproduced, nor is it every animal that has reproductive powers. The worm, or the mollusc, seems capable of reproducing every part; the crab will reproduce its claws, but not its head or tail; the perfect insect of the higher orders will reproduce no part (indeed the amputation of its antennæ only is fatal), the salamander will reproduce its leg, the frog not. In human beings a muscle is said never to be reproduced; but this is not the case in the rare examples of supplementary fingers and toes, which have been known to grow again after amputation. The explanation of this difference in the reproductive powers of different animals is usually assigned to the degree in which their organisms retain the embryonic condition; and this explanation is made plausible by the fact that the animals which when adult have no power of replacing lost limbs

* BRONN: *Morphologische Studien über die Gestaltung-Gesetze*, 1858. Compare the note on § 11.

† DARWIN: *On Domestication*, ii. 340. In the *Annales des Sciences*, 1862, p. 358, M. MALM describes a fish in his collection, the tail of which had been broken, and the bone which grew out at the injured spot had formed a second tail with terminal fin.

have the power when in the larval state. But although this may in some cases be the true explanation, there are many in which it fails, as will be acknowledged after a survey of the extremely various organisms at widely different parts of the animal series which possess the reproductive power. Even animals in the same class, and at the same stage of development, differ in this respect. I do not attach much importance to the fact that all my experiments on marine annelids failed to furnish evidence of their power of reproducing lost segments; because it is difficult to keep them under conditions similar to those in which they live. But it is significant that, among the hundreds which have passed under my observation, not one should have been found with a head-segment in the process of development, replacing one that had been destroyed; and this is all the more remarkable from the great tenacity of life which the mutilated segments manifest. Quatrefages had observed portions of a worm, after gangrene had destroyed its head and several segments, move about in the water and avoid the light!*

115. A final argument to show that the reproduction is not determined by any ruling Idea, but by the organic conditions and the necessary stages of evolution, is seen in the reappearance of a tumour or cancer after it has been removed. We find the new tissue appear with all the characters of the

* In the memoir on the *Anatomy and Physiology of the Nematoids*, by Dr. CHARLTON BASTIAN, which appeared in the *Philosophical Transactions* for 1866, we read that even these lowly-organised worms have little power of repair. Speaking of the "paste eels" (*Anguilulidæ*), he says, "I may state as the result of many experiments with these that the power they possess of repairing injuries seems very low. I have cut off portions of the posterior extremity, and though I watched the animal for days after, could never recognise any attempt at repair." Perhaps, however, the season may have some influence; and Dr. WILLIAMS's denial respecting the Naïs may be thus explained. [What is said above was written in 1868, and published in the June number of the *Fortnightly Review*. In the August of that year the question of reproduction of lost limbs was treated by Prof. ROLLESTON in his *Address to the British Medical Association*, in which he showed cogent evidence for the conclusion that the reproduction of limbs only exists in animals that have feeble respiration, and consequently slow vital processes.]

normal tissue of the gland, then rapidly assume one by one the characters of the diseased tissue which had been removed and the reason is, that the regeneration of the tissue is accompanied by the same abnormal conditions which formerly gave rise to the tumour: the directions of "crystallisation" are similar because the conditions are similar. In every case of growth or regrowth the conditions being the same, the result must be the same.

116. It seems a truism to insist that similarity in the results must be due to similarity in the conditions; yet it is one which many theorists disregard; and especially do we need to bear it in mind when arguing about Species. I will here only touch on the suggestive topic of the analogies observed not simply among animals at the extreme ends of the scale, but also between animals and plants where the idea of a direct kinship is out of the question.

My very imperfect zoological knowledge will not allow me to adduce a long array of instances, but such an array will assuredly occur to every well-stored mind. It is enough to point to the many analogies of Function, more especially in the reproductive processes—to the existence of burrowers, waders, flyers, swimmers in various classes—to the existence of predatory mammals, predatory birds, predatory reptiles, predatory insects by the side of herbivorous congeners,—to the nest-building and incubating fishes; and in the matter of Structure the analogies are even more illustrative when we consider the widely-diffused spicula, setæ, spines, hooks, tentacles, beaks, feathery forms, nettling-organs, poison-sacs, luminous organs, &c.; because these have the obvious impress of being due to a community of substance under similar conditions rather than to a community of kinship. The beak of the tadpole, the cephalopod, the male salmon, and the bird, are no doubt in many respects unlike; but there is a significant likeness among them, which constitutes a true analogy. I think there is such an analogy between the air-bladder of fishes and the tracheal rudiment which is found in the gnat-larva (*Corethra plumicornis*).* Very remarkable also is the resemblance of the *avicularium*, or "bird's-head process," on the polyzoon known popularly as the Corkscrew Coralline (*Bugula avicularia*), which presents us in miniature with a vulture's head—two mandibles, one fixed, the other moved by muscles visible within the head. No one can watch this organ snapping incessantly, without being reminded of a vulture, yet no one would suppose for a moment that the resemblance has anything to do with kinship.

117. Such cases are commonly robbed of their due significance by being dismissed as coincidences. But what determines the coincidence? If we assume, as we are justified in assuming, that the *possible directions* of Organic Combination, and the resultant forms, are limited, there must inevitably occur such coincident lines: the hooks on a Climbing Plant will resemble the hooks on a Crustacean or the claws of a Bird, as the one form in which under similar external forces the more solid but not massive portions of the integument tend to develop. I am too ill acquainted with the anatomy of plants to say how the hooks so common among them arise; but from examination of the Blackberry, and comparison of its thorns with the hooks and spines of the Crustacea, I am led to infer that in each case the mode of development is identical—namely, the secretion of chitine from the cellular matrix of the integument.

Another mode of evading the real significance of such

* This beautiful and transparent larva reminds one in many respects of the Pike as it poises itself in the water awaiting its prey. It is enabled to do so without the slightest exertion by the air-bladders which it possesses in the two kidney-shaped rudiments of tracheæ, and which in the gnat become developed into the respiratory apparatus. The resemblance to the air-bladder of fishes is not simply that it serves a similar purpose of sustaining the body in the water, it is in both cases a rudiment of the respiratory apparatus, which in the fish never becomes developed. WEISMANN calls attention to an organ in the larvæ of certain insects (the *Culicidæ*), which have what he calls a tracheal *gill*, which gill has this striking analogy with the fish-gill that it separates the air from the water, and not, as a trachea, direct from the atmosphere. See his remarkable memoir *Die nachembryonale Entwickelung des Muscidens*, in *Siebold und Kölliker's Zeitschrift*, 1864, p. 223.

resemblances is to call them analogies, not homologies. There is an advantage in having two such terms, but we ought to be very clear as to their meaning and their point of separation. Analogy is used to designate similarity in Function with dissimilarity in Structure. The wing of an insect, the wing of a bird, and the wing of a bat, are called analogous, but not homologous, because their anatomical structure is different: they are not constructed out of similar anatomical parts. The fore-leg of a mammal, the wing of a bird, or the paddle of a whale, are called homologous, because in spite of their diverse uses they are constructed out of corresponding anatomical parts. To the anatomist such distinctions are eminently serviceable. But they have led to some misconceptions, because they are connected with a profound misconception of the relation between Function and Organ. Embryology teaches that the wing of the bird and the paddle of the whale are developed out of corresponding parts, and that these are not like the parts from which the wing of an insect or the flying-fish will be developed; nevertheless, the most cursory inspection reveals that the wing of a bird and the paddle of a whale are very unlike in structure no less than in function, and that their diversities in function correspond with their diversities in structure; whereas the wing of the insect, of the bird, and of the bat, are in certain characters very similar, and correspondingly there are similarities in their function. It is, however, obvious that the resemblance in function is strictly limited to the resemblance in anatomical structure; only in loose ordinary speech can the flight of an insect, a bird, or a bat be said to be "the same:" it is different in each—the weight to be moved, the rapidity of the movement, the precision of the movements, and their endurance, all differ.

NATURAL SELECTION AND ORGANIC AFFINITY.

118. It is impossible to treat of Evolution without taking notice of that luminous hypothesis by which Mr. Darwin has revolutionised Zoology. There are two points needful to be clearly apprehended before the question is entered upon. The first point relates to the lax use of the phrase "conditions," sometimes more instructively replaced by "conditions of existence." Inasmuch as Life is only possible under definite relations of the organism and its medium, the "conditions of existence" will be those physical, chemical, and physiological changes, which *in* the organism, and *out* of it, *co-operate* to produce the result. There are myriads of changes in the external medium which have no corresponding changes in the organism, not being in any direct relation to it (see § 54). These, not being co-operant conditions, must be left out of the account; they are not conditions of existence for the organism, and therefore the organism does not vary with their variations. On the other hand, what seem very slight changes in the medium are often responded to by important changes in the vital chemistry, and consequently in the structure of the organism. Now the nature of the organism at the time being, that is to say, its structure and the physico-chemical state of its tissues and plasmodes, is the main *condition* of this response; the same external agent will be powerful, or powerless, over slightly different organisms, or over the same organism at different times. Usually, and for convenience, when biologists speak of conditions, they only refer to external changes. This usage has been the source of no little confusion in discussing the Development Hypothesis. Mr. Darwin, however, while following the established usage, is careful in several places to declare that of the two factors in Variation—the nature of the organism and the nature of the conditions—the former is by far the more important.

118*a*. A still greater modification of terms must now be made. Instead of confining the "struggle for existence" to the competition of rivals and the antagonism of foes, we must extend it to the competition and antagonism of tissues and organs. The existence of an organism is not only dependent on the external existence of others, and is the outcome of a struggle; but also on the internal conditions which co-operate in the formation of its structure, this structure being the outcome of a struggle. The organism is this *particular* organism, differing from others, because of the particular conditions which have co-operated. The primary and fundamental struggle must be that of the organic forces at work in creating a structure capable of pushing its way amid external forces. The organism must find a footing in the world, before it can compete with rivals, and defend itself against foes. Owing to the power of reproduction, every organism has a potential indefiniteness of multiplication; that potential indefiniteness is, however, in reality restricted by the supply of food, and by the competition of rivals for that supply. The multiplication of any one species is thus kept down by the presence of rivals and foes: a balance is reached, which permits of the restricted quantities of various species. This balance is the result of a struggle.

Now let me call attention to a similar process in the formation of the organism itself. Every organite, and every tissue, has a potential growth of indefinite extent, but its real growth is rigorously limited by the competition and antagonism of the others, each of which has its potential indefiniteness, and its real limits. Something, in the food assimilated, slightly alters the part which assimilates it. This change may be the origin of other changes in the part itself, or in neighbouring parts, stimulating or arresting the vital processes. A modification of structure results. Or there may be no new substance assimilated, but external forces may call a part into increased activity—which means increased waste and repair; and this increase here is the cause of a corresponding decrease somewhere else. Whatever the nature of the change, it finds its place amid a complex of changes, and its results are compounded with theirs. When organites and tissues are said to have a potential indefiniteness of growth, there is assumed a potential indefiniteness in the pabulum supplied: *if* the pabulum were supplied, and *if* there were no antagonism thwarting its assimilation, growth would of course continue without pause, or end; but in reality this cannot be so. For, take the blood as the vehicle of the pabulum—not only is its quantity limited, and partly limited by the very action of the tissues it feeds, but even in any given quantity there is a limit to its composition—it will only take up a limited quantity of salts, iron, albumen, &c.; no matter how abundant these may be in the food. So again with the plasmodes of the various tissues—they have each their definite capacities of assimilation. What has already been stated respecting chemical affinity (§ 20) is equally applicable to organic affinity; as the presence of fused iron in the crucible partially obstructs the combination of sulphur and lead, so the presence of connective tissue partially obstructs the combination of muscle protoplasm with its pabulum.

118*b*. Owing to the action and reaction of blood and plasmode, of tissues on tissues, and organs on organs, and their mutual limitations, the growth of each organism has a limit, and the growth of each organ has a limit. Beyond this limit, no extra supply of food will increase the size of the organism; no increase of activity will increase the organ. "Man cannot add a cubit to his stature." The blacksmith's arm will not grow larger by twenty years of daily exercise, after it has once attained a certain size. Increase of activity caused it to enlarge up to this limit; but no increase of activity will cause it to pass this limit. Why? Because here a balance of the co-operating formative forces has been reached. Larger muscles, or more muscle-fibres, demand arteries of larger calibre, and these a heart of larger size; with the increase of muscle would come increase of connective tissue; and this tissue would not only compete with the muscle for pabulum, but by mechanical pressure would diminish the flow of that pabulum. And why would connective tissue increase? Because, in the first place, there is a formative association between the two, so that owing to a law, not yet understood, the one always accompanies the other; and, in the second place, there is a functional association between the two, a muscle fibre being *inoperative* unless it be attached to a tendon, or connective tissue; it will contract *out* of the body although separated from its tendon or other attachment; but *in* the body its contraction would be useless without this attachment. We must bear in mind that muscle-fibres are very much shorter than ordinary muscles; according to the measurements of W. Krause they never exceed 4 *cm* in length, and usually range between 2 and 3 *cm;* their fine points being fixed to the interstitial connective tissue, as the whole muscle is fixed to its tendon. The function of the muscle is thus dependent on a due balance of its component tissues; if that balance is disturbed the function is disturbed. Should, from any cause, an excess of muscle-fibre arise, the balance would be disturbed; should an encroachment of connective tissue, or of fat, take place, there would be also a defect of function.

Here we have the co-operation and limitation of the tissues illustrated; let us extend our glance, and we shall see how the co-operation and limitation of the organs come into play, so that the resulting function depends on the balance of their forces. The contractile power of each individual muscle is always limited by the resistance of antagonists, which prevent the muscle being contracted more than about a third of its *possible* extent, *i.e.*, possible when there are no resistances to be overcome. Not only the increasing tension of antagonist muscles, but the resistance of tendons, bones, and softer parts must be taken into account. Thus, the increase of the blacksmith's muscular power would involve a considerable increase in all the tissues of the arm; but such an increase would involve a reconstruction of his whole organism.

Whenever there is an encroachment of one tissue on another, there is a disturbance of the normal balance, which readily passes into a pathological state. If the brain is overrun with connective tissue, or the heart with fatty tissue, we know the consequences. If connective tissue is deficient, epithelial runs to excess, no longer limited by its normal antagonist, and pus, or cancer result.

118*c*. It is unnecessary here to enlarge on this point. I have adduced it to show that we must extend our conception of the struggle for existence beyond that of the competition and antagonism of organisms—the external struggle; and include under it the competition and antagonism of tissues and organs—the internal struggle. Variability is inherent in organic substances, as the result of their indefiniteness of composition (§ 45*b*). This variability is indefinite, and is rendered definite by the competition and antagonism, so that every particular variation is the resultant of a composition of forces. The forces in operation are the internal and external conditions of existence—*i.e.*, the nature of the organism, and its response to the actions of its medium. A change may take place in the medium without a corresponding response from the organism; or the change may find a response and the organism become modified. Every modification is a selection, determined by laws of growth; it is the resultant of a struggle between what, for want of a better term, may be called the *organic affinities*—which represent in organised substances what chemical affinities are in the anorganised. Just as an organism which has been modified and thereby gained a superiority over others, has by this modification been *selected* for survival—the selection being only another aspect of this modification—so one tissue, or one organ, which has surpassed another in the struggle of growth, will thereby have become selected. Natural Selection, or survival of the fittest, therefore, is simply the metaphorical expression of the fact that any balance of the forces which is best adapted for survival will survive. Unless we interpret it as a shorthand expression of *all* the internal and external conditions of existence, it is not acceptable as the origin of species.

118*d*. Mr. Darwin has so patiently and profoundly meditated on the whole subject, that we must be very slow in presuming him to have overlooked any important point. I know that he has not altogether overlooked this which we are now considering; but he is so preoccupied with the tracing out of his splendid discovery in all its bearings, that he has thrown the emphasis mainly on the external struggle, neglecting the internal struggle; and has thus in many passages employed language which implies a radical distinction where—as I conceive—no such distinction can be recognised. "Natural Selection," he says, "depends on the survival under various and complex circumstances of the best-fitted individuals, but has no relation whatever to the primary cause of any modification of structure."* On this we may remark, First, that selection does not *depend* on the survival, but *is* that survival; secondly, that the best-fitted individual survives because of that modification of its structure which has given it the superiority; therefore if the primary cause of this modification is not due to selection, then selection cannot be the cause of species. He separates Natural Selection from all the primary causes of variation, either internal or external—either as results of the laws of growth, of the correlations of variation, of use and disuse, &c., and limits it to the slow accumulations of such variations as are profitable in the struggle with competitors. And for his purpose this separation is necessary. But biological philosophy must, I think, regard the distinction as artificial, referring only to one of the great factors in the production of species. And for this reason: Selection only comes into existence in the modifications produced either by external or internal changes; and the selected change cannot be developed further by mere inheritance, unless the successive progeny have such a disposition of the organic affinities as will repeat the primary change. Inherited superiority will not by mere transmission become greater. The facts which are relied on in support of the idea of "fixity of species," show at any rate that a given superiority will remain stationary for thousands of years; and no one supposes that the progeny of an organism will vary unless some external or internal cause of variation accompanies the inheritance. Mr. Darwin agrees with Mr. Spencer in admitting the difficulty of distinguishing between the effects of some definite action of external conditions, and the accumulation through natural selection of inherited variations serviceable to the organism. But even in cases where the distinction could be clearly established, I think we should only see an *historical* distinction, that is to say, one between effects produced by particular causes now in operation, and effects produced by very complex and obscure causes in operation during ancestral development.

118*e*. The reader will understand that my criticism does

* *The Variation of Animals and Plants*, 1868, ii. p. 272.

not pretend to invalidate Mr. Darwin's discovery, but rather to enlarge its terms, so as to make it include all the biological conditions, and thus explain many of the variations which Natural Selection—in the restricted acceptation—leaves out of account. Mr. Darwin draws a broad line of distinction between Variation and Selection, regarding only those variations that are favourable as selected. I conceive that all variations which survive are by that fact of survival, *selections*, whether favourable or indifferent. A variety is a species in formation; now Selection itself is not a cause, or condition, of variation, it is the *expression* of variation. Mr. Darwin is at times explicit enough on this head: "It may metaphorically be said that Natural Selection is daily and hourly scrutinising throughout the world the slightest variations; rejecting those that are bad, preserving and adding up all that are good; silently and insensibly working, whenever and wherever opportunity offers, at the improvement of each organic being in relation to its organic and inorganic conditions of life."* But the metaphorical nature of the term is not always borne in mind, so that elsewhere Natural Selection is said to "act on and modify organic beings," as if it were a positive condition and not the expression of the modifying processes. Because grouse are largely destroyed by birds of prey, any change in their colour which would render them less conspicuous, would enable more birds to escape; but it is obvious that this change of colour will be due to Organic Affinity; and only when the change is *effected* will there have been that selection which *expresses* it. Mr. Darwin's language, however, is misleading. He says: "Hence Natural Selection might be most effective in *giving* the proper colour to each kind of grouse, and in *keeping* that colour when once acquired." This is to make Selection an agent, a condition of the development of colour; which may be accepted if we extend the term so as to include the organic changes themselves. Again: "Some writers have imagined that Natural Selection *induces variability*, whereas it only implies the *pre-*

* *Origin of Species*, 5th ed. p. 96.

servation of such variations as are beneficial to the being under its conditions of life." It, however, is made to imply more than this, namely, the accumulation and further modification of such variations. "The mere existence of individual variability and of some well-marked varieties, though necessary as the foundation, helps us but little in understanding how species arise in nature. How have all those exquisite adaptations of one part of the organisation to another part, and to the conditions of life, and of one organic being to another being, been perfected?" My answer to this question would be: By Organic Affinity, and the resulting struggle of the tissues and organs, the consequences of which are that very *adaptation* of the organism to external conditions, which is expressed as the *selection* of the structures best adapted. The selections are the results of the struggle, according to my proposed extension of the term "struggle." Mr. Darwin defines the struggle: "The dependence of one being on another, and including (what is more important) not only the life of the individual but success in leaving progeny." This definition seems defective, since it omits the primary and more important struggle which takes place between the organic affinities in operation. To succeed in the struggle with competitors, the organism must have first acquired—by selection—a superiority in one or more of its organs.

118*f*. A little reflection will disclose the importance of keeping our eyes fixed on the internal causes of variation, as well as on the external conditions of the struggle. Mr. Darwin seems to imply that the external conditions which cause a variation, are to be distinguished from the conditions which accumulate and perfect such variation, that is to say, he implies a radical difference between the process of variation, and the process of selection. This, I have already said, does not seem to me acceptable; the selection, I conceive, to be simply the variation which has survived.*

* Mr. Darwin has himself, in the following passage, stated a somewhat similar view, and rejected it:—"In one sense the conditions of life may be said not only to cause variability, but likewise to include Natural Selection, for *the conditions determine whether this or that variety shall survive*. But when man is the selecting agent, we clearly see that the

If it be true that a Variety is an incipient Species and shows us Species in formation, it is in the same sense true that a variation is an incipient organ. A species is the result of a slowly accumulating divergence of structure; an organ is the result of a slowly accumulating differentiation. At each stage of differentiation there has been a selection, but we cannot by any means say that this selection was determined by the fact of its giving the organism a superiority over rivals, inasmuch as during all the early stages, while the organ was still in formation, there could be no advantage accruing from it. One animal having teeth and claws developed will have a decided superiority in the struggle over another animal that has no teeth and claws; but so long as the teeth and claws are in an undeveloped state of mere preparation they confer no superiority.

118*g*. Natural Selection is only the expression of the results of obscure physiological processes; and for a satisfactory theory of such results we must understand the nature of the processes. In other words to understand Natural Selection we must recognise not only the facts thus expressed, but the factors of these facts—we must analyse the "conditions of existence." As a preliminary analysis we find *external conditions*, among which are included not only the dependence of the organism on the inorganic medium, but also the dependence of one organism on another—the competition and antagonism of the whole organic world; and *internal conditions*, among which are included not only the dependence of the organism on the laws of composition and decomposition whereby each organite and each tissue is formed, but also the dependence of one organite and one tissue on all the others—the competition and antagonism of all the elements.

The changes wrought in an organism by these two kinds of conditions determine Varieties and Species. Although

two elements of change are distinct; the conditions cause the variability, the will of man acting either consciously or unconsciously accumulates the variations in certain directions, and this answers to the survival of the fittest under nature" (p. 168.)

many of the changes are due to the process of natural selection brought about in the struggle with competitors and foes, many other changes have no such relation to the external struggle, but are simply the results of the organic affinities. They may or they may not give the organism a greater stability, or a greater advantage over rivals; it is enough that they are no disadvantage to the organism, they will then survive by virtue of the forces which produced them.

119. The position thus reached will be important in our examination of the Theory of Descent by which Mr. Darwin tentatively, and his followers boldly, explain the observed resemblances in structure and function as due to blood-relationship. The doctrine of Evolution affirms that all complex organisms are evolved by differentiation from simpler organisms, as we see the complex organ evolved from simpler forms. But it does not necessarily affirm that the vast variety of organisms had one starting-point—one ancestor; on the contrary, I conceive that the principles of Evolution are adverse to such a view, and insist rather on the necessity of innumerable starting-points. Let us consider the question.

That the Theory of Descent explains many of the facts must be admitted; but there are many which it leaves obscure; and Mr. Darwin, with that noble calmness which distinguishes him, admits the numerous difficulties. Whether these will hereafter be cleared away by an improvement in the Geological Record, now confessedly imperfect, or by more exhaustive exploration of distant countries, none can say; but, to my mind, the probability is, that we shall have to seek our explanation by enlarging the idea of Natural Selection, subordinating it to the laws of Organic Affinity. It does not seem to me, at present, warrantable to assume Descent as the sole principle of morphological uniformities; there are other grounds of resemblance beyond those of blood-relationship; and these have been too much overlooked; yet a brief consideration will disclose that similarity in the physiological laws and the conditions of Organic Affinity must produce similarity in organisms, independently of relationship; just as similarity in the laws and conditions of inorganic affinity will produce identity in chemical species. We do not suppose the carbonates and phosphates found in various parts of the globe, or the families of alkaloids and salts, to have any nearer kinship than that which consists in the similarity of their elements and the conditions of their combination. Hence, in organisms, as in salts, morphological identity may be due to a community of conditions, rather than community of descent. Mr. Darwin justly holds it to be "incredible that individuals identically the same should have been produced through Natural Selection from parents *specifically distinct*," but he, since he admits analogous variations, will not deny that identical forms might issue from parents having widely different origins, provided that these parent forms and the conditions of their reproduction were identical, as in the case of vegetable and animal resemblances. To deny this would be to deny the law of causation. And that which is true of identical forms under identical conditions is true of similar forms under similar conditions. When History and Ethnology reveal a striking uniformity in the progression of social phases, we do not thence conclude that the nations are directly related, or that the social forms have a common parentage; we conclude that the social phases are alike because they have had common causes. When chemists point out the uniformity of type which exists in compounds so diverse in many of their properties as water and sulphuretted or selenetted hydrogen, and when they declare phosphoretted hydrogen to be the congener of ammonia, they do not mean that the one is descended from the other, or that any closer link connects them than that of resemblance in their elements.

In the case of vegetal and animal organisms, we observe such a community of elementary substance as of itself to imply a community in their laws of combination; and under similar conditions the evolved forms must be similar. With this community of elementary substance, there are also diversities of substance and of co-operant conditions; corresponding with these diversities, there must be differences of form. Thus, although observation reveals that the bond of kinship does really unite many widely divergent forms, and the principle of Descent with Natural Selection will account for many of the resemblances and differences, there is at present no warrant for assuming that all resemblances and differences are due to this one cause, but, on the contrary, we are justified in assuming a deeper principle which may be thus formulated: All the complex organisms are evolved from organisms less complex, as these were evolved from simpler forms; the link which unites all organisms is not always the common bond of heritage, but the uniformity of organised substance acting under similar conditions.

It is therefore consistent with the hypothesis of Evolution to admit a variety of origins or starting-points, though not consistent to admit the sudden appearance of complex Types, such as is implied in the hypothesis of specific creations.

119*a*. The analogies of organic forms and functions demand a more exhaustive scrutiny than has yet been given them. Why is it that vessels, nerves, and bones *ramify* like branches, and why do these branches take on the aspect of many crystalline forms? Why is it that cavities are constantly prolonged in ducts, *e.g.*, the mouth succeeded by the œsophagus, the stomach by the intestines, the bladder by the urethra, the heart by the aorta, the ovary by the oviduct, and so on? Why are there never more than four limbs attached to a vertebral column, and these always attached to particular vertebræ? Why is there a tendency in certain tissues to form tubes, and in these tubes commonly to assume a muscular coat?* To some of these queries an answer might be suggested which would bring them under known physical laws. I merely notice them here for the sake of emphasising the fact that such analogies lie deeply embedded in the laws of evolution, and that what has been metaphorically called organic crystallisation, will account for many similarities in form, without forcing us to have recourse to kinship. To take a very simple case. No

* Even in the nerve-sheaths of some Annelids there are muscles.

one will maintain that the crystalline forms of snow have any kinship with the plants which they often resemble. Mr. Spencer has noticed the development of a wing-bearing branch from a wing of the *Ptilota plumosa*, when its nutrition is in excess. "This form, so strikingly like that of the feathery crystallisations of many inorganic substances, proves to us that in such crystallisations the simplicity or complexity of structure at any place depends on the quantity of matter that has to be polarised at that place in a given time. How the element of time modifies the result, is shown by the familiar fact that crystals rapidly formed are small, and that they become larger when they are formed more slowly." *

It may be objected, and justly, that in the resemblance between crystals and organisms the analogy is purely that of form, and usually confined to one element, whereas between organisms there is resemblance of substance no less than of form, and usually the organisms are alike in several respects. The answer to this objection is, that wherever there is a similarity in the causal conditions (substance and history) there must be a corresponding similarity in the results; if this similarity extends to only a few of the conditions, the analogy will be slight; if to several, deep. But whether slight or deep we are not justified, simply on the ground of resemblance, in assuming, short of evidence, that because they are alike, two organisms are related by descent from a common ancestor.

120. Let us glance at a few illustrations. It has been urged as a serious objection to Mr. Darwin's hypothesis,† that it fails to explain the existence of phosphorescent organs in a few insects; and certainly, when one considers the widely-different orders in which these organs appear, and their absence in nearly-related forms, it is a difficulty. In noctilucæ, earthworms, molluscs, scolopendra, and fire-flies, we may easily suppose the presence of similar organic conditions producing the luminosity; but it requires a strong faith to assign

* SPENCER, *Principles of Biology*, ii. 72.

† FAIVRE, *Variabilité de l' Espèce*, p. 15.

Descent as the cause.* We may say the same of the electric organs possessed by seven species of fish, belonging to five widely-separated genera. Although each species appears to have a limited geographical range, one or the other is found in almost every part of the globe. These organs occupy different positions, being now on each side of the head, now along the body, and now along the tail; and in different species they are innervated from different sources. Their intimate structure also varies; as appears from the remarkable investigations of Max Schultze.† They cannot, therefore, be homologous. How could they have arisen? Not by the slow accumulations of Natural Selection, because, until the organs were fully formed, they could be of no advantage in the struggle; hence the slow growth of the organ must have proceeded without the aid of an advantage in the struggle—in each case from some analogous conditions which produced a differentiation in certain muscles. The fundamental resemblance to muscles was pointed out by Carus long ago. It has been insisted on by Leydig:‡ and Owen says, "The

* These luminous organs would furnish an interesting digression if space permitted it. The student is referred to the chapter in MILNE EDWARD'S *Leçons sur la Physiologie et l'Anatomie Comparée*, 1863, viii. 94, sq. LEYDIG: *Histologie*, 1857, p. 343. KÖLLIKER: *Microscopical Journal*, 1858, viii. 166, and MAX SCHULTZE, *Archiv für mikros. Anat.*, 1865, p. 124. My friend SCHULTZE was kind enough to show me some of his preparations of the organs of *Lempyris splendidula*, from which the drawings in his memoir were made. They reminded me of the electric organs in fishes by a certain faint analogy, the trachea in the one holding the position of nerves in the other. I may remark, in passing, that it is not every phosphorescent animal that has distinct luminous organs. There is a lizard (*Pterodactylus Gecko*) which occasionally becomes luminous. "A singular circumstance occurred to the colonial surgeon, who related it to me. He was lying awake in bed when a lizard fell from the ceiling upon the top of his mosquito-curtain; at the moment of touching it the lizard became brilliantly luminous, illuminating the objects in the neighbourhood, much to the astonishment of the doctor." COLLINGWOOD, *Rambles of a Naturalist*, 1868, p. 169.

† MAX SCHULTZE: *Zur Kenntniss der electrischen Organe der Fische*, 1858–9.

‡ LEYDIG: *Histologie*, 1857, p. 45.

row of compressed cells constituting the electric prism of the Torpedo offers some analogy to the row of microscopic discs of which the elementary muscle fibre appears to consist." * We must not, however, forget that these resemblances are merely such as suggest that the electric organ is a *differentiation* of the substance which elsewhere becomes muscular, and that Dr. Davy was justified in denying the organ to be muscular.† That it is substituted for muscle cannot be doubted. Now, although we are entirely ignorant of the conditions which cause this differentiation of substance which elsewhere becomes muscular, but here becomes electric organs, we can understand that, when once such a development had taken place, if it in any way profited the fish in its struggle for existence, Natural Selection would *tend* to its further increase and propagation. So far Mr. Darwin carries us with him; but we decline proceeding further. The development of these organs in fishes so widely removed, does not imply an ancestral community. It is interpretable as mere growth on a basis once laid; and therefore would occur with or without any advantage in the struggle with rivals. The similarity in concurrent conditions is quite enough to account for the resemblance in structure. This, with his accustomed candour, Mr. Darwin admits. "If the electric organs," he says, "had been inherited from one ancient progenitor thus provided, we might have expected that all electric fishes would be specially related to each other. Nor does Geology at all lead to the belief that formerly most fishes had electric organs which most of their modified descendants have lost."

121. It may seem strange that he should urge a difficulty against his hypothesis when it could be avoided by the simple admission that even among nearly allied animals great differences in development are observable, and the electric organs might be ranged under such diversities. But Mr. Darwin has so thoroughly wrought out his scheme, that he foresees most objections, and rightly suspects that if this principle of divergent development be admitted, it will cut the ground from

* OWEN: *Anatomy of the Vertebrates*, 1866, i. 358.

† DAVY: *Researches, Physiological and Anatomical*, 139, i. 33.

under a vast array of facts which his hypothesis of Descent requires.

The sudden appearance of new organs, not a trace of which is discernible in the embryo or adult form of organisms lower in the scale,—for instance, the phosphorescent and electric organs — is like the sudden appearance of new instruments in the social organism, such as the printing-press and the railway, wholly inexplicable on the theory of Descent,* but is explicable on the theory of Organic Affinity. For observe: if we admit that differentiations of structure, and the sudden appearance of organs, can have arisen spontaneously—*i.e.*, not hereditarily—as the outcome of certain changed physical conditions, we can hardly refuse to extend to the whole organism what we admit of a particular organ. If, again, we admit that organs very similar in structure and function spontaneously appear in organisms of widely different kinds—*e.g.*, the phosphorescent and electric organs—we must also admit that similar resemblances

* "If it could be demonstrated that any complex organ existed which could not possibly have been formed by numerous successive slight modifications, my theory would absolutely break down." Darwin.—*Origin of Species*, 5th ed. p. 227. In several passages insistence is made on this. "Natura non facit saltum" may be perfectly true; but without impugning the Law of Continuity we may urge that the Law of Discontinuity is equally true. The one is an abstract ideal conception; the other is a concrete ideal conception. According to the one, every change from rest to motion, or from one state to another, must pass through infinites; according to the other every change is abrupt. In my First Series, vol. i. p. 302, I have shown how, on mechanical principles, every change in an organism must be abrupt. A glance at the metamorphoses of the embryo, or the stages of insect-development, will show very sudden and abrupt changes. Let me also cite Mr. Darwin against himself: "When we remember such cases as the formation of the more complex galls, and certain monstrosities, which cannot be accounted for by reversion, cohesion, &c., and *sudden, strongly-marked deviations of structure*, such as the appearance of a moss-rose on a common rose, we must admit that the organisation of the individual is capable through *its own laws of growth, under certain conditions*, of undergoing great modifications, independent of the gradual accumulation of slight inherited modifications."—*Origin*, p. 151. See also note to § 130, further on, p. 125.

may present themselves in organisms having a widely-different parentage; and thus the admission of the spontaneous evolution of closely-resembling organs carries with it the admission of the spontaneous evolution of closely-resembling organisms: that the protoplasm of muscular tissue should, under certain changed conditions, develop into the tissue of electric organs, is but one case of the law that organised substance will develop into organisms closely resembling each other when the conditions have been similar.

122. It is to be remarked that Mr. Darwin fixes his attention somewhat too exclusively on the adaptations which arise during the external struggle for existence, and to that extent neglects the laws of organic affinity; just as Lamarck too exclusively fixed his attention on the influence of external conditions and of wants. Not that Mr. Darwin can be said to overlook the organic laws; he simply under-estimates the part they play. Occasionally he seems arrested by them, as when instancing the "trailing palm in the Malay Archipelago, which climbs the loftiest trees by the aid of exquisitely constructed hooks, clustered around the ends of the branches, and this contrivance no doubt is of the highest service to the plant; but as there are nearly similar hooks on many trees which are not climbers, the hooks on the palm may have arisen from unknown laws of growth, and have been subsequently taken advantage of by the plant undergoing further modification and becoming a climber."

123. I come round to the position from which I started, that the resemblances traceable among animals are no proof of kinship; even a resemblance so close as to defy discrimination would not, in itself, be such a proof. The absolute identity of chalk in Australia and in Europe is a proof that there was absolute identity in the formative conditions and the constituent elements, but no proof whatever that the two substances were originally connected by genesis. In like manner the similarity of a plant or animal in Africa and Europe may be due to a common kinship, but it may also be due to a *common history*. It is indeed barely conceivable that the history, from first to last, would ever be so rigorously identical in two parts of the globe as to produce complex identical forms in both; because *any* diversity either in structure or external conditions may be the starting-point of a wide diversity in subsequent development; and the case of organic combinations is so far unlike the inorganic, that while only one form is possible to the latter (chalk is either formed or not formed), many forms are possible to organic elements owing to the complexity and indefiniteness of organic composition. But although forms so allied as those of Species are not readily assignable to an identical history in different quarters of the globe, it is not only conceivable, but is eminently probable, that Orders and Classes have no nearer link of relationship than is implied in their community of organised substance and their common history. The fact that there is not a single mammal common to Europe and Australia is explicable, as Mr. Darwin explains it, on the ground that migration has been impossible to them; but it is also explicable on the laws of Evolution—to have had mammals of the same species and genera would imply a minute coincidence in their history; which is against the probabilities. Again, in the Oceanic Islands there are no Batrachians; but there are Reptiles, and these conform to the reptilian type. Mr. Darwin suggests that the absence of Batrachia is due to the impossibility of migration, their ova being destroyed by salt water. But may it not be due to the divergence from the reptilian type, which was effected elsewhere, not having taken place in these regions? When we find the metal Tin in Prussia and Cornwall, and nowhere else in Europe, must we not conclude that in these two countries, and nowhere else, a peculiar conjunction of conditions caused this peculiar evolution?

124. The question at issue is, Are the resemblances observable among organic forms due to remote kinship, and their diversities to the divergences caused by adaptation to new conditions? or are the resemblances due to similarities, and the diversities to dissimilarities in the *substance and history* of organic beings? Are we to assume one starting-point and one centre of creation, or many similar starting-

points at many centres? So far from believing that all plants and animals had their origin in one primordial cell, at one particular spot, from which descendants migrated and became diversified under the diverse conditions of their migration, it seems to me more consistent with the principle of Evolution to admit a vast variety of origins more or less resembling each other; and this initial resemblance will account for the similarities still traceable under the various forms; while the *early differences*, becoming intensified by development under different conditions, will yield the diversities. The evolution of organisms, like the evolution of crystals, or the evolution of islands and continents, is determined, 1st, by laws *inherent in the substances evolved*, and, 2d, by relations to the medium in which the evolution takes place. This being so, we may *à priori* affirm that the resultant forms will have a community strictly corresponding with the resemblance of the substances and their conditions of evolution, together with a diversity corresponding with their differences in substance and conditions. It is usually supposed that the admission of separate "centres of creation" is tantamount to an admission of "successive creations" as interpreted by the majority of those who invoke "creative fiats." But the doctrine of Evolution, which regards Life as making its appearance *consequent upon a concurrence of definite conditions*, and regards the specific forms of Life as the necessary consequences of special circumstances, must also accept the probability of similar conditions occurring at different times and in different places. Upon what grounds, cosmical or biological, are we to assume that on only *one* microscopic spot of this developing planet such a group of conditions was found—on only one spot a particle of protein substance was formed out of the abundant elements, and under conditions which caused it to grow and multiply, till in time its descendants overran the globe? The hypothesis that all organic forms are the descendants of a single germ, or of even a few germs, and are therefore united by links of kinship more or less remote, is not more acceptable than the hypothesis that all the carbonates and phosphates, all the crystals, and all the strata found in different parts of the globe, are the *descendants of a single molecule,* or a few molecules; or,—since this may seem too extravagant,—than that the various maladies which afflict organic beings are, in a literal sense, members of *families* having a nearer relationship than that of being the phenomena manifested by similar organs under similar conditions—a conception which might have been accepted by those metaphysical pathologists who regarded Disease as an entity. Few philosophers have any hesitation in supposing that other planets besides our own are peopled with organic forms, though, from the great differences in the conditions, these forms must be extremely unlike those of our own planet. If separate worlds, why not separate centres? The conclusion seems inevitable that wherever and whenever the state of things permitted that peculiar combination of elements known as organised substance, there and then a centre was established—Life had a root. From roots closely resembling each other in all essential characters, but all more or less different, there have been developed the various stems of the great tree. Myriads of roots have probably perished without issue; myriads have developed into forms so ill-adapted to sustain the fluctuations of the medium, so ill-fitted for the struggle of existence, that they became extinct before even our organic record begins; myriads have become extinct since then; and the descendants of those which now survive are like the shattered regiments and companies after some terrific battle.

125. There seems to me only one alternative logically permissible to the Evolution Hypothesis, namely, that all organic forms have had either a single origin, or else numerous origins; in other words, that a primordial cell was the starting-point from which all organisms have been successively developed; or that the development issued from many independent starting-points, more or less varied. This is apparently not the aspect presented by the hypothesis to many of its advocates; they seem to consider that if all organic forms are not the lineal descendants of one progenitor, they must at any rate be the descendants of not more than four or five.

The common belief inclines to one. Mr. Darwin, whose caution is as remarkable as his courage, and whose candour is delightful, hesitates as to which conclusion should be adopted: "I cannot doubt," he says, "that the theory of descent, with modifications, embraces all the members of the same class. I believe that animals have descended from, at most, only four or five progenitors, and plants from an equal or lesser number. Analogy would lead me one step further, namely, to the belief that all animals and plants have descended from some one prototype. But analogy may be a deceitful guide."

126. I cannot see the evidence which would warrant the belief that Life originated solely in one microscopic lump of protoplasm on one single point of our earth's surface; on the contrary, it is more probable that from innumerable and separate points of this teeming earth, myriads of protoplasts sprang into existence, *whenever* and *wherever* the conditions of the formation of organised substance were present. It is probable that this has been incessantly going on, and that every day new protoplasts appear, struggle for existence, and serve as food for more highly organised rivals; but whether an evolution of the lower forms is, or is not, still going on, there can be no reluctance on the part of every believer in Evolution to admit that when organised substance was first evolved, it was evolved at many points. If this be so, the community observable in organised substance, wherever found, may as often be due to the fact of a common elementary composition as to the fact of inheritance. If this be so, we have a simple explanation both of the fundamental resemblances which link all organisms together, and of the characteristic diversities which separate them into kingdoms, classes, and orders. The resemblances are many, and close, because the forms evolved had a similar elementary composition, and their stages of evolution were determined by similar conditions. The diversities are many, because the forms evolved had from the first some diversities in elementary composition, and their stages of evolution were determined under conditions which, though similar in general, have varied in particulars. Indeed, there is no other ground for the resemblances and differences among organic beings than the similarities and dissimilarities in their Substance and History; and, whether the similarities are due to blood-relationship, or to other causes, the results are the same. There is something seductive in the supposition that Life radiated from a single centre in ever-increasing circles, its forms becoming more and more various as they came under more various conditions, until at last the whole earth was crowded with diversified existences. "From one cell to myriads of complex organisms, through countless æons of development," is a formula of speculative grandeur, but I cannot bring myself to accept it; and I think that a lingering influence of the tradition of a "creative fiat" may be traced in its conception. May we not rather assume that the earth at the dawn of Life was a vast germinal membrane, every slightly diversified point producing its own vital form; and these myriads upon myriads of forms—all alike and all unlike—urged by the indwelling tendencies of development, struggled with each other for existence, many failing, many victorious, the victors carrying their tents into the camping ground of the vanquished? The point raised is the immense improbability of organised substance having been evolved only in one microscopic spot; if it were evolved at more than one spot, and under slightly varying conditions, there would necessarily have arisen in these earliest formations the *initial* diversities which afterwards determined the essential independence and difference of organisms.

129. Let us for a moment glance at the resemblances and diversities observable in all organisms. All have a *common basis,* all being constructed out of the same fundamental elements: carbon, hydrogen, nitrogen, and oxygen; these (the organogens, as they are named), with varying additions of some other elements, make up what we know as Organic Substance, vegetal and animal. Another peculiarity all organisms have in common, namely, that their matter is neither solid nor liquid, but viscid. Beside this community of *Substance* we must now place a community of *History.*

All organisms grow and multiply by the same process; all pass through metamorphic stages ending in death; all, except the very simplest, differentiate parts of their substance for special uses, and these parts (cilia, membranes, tubes, glands, muscles, nerves), have similar characters in whatever organism they appear, and their development is always similar, so that the muscles or nerves of an intestinal worm, a lobster, or a man, are in structure and history fundamentally alike. When, therefore, we see that there is no biological character of fundamental importance which is not universal throughout the organic world, when we see that in Structure and History all organisms have a community pervading every variety, it is difficult not to draw the conclusion that some hidden link connects all organisms into one; and when, further, it is seen that the most divergent forms may be so arranged by the help of intermediate forms only slightly varying one from the other, that the extreme ends—the monad and the man—may be connected, and a genealogical tree constructed, which will group all forms as modified descendants from a single form, the hypothesis that kinship is the hidden link of which we are in search becomes more and more cogent.

130. But now let the other aspect be considered. If there is an unmistakable uniformity, there is also a diversity no less unmistakable. The chemical composition of organic substances is various. Unlike inorganic substances, the composition of which is rigorously definite, organic substances are, within narrow limits, variable in composition (§ 45).

I pass over the resemblances and differences observed in the earliest stages of development, marked as they are, and direct attention to the fact, that down at what must be considered the very lowest organic region, we meet with differences not less striking than those met with in the highest, we find structures (if structures they may be called), which cannot be affiliated, so widely divergent is their composition. The structureless vibrio, for example, is not only capable of living in a medium destitute of oxygen, but is, according to M. Pasteur, actually killed by oxygen; whereas the equally simple bacteria can no more dispense with oxygen than other animals can. Consider for a moment the differences implied in the fact that one organism cannot even form an enveloping membrane to contain its protoplasm, whereas another contrives to secrete an exquisite shell; yet between the naked Rhizopod and the shelled Rhizopod our lenses and reagents fail to detect a difference. One Monad can assimilate food of only one kind, another Monad assimilates various kinds.* What a revelation of chemical differences appears in the obervations of M. Pasteur respecting the vibrio and bacteria, in a fermentescible liquid—the former beginning the putrid fermentation which the latter completes! We cannot doubt that some marked difference must exist between the single-celled organism which produces alcoholic fermentation, and that which produces acetic fermentation, and that again which produces butyric fermentation; and if we find distinctions thus established at the lowest region of the organic series, we need not marvel if the distinctions become wider and more numerous as the series becomes more diversified. The structure and development of an organism are dependent on the affinities of its constituent molecules, and it is a biological principle of great importance which Sir James Paget insists on, when he shows how "the existence of certain materials in the blood may determine the formation of structures in which they may be incorporated." † *Any* initial diversity may thus become the starting point of a considerable variation in subsequent evolution. ‡ Thus,

* On the Nutrition of Monads, see the remarkable memoir by CIENKOWSKI, in the *Archiv für mikros. Anatomie*, i. 221, sq.

† PAGET: *Lectures on Surgical Pathology*, edited by TURNER, 1865, p. 19.

‡ It has recently been shown that certain Crustacea vary not only from species to species, but from genus to genus, when living in water of different degrees of saltness. By continued dilution of the salt water an *Artemia* was developed into another species, and this again into a *Branchipus*—a genus of large dimensions, with an extra abdominal segment, and a different tail; a genus, moreover, which is propagated sexually, whereas the *Artemia* is parthenogenetic, as a rule. See *Nature* 1876, June 8, p. 133.

The exceeding importance of this fact is, that it proves specific and even generic differences to originate simply through the gradual supposing that on a given spot there are a dozen protoplasts closely resembling each other, yet each in some one detail slightly varying; if this variation is one which, by its relations to the external medium, admits of a difference in the assimilation of materials present in the medium, it may be the origin of some *new direction* in development, and the ultimate consequence may be the formation of a shell, an internal skeleton, a muscle, or a nerve. Were this not so, it would be impossible to explain such facts as that chitine is peculiar to the Articulata, cellulose to Molluscoida, carbonates of lime to Mollusca and Crustacea, and phosphates to Vertebrata—all assimilated from the same external medium. But we see that from this medium one organism selects the materials which another rejects; and this selection is determined by the nature of the structure: which assimilates only those materials it is *fitted* to assimilate. We hear a great deal of Adaptation determining changes of structure and function, and are too apt to regard this process as if it were not intimately dependent on a corresponding structural change. By no amount of external influence which left the elementary composition of the structure unchanged, could an organism with only two tissues be developed into an organism with three or four. By no supply or stimulus, could an animal incapable of assimilating peroxide of iron acquire red blood corpuscles, although it might have the iron without the corpuscles; nor could an oyster form its shell unless capable of assimilating carbonate of lime. For myriads of years, in seas and ponds, under endless varieties of external conditions, the amœbæ have lived and died without forming a solid envelope, although the materials were abundant, and other organisms equally simple have formed envelopes of infinite variety. In all the seas, and from the earliest ages, zoophytes have lived, and

changes of the medium and the adaptation of the organism to these new conditions. It also disproves the very common notion—adopted even by Mr. Darwin himself—that "organic beings must be exposed *during several generations* to new conditions to cause any appreciable amount of variation." Again, "Natural Selection, if it be a true principle, will banish the belief of any great and sudden modification of structure."—Comp. note to § 121, p. 117.

assumed a marvellous variety of shapes and specialisation of functions; but although some of them have acquired muscles, none have acquired true nerves, none bone. Ages upon ages rolled on before fishes were capable of forming bone; and thousands are still incapable of forming it, though living in the same waters as the osseous fishes.

131. "Looking to the dawn of life," says Mr. Darwin (repeating an objection urged against his hypothesis), "when all organic beings, as we imagine, presented the simplest structure, how could the first steps in advancement, or in the differentiation and specialisation of parts have arisen? I can make no sufficient answer; and can only say that, as we have no facts to guide us, all speculation would be baseless and useless."

Where Mr. Darwin hesitates, lesser men need extra caution; but I must risk the danger of presumption, at least so far as to suggest that while an answer to this question is difficult on that dynamical view of Evolution which regards Function as determining Structure, it is less difficult on the statico-dynamical view propounded in these pages; the difficulty which besets the explanation when all the manifold varieties of organic forms are conceived as the successive divergences from an original starting-point, is lessened when a variety of different starting-points is assumed, in each of which some initial diversity prepared the way for subsequent differentiations; just as we know that between the ovum of a vertebrate and the ovum of an invertebrate, similar as they are, there is a diversity which manifests itself in their subsequent evolution. If Function is determined by Structure, and Evolution is the product of the two, it is clear that the different directions in the lines of development will have their origin in structural differences, and not in the action of external circumstances, unless these previously bring about a structural change. The action of the medium on the organism is assuredly a potent factor which Biology cannot ignore: but the organism itself is a factor, and according to its nature the influence of the medium is defined. (§ 118).

132. Quitting for a moment the track of this argument, let us glance at the resemblances and differences observable in Plants and Animals, because most people admit that these have separate origins. The resemblances are scarcely less significant than those existing among animals. Both have a similar basis of elementary composition; not only are both formed out of protoplasts with similar properties, but in both the first step from the protoplasm to definite structure is the Cell. And the life of this Cell is remarkably alike in both, its phases of development being in many respects identical; nay, even such variations as obtain in the cell-membranes are curiously linked together by a community in the formative process.* In both Plants and Animals we find individuals constituted—1st, by single cells; 2nd, by groups of cells undistinguishable among each other; and 3rd, by groups of differentiated cells. In both we find colonies of individuals leading a common life. In both the processes of Nutrition and Reproduction are essentially similar; both propagate sexually and asexually; both exhibit the surprising phenomena of parthenogenesis and alternate generations. In both there are examples of a free-roving embryo which in maturity becomes fixed to one spot, losing its locomotive organs and developing its reproductive organs. In both the development of the reproductive organs is the climax which carries Death. So close is the analogy between plant-life and animal-life, that it even reaches the properties usually held to be exclusively animal; I mean that even should we hesitate to accept Cohn's discovery of the muscles in certain plants,† we cannot deny that plants exhibit Contractility;

* Compare LEYDIG: *Vom Bau des thierischen Körpers*, 1864, p. 27.

† FERDINAND COHN: *Die contractile Gewebe im Pflanzenreich*, 1862. By a series of numerous well-devised experiments, Cohn found that in the stamen of the *centauria* a tissue exists which is excitable by the same stimula as muscle is, and which reacts like muscle, describing a similar curve when excited, and, after reaching its maximum, relaxing. Like the muscle it becomes fatigued by repeated contraction, and recovers it powers by repose. Like the muscle it may be rendered tetanic. (The researches of Dr. BURDON SANDERSON and Mr. DARWIN have since placed beyond a doubt the Contractility and Sensibility of certain plants.)

and should we refuse to interpret as Sensibility the phenomena exhibited by the Sensitive Plants, we cannot deny that they present a very striking analogy to the phenomena of Sensibility exhibited by animals.

133. It is unnecessary to continue this enumeration, which might easily be carried into minute detail. A chapter of such resemblances would only burden the reader's mind, without adding force to the conclusion that a surprising community in Substance and Life-history must be admitted between Plants and Animals. This granted, we turn to the differences, and find them no less fundamental and detailed. Chemistry tells us nothing of the differences in the protoplasms from which animals and plants arise; but that initial differences must exist is proved by the divergence of the products. The vegetable cell is not the animal cell; and although both plants and animals have albumen, fibrine, and caseine, the *derivatives* of these are unlike. Horny substance, connective tissue, nerve tissue, chitine, biliverdine, creatine, urea, hippuric acid, and a variety of other products of evolution or of waste, never appear in plants; while the hydrocarbons so abundant in plants are, with two or three exceptions, absent from animals. Such facts imply differences in elementary composition; and this result is further enforced by the fact that where the two seem to resemble, they are still different: the plant protoplasm forms various cells, but never forms a cartilage-cell or nerve-cell; fibres, but never a fibre of elastic tissue; tubes, but never a nerve tube; vessels, but never a vessel with muscular coatings; solid "skeletons," but always from an organic substance (*cellulose*), not from phosphates and carbonates. In no one character can we say that the plant and the animal are identical; we can only point throughout the two kingdoms to a great similarity accompanying a radical diversity.

134. Having brought together the manifold resemblances, and the no less marked diversities, we must ask what is their significance? Do the resemblances imply a community of origin, an universal kinship? If so, the diversities will be nothing more than the divergences which have been pro-

duced by variations in the Life-history of the several groups. Or—taking the alternative view—do the diversities imply radical differences of origin? If so, the resemblances will be nothing more than the inevitable analogies resulting from Organised Substance being everywhere somewhat similar in composition, and similar in certain phases of evolution. To state the former position in the simplest way, we may assume that of two masses of protoplasm having a common parentage, one, by the accident of assimilating a certain element not brought within the range of the other, thereby becomes so differentiated as to form the starting-point of a series of evolutions widely divergent from those possible to its congener; and at each stage of evolution the introduction of a new element (made possible by that stage) will form the origin of a new variation. It is thus feasible to reduce all organic forms to a primordial protoplasm, in the evolutions of which successive differentiations have been established. On the other hand, it is equally feasible to assume that the existence of radical differences must be invoked to account for the possibility of the successive differentiations.

135. The hunt after resemblances has led to much mistaken speculation; and with reference to the topic now before us, it may be urged, that although by attaching ourselves to the points of community, in disregard of the diversities, we may make it appear that all animals have a common parentage, and that plants and animals are merely divergent groups of the same prototype, a rigorous logic will force us onwards, and compel us to admit that a kinship no less real unites the organic with the inorganic world. For upon what principle are we to pause at the cell or protoplasm? If by a successive elimination of differences we reduce all organisms to the cell, we must go on and reduce the cell itself to the chemical elements out of which it is constructed; and inasmuch as these elements are all common to the inorganic world, the only difference being one of synthesis, we reach a result which is the stultification of all classification, namely, the assertion of a kinship which is universal. We must bear in mind that all things may be reduced to a common root by simply disregarding their differences. All things are alike when we set aside their unlikeness.

136. Suppose, for the sake of illustration, we regard an Orchestra in the light of the Development Hypothesis. The various instruments of which it is composed have general resemblances and particular differences, not unlike those observable in various organisms; and as we proceed in the work of classification we quickly discover that they may be arranged in groups analogous to the Sub-kingdoms, Classes, Orders, Genera, and Species of the organic world. Each group has its cardinal distinction, its initial point of divergence. All musical instruments resemble each other in the fundamental character of producing Tone by the vibrations of their substance. This may be called their organic basis. The first marked difference which determines the character of two sub-kingdoms (namely, instruments of Percussion and Wind instruments) arises from a difference in the method of impressing the vibrations; and the grand divisions of these sub-kingdoms arise from the nature of the vibrating substances. Each type admits of many modifications, but the primary distinction is ineffaceable. We can conceive the Pipe modified into a Flute, a Flageolet, a Clarionet, a Hautbois, a Bassoon, or a Fife, by simple accessory changes; to modify the Pipe into a Trumpet, and thus produce the peculiar *timbre* of the trumpet, would be impossible except by the *substitution* of a new material; by replacing the wood with metal we may adhere to the old Type, but we have created a new Class. (Attention is requested to this point, because the current views respecting the transmutation of tissues, which seem to lend a decisive support to the hypothesis of the transmutation of species are very commonly vitiated by the confusion of transformation with substitution. No anatomical element is *transformed* into another specifically different—an epithelial-cell into a nerve-cell, for instance—but one anatomical element is frequently *substituted* for another.) To convert the Pipe or the Trumpet into a Violin or a Drum would be impossible. We can follow the modifications of a Tambourine into a Drum or Kettle-drum, but no modifications of these will yield the Cymbals

That is to say, the vibrating materials—wood, metal, parchment, and the combination of wood and strings—have peculiar properties, and the instruments formed of such materials must necessarily from the very first belong to different groups, each subdivision of the groups being dependent on some characteristic difference in methods of impressing the vibrations, or in the materials. Although all musical instruments have a common property and a common purpose, we do not regard them as transformations of one primitive instrument; their kindred nature is a subjective conception; the analogies are numerous and close, but we know their origin. It is obvious that men being pleased by musical tones, have been led by their delight to construct instruments whenever they have discovered substances capable of musical vibrations, or methods of impressing such vibrations. By substituting the bow for the plectrum or the fingers, they may have changed the Lyre into the Violin, Viola, Violoncello, and Bass. (It seems historically probable that the real origin of the Violin class was an instrument with one string played on by a bow.) By grouping together Pipes of various sizes they got the Pan-pipes; by substituting metal and enlarging the blowing apparatus they got the Organ. By beating on stretched parchment with the finger, they got the Tambourine and Tom-Tom; by doubling this and using a stick they got the Drum. By beating metal with metal they got the Cymbals; by beating wood they got the Castanets.

137. The application of this illustration is plain. Just as a wind-instrument is incapable of becoming a Stringed instrument, so a Mollusc, with all its muscles unstriped, and its nervous system unsymmetrical, is incapable of becoming a Crustacean, with all its muscles striped and its nervous system symmetrical. Indeed there are probably few biologists of the present day who imagine the transmutation of one kind into the other to be possible; but many biologists assume that both may have been evolved from a common root. The point is beyond proof; yet I think there is a greater probability in the assumption that both were evolved from different roots. At any rate, one thing is certain; a divergence could only have been effected by a series of *substitutions;* and the question when and how these substitutions took place is unanswerable: one school believes them to have been creative fiats, the other school believes them to have been transmutations.

138. When we see an annelid and a vertebrate resembling each other in some special point which is not common either to their classes or to any intermediate classes—as when we see the woodlouse (*Oniscus*) and the hedgehog defend themselves in the same strange way by rolling up into a ball—we cannot interpret this as a trace of distant kinship. When we see a breed of pigeons and a breed of canaries turning somersaults, and one of the Bear family (*Ratel*) given to the same singular habit, we can hardly suppose that this is in each case inherited from a common progenitor. When we see one savage race tipping arrows with iron, and another ignorant of iron, using poison, there is a community of object effected by diversity of means, but the analogy does not necessarily imply any closer connection between the two races than the fact that men with similar faculties and similar wants find out similar methods of supplying their wants. Even those who admit that the human race is one family, and that the various peoples carried with them a common fund of knowledge when they separated from the parent stock, may still point to a variety of new inventions and new social developments which occurred quite independently of each other, yet are strikingly alike. Their resemblance will be due to resemblance in the conditions. The existence, for example, of a religious worship, or a social institution, in two nations widely separated both in time and space, and under great historical diversities, is no absolute proof that these two nations are from the same stock, and that the ideas have the same parentage. It may be so; it may be otherwise. It may be an analogy no more implying kinship than the fact of ants making slaves of other ants (and these the black ants!) implies a kinship with men. Given an organisation which in the two nations is alike, and a history which is in certain characteristics analogous, there

must inevitably result religious and social institutions having a corresponding resemblance. I do not wish to imply that the researches of philologists and ethnologists are misdirected, or that their conclusions respecting the kinship of mankind are to be rejected; I only urge the consideration that perhaps too much stress is laid on community of blood, and not enough on community of conditions.

RECAPITULATION.

139. The various lines of argument may here be recapitulated. The organic world presents a spectacle of endless diversity, accompanied by a pervading uniformity. The general resemblances in forms and functions are more or less masked by particular differences. The resemblances, it is said, may be all due to kinship, all the living individuals having descended from a primordial cell; and at each stage of the descent the adaptations to new conditions may have issued in deviations from the ancestral form, while the process of Natural Selection giving stability to those variations which best fitted the organism in the struggle of existence, has made greater and greater gaps, and produced more marked diversities among the descendants. This is the Darwinian Theory: "On my theory unity of Type is explained by unity of Descent."

140. By the general consent of biologists, this theory is held to explain many if not all the observed facts. It is a very luminous suggestion; but it requires an enlargement so as to include Organic Affinity; and when once this fundamental principle is admitted, it brings with it very serious doubts as to the theory of Descent. We are then entitled to assume that many of the most striking resemblances, instead of being due to kinship, are due simply to the general principle that similar causes must have similar effects, and that organic substances having a very close resemblance, organised substances must have similar stages of evolution under similar conditions; and thus organs will necessarily take on very similar forms in very different organisms (for example, the eye of the cephalopod and the eye of the vertebrate), and organisms having widely different parentage may closely resemble each other. If we are entitled to assume that protoplasm appeared not in one microscopic spot alone, but in many places and in vast quantities—and this is surely the more justifiable assumption—then we must also admit that these germinal starting-points were from the first, or very shortly afterwards, differentiated by variations in their elementary composition. Now we know that a very minute change in composition may lead to immense differences in evolution. Thus the descendants of two slightly different progenitors may, by continual differentiation, become very markedly unlike; yet, because of the original resemblance of their substances, they will reveal a pervading similarity.

While it is thus conceivable that all organisms may resemble each other, and all differ, owing to the similarities and diversities in the "conditions of existence" (and among those conditions that of descent is of wide range), it is not very readily conceivable how advantage in the external struggle could have determined the varieties of form and function, because many differentiations give no superiority in the struggle. As Mr. St. George Mivart urges, "Natural Selection utterly fails to account for the conservation and development of the minute and rudimentary beginnings, the slight and infinitesimal commencements of structures, however useful those structures may afterwards become."* And this is undeniable on the supposition that Natural Selection is an agency not identical with the variations of growth, but exclusively confined to the accumulation of favourable variations.

141. In estimating the two hypotheses—First, of Descent from one primordial germ, and the modifications *due* to Natural Selection, or as I should say *expressed* in Selection; and Secondly, of Descent from innumerable germs having initial differences, which differences radiated into the marked modi-

* MIVART: *The Genesis of Species*, 1871, p. 23.

fications, there is this superiority to be claimed for the first, that it is more easily handled as an aid to research, and is therefore more decidedly useful. The laws of Organic Affinity are at present too obscure for any successful application. I only wish to point out that the theory of Descent is an imaginary construction of what *may have been* the process of species-formation, not a transcription of the process observed. It constructs an imaginary Type as progenitor of a long line of widely different descendants. The annelid which is taken as the ancestor of the vertebrates is not any annelid known either to zoologists or geologists, but a generalised and imaginary type. So daringly liberal is the imagination in endowing the ancestor with whatever may be required for the descendants, that Mr. Darwin thinks it *probable,* from what we know of the embryos of vertebrates, that these animals "are the modified descendants of some ancient progenitor which was furnished in its adult state with branchiæ, a swim-bladder, four simple limbs, and a long tail, all fitted for an organic life," (p. 533); and Dr. Dohrn conceives the original type to have contained within itself all that has been subsequently evolved in the highest vertebrate, the other and less elaborate organisms being mere degradations from this type.* This use of the imagination although not without advantages is also not without dangers. It may direct research, it must not be suffered to replace research.

* DOHRN: *Der Ursprung der Wirbelthiere und das Princip des Functionswechsels,* 1875, p. 74.

PROBLEM II.

THE NERVOUS MECHANISM.

"All the functions of the nervous system are as dependent upon its structure and nature, as the accurate indication of time upon the construction of the chronometer."

PROCHASKA.

"Unser Wissen wird nie vollendet, ist und bleibt Stückwerk; dessen Ergänzung das Streben und Hoffen der forschenden Denker bleiben wird für alle Zeit."

RADENHAUSEN: *Osiris.*

"Our nimble souls
Can spin an insubstantial universe
Suiting our mood, and call it possible,
Sooner than see one grain with eye exact,
And give strict record of it."

GEORGE ELIOT: *The Spanish Gypsy.*

"If we compare the teachings of our books with what Nature is constantly showing, we find there is no agreement between those two sources of learning."

BROWN SÉQUARD.

THE NERVOUS MECHANISM.

CHAPTER I.

SURVEY OF THE SYSTEM.

1. OUR knowledge of mental processes is derived from reflection on our personal experiences, combined with inferences from our observation of other men and animals, under similar conditions. The processes are complex and variable; so complex and variable, that knowledge of their component factors can only be gained through long tentative study, aided by fortunate circumstances which present these factors separately, or at any rate in such marked predominance as to fix attention. This subjective analysis of the *processes* has to be supplemented by, and confirmed by an objective analysis of, the *conditions*, external and internal: the facts of Feeling have to be traced to facts of Physiology, which will exhibit that Physical Basis of Mind so earnestly sought by the inquirer.

Both the subjective and the objective analysis are at present in a very imperfect state. Although there is much confident assertion and "false persuasion of knowledge" in both regions, there is, unhappily, little that can be seriously accepted as demonstrated. In the present volume we shall concern ourselves almost exclusively with the objective analysis, and do our utmost to mark what is mere inference from what is verified observation. It is only by Observation that facts can be *settled*; however Analogy and Inference may suggest where the truth may lie, they are finger-posts, not goals. At the best they only tell us what Observation *would* reveal could the processes be submitted to Sense.

In a loose and general way every one knows that the Nervous System is a dominant agent in all sentient processes; although not by any means the only agent, yet, because of its predominance, it is artificially accepted as the only one. With the greater complexity of this system, there is observed a corresponding increase in the variety of sentient phenomena. The labours of anatomists have secured a tolerably exact plan of the topographical distribution of this system; a somewhat chaotic mass of observation and inference passes as a description of its elementary structure. The labours of physiologists have succeeded to a small extent in localising certain functions in certain organs of this system. But imperfect as our knowledge of the elementary structures is, our knowledge of the functions is still more so. I wish I could say otherwise, and that I could ask my readers to accept with confidence what teachers confidently propound. The attitude of scepticism is always repulsive; the sceptic is seldom received without disfavour, because he throws on us the labour of investigation there where we wish for the confidence of knowledge. Yet it is only by facing the facts that we can hope one day to solve the great questions.

2. The nervous system has, in our artificial view of it, two divisions: the Peripheral, which connects the organism with the external world; and the Central, which connects each part of the organism with all the other parts. Although the system is constituted by various tissues—neural, connective, vascular, and elastic—it receives its characteristic designation from nerve-fibrils, nerve-fibres, and nerve-cells; just as the muscular system receives its designation from contractile cells and fibres. This neural tissue assumes three well-marked forms: 1°, *nerves,* which are bundles of fibres and fibrils, enclosed in a membranous sheath; 2°, *ganglia,* which are clusters of cells, fibres, and fibrils, sometimes enclosed in a sheath, sometimes not; 3°, *centres,* which are artificial divisions of the neural axis, serving as points of union for different organs.

In the Invertebrata the neural axis is the chain of ganglionic masses running along the ventral side, and giving off the nerves to organs of sense, and to the muscles. It may be seen represented in Fig. 1.

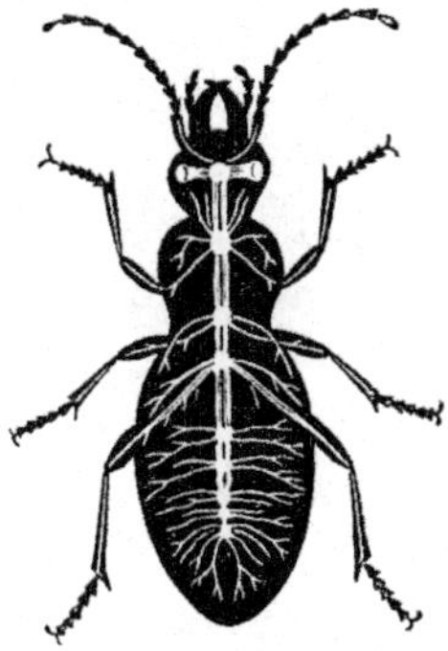

Fig. 1.—*Nervous system of a beetle.* The small round masses, or *ganglia*, are seen to be connected by longitudinal fibres, and from the ganglia issue fibres to the limbs, organs of sense, and viscera.

In the Vertebrata the axis is dorsal, and is called the *cerebro-spinal axis*, including brain and spinal cord. When we look at this structure superficially we see various nerves radiating *from* it to skin, glands, and muscles; but a closer examination, enlightened by knowledge of function, shows that some of these nerves pass *into* it from the various surfaces and sense-organs, and are therefore called *afferent* or *sensory*; whereas another set passes out of it to glands and muscles, and these nerves are therefore called *efferent* or *motory*. There are also fibres which, passing from one part of the great centre to another, are called *commissural*.

To this brief account of the cerebro-spinal system may be added a word on the connected chain of ganglia and nerves known as the Sympathetic, because it was formerly supposed to be the organ through which the various "sympathies" were effected. It is now held to be the system devoted to the viscera and blood-vessels; but there is still great want of agreement among physiologists as to whether it is an independent system, having a special structure somewhat different from that of the cerebro-spinal, or whether it is simply a great plexus of nerves and ganglia, only topographically distinguishable from the rest of the nervous system. Into this point it is unnecessary for me to enter here. Enough to say, that I entirely agree with Sigmund Mayer in adopting the second view.* In no histological character, yet specified, are the sympathetic nerves and ganglia demarcated from the others. There are, indeed, *more* non-medullary

* Sigmund Mayer: *Die peripherische Nervenzelle und die sympathische Nervensystem*, 1876.

fibres (the grey fibres of Remak) in the sympathetic; but the same fibres are also abundant in the cerebro-spinal system; and the sympathetic has also its large medullary fibres.

3. The Centres are composed of two substances: the grey and the white. The grey substance is often called the vesicular because of its abundant cells; but it has even more fibres than cells, and the white substance has also a few cells.* The grey substance is distributed over the surface of the brain—in the convolutions; and in various other parts of the encephalon. It surrounds the central canal which forms the ventricles of the brain and is continued as a very small cavity all down the spinal cord. Besides entering into the important and conspicuous masses known as the cerebral ganglia—(the *optic thalami*, and *corpora striata*)—the grey substance is massed in the *corpora quadrigemina*, *crura cerebri pons varolii*, and *medulla oblongata*. We shall have occasion to refer to each of those parts. Until modern times all the masses included in the skull under the familiar term Brain (or the technical term Encephalon) were regarded as the only centre, and also as the origin of all the nerves. Nor has this notion even yet entirely disappeared, although the spinal cord is known not to be a large nerve trunk, but a centre or connected chain of centres, structurally and functionally similar to the cranial centres. The shadow of the ancient error still obscures interpretation of the part this spinal cord plays in the sentient mechanism; and thus although the cord is universally admitted to be a centre for "sensitive impressions," it is usually excluded from Sensation. This widespread and misleading notion will be critically examined in a future problem.

4. Beginning our survey of the cerebro-spinal axis with the Spinal Cord, we observe it to consist: 1°, of *central grey substance* surrounding the scarcely visible canal, which is all that remains of the primitive groove in the germinal membrane (§ 9); 2°, irregular grey masses, called the *anterior and posterior horns*,† connected with the anterior and posterior

* On these cells see note to § 140.

† These terms designate the surface aspect of a transverse section, of what more correctly should be called the grey columns. See figs. 3 to 6.

roots of the spinal nerves; and 3°, strands of white fibres enclosing this central substance, and called the *anterior lateral and posterior columns.*

Like the Cerebrum, it is a double organ formed by two symmetrical halves, as the cerebrum is of two hemispheres. Each half innervates the corresponding half of the body. The cord is unlike the cerebrum in external form, though very like it in internal structure. The grey structure is mainly external in the cerebrum, and is internal in the cord.

From the anterior side of the cord (that which in animals is the under side) the motor nerves issue; from the posterior (in animals the upper) side, issue the sensory nerves. On each of the sensory nerves there is a ganglion. The *roots* of each nerve, formed of several rootlets issuing from the anterior and posterior columns, subsequently unite together, and proceed in a single sheath to muscles and skin, separating again, however, before they reach muscles and skin. Fig. 2 represents this arrangement.

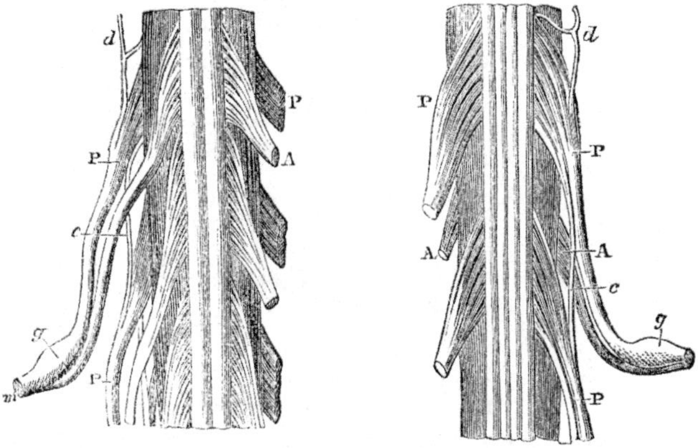

Fig. 2.—*A portion of the spinal cord with its nerves* (after Bernard). The left-hand figure shows the anterior side; the right hand the posterior. A the anterior, and P, the posterior root, they meet at *g*, the ganglion; c and *d* are filaments connecting two posterior roots.

5. There are thirty-one pairs (sometimes thirty-two) of such nerves—namely, eight cervical, twelve thoracic, five lumbar, five sacral, and one (or two) coccygeal. Figs. 3 to 6

represent transverse sections, which display the entrance of the roots of the nerves into the anterior and posterior horns.

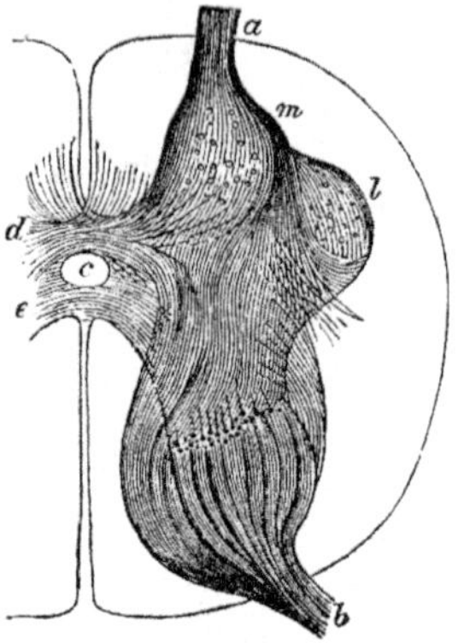

Fig. 3.—*Transverse section of one half of the spinal cord in the lumbar region* (after Kolliker). *a*, anterior root entering the anterior grey horns, *m* and *l*, where cells are clustered ; *c*, central canal ; *d* and *e*, the anterior and posterior commissures uniting the two halves of the cord ; *b*, posterior root entering the posterior grey horn.

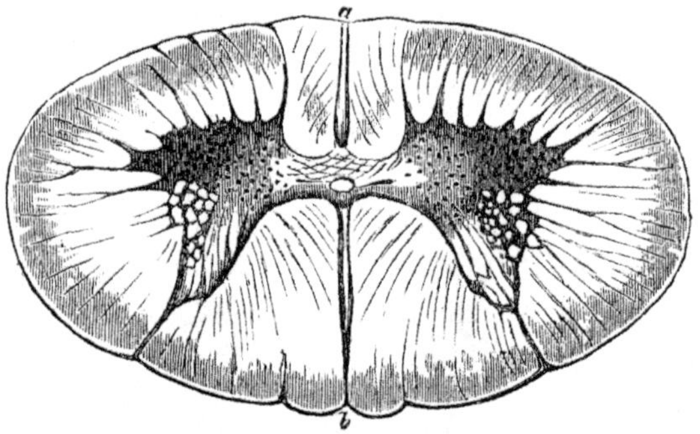

Fig. 4.—*Tranverse section of both halves of the cord, cervical region.* *a*, Fissure separating the anterior columns ; *b*, fissure of the posterior.

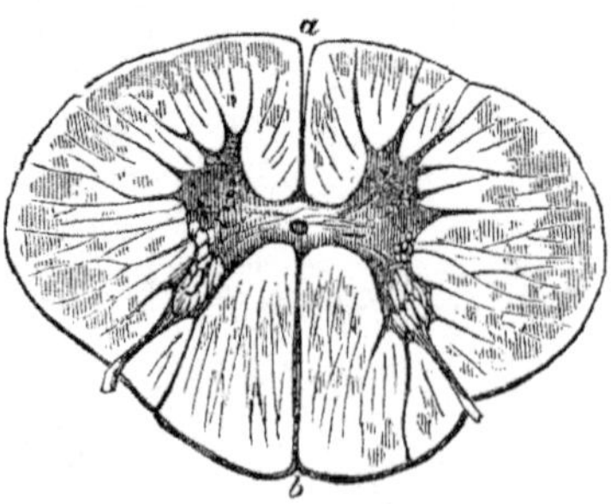

Fig. 5.—*Transverse section of the cord in the dorsal region.*

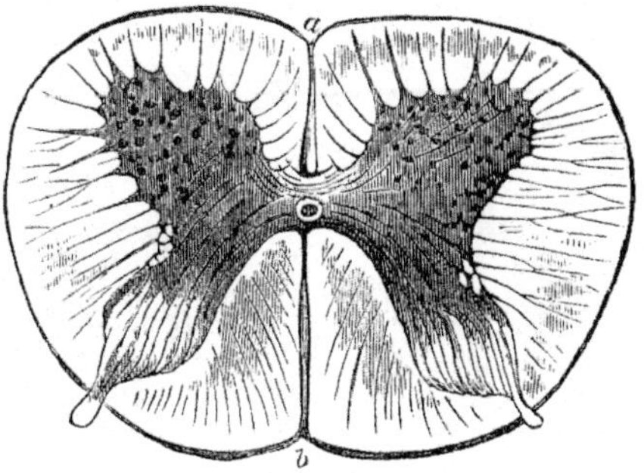

Fig 6.—*Transverse section in the lumbar region.*

6. Similar masses of grey substance in the *Medulla Oblongata* (which is the name given to the cord when it passes into the skull)* are supposed to be the origins of some other nerves (the cranial).

Although the Medulla Spinalis is unquestionably continued as the Medulla Oblongata, the arrangement of its tissues here becomes gradually changed, and so complicated that it baffles the scalpel. Anatomists are, however, agreed on the one point of fundamental importance to us here—namely, that there is only a re-arrangement, not a new tissue. Accepting the artificial division into two organs, we may say that their functions are different, inasmuch as they are different in their anatomical connections—they innervate different parts; but as nerve-centres they have one and the same property.

On its posterior surface the Medulla Oblongata opens as the *fourth ventricle.* It is then no longer a closed canal, but an expansion of the spinal canal, which is covered by the Cerebellum. On its anterior surface projects the *pons varolii.* Figs. 7 and 8 represent these.

While thus on the one hand continuing the Medulla Spinalis, the Medulla Oblongata is seen on the other hand to

* But this only in the higher animals. In reptiles and amphibia the medulla descends into the cervical region, as far as the second and third cervical vertebræ. This should be remembered in experimenting.

K

be continuous with the Brain—its white columns passing upwards in the *crura cerebri*, its cavity repeated in the other

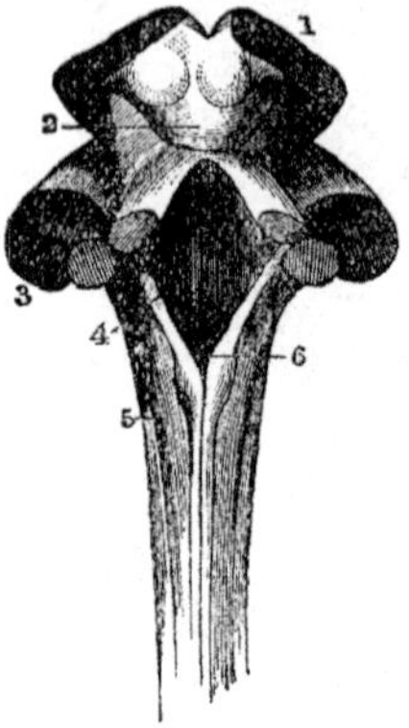

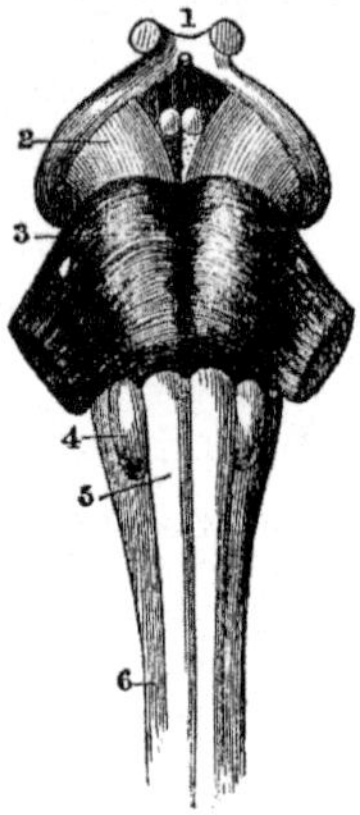

Fig. 7.—*Back, or upper view of the Medulla Oblongata as it continues the Med. Spinalis.* 1, Section of the thalami; 2, corpora quadrigemina (the two lower bodies are imperfectly represented in the engraving); 3, section of the crura cerebelli; 4, the fourth ventricle; 5, the restiform bodies; 6, the calamus scriptorius.

Fig. 8.—*Front, or under view of the Med. Oblong.* 1, Optic nerves cut off at the chiasma; 2, crura cerebri; 3, pons varolii; 4, olivary bodies; 5, anterior pyramids; 6, spinal columns.

ventricles. Above it lie the ganglionic masses the *corpora quadrigemina, optic thalami*, and *corpora striata.* Crowning these are the big and little brains, Cerebrum and Cerebellum. Figs. 9 and 10 represent this relation of Medulla Spinalis, Medulla Oblongata, and Brain. Fig. 11 is a purely artificial

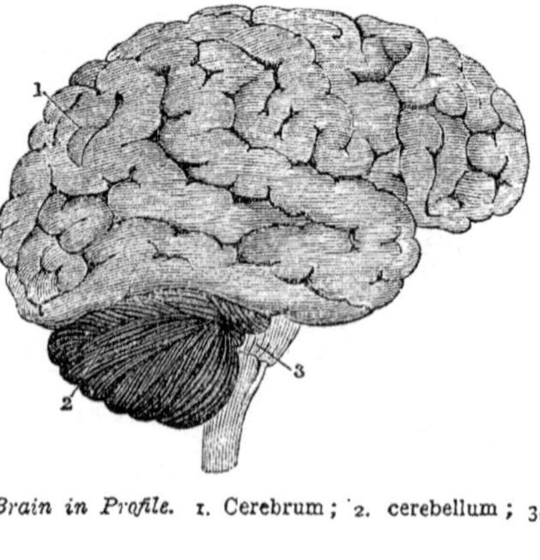

Fig. 9.—*Human Brain in Profile.* 1. Cerebrum; 2. cerebellum; 3, pons varolii and medulla oblongata.

diagram which will give the reader some idea of the disposition of the white and grey substances.

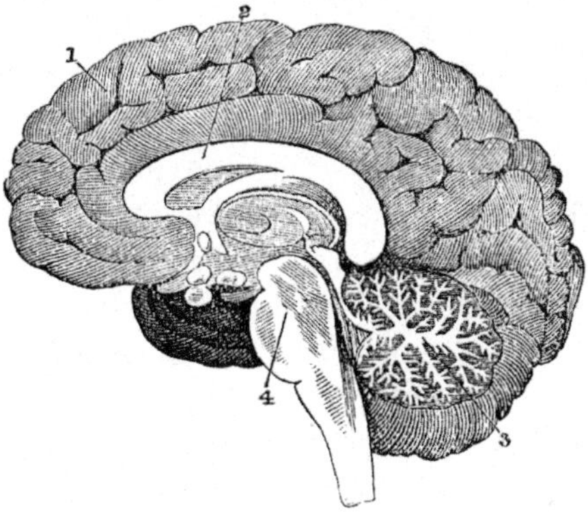

Fig. 10.—*One half of the Brain in Profile, from the inside.* 1, Convolutions of the cerebrum; 2, corpus callosum or great commissure uniting the two hemispheres; 3, arbor vitæ or branching arrangement of grey and white matter in the cerebellum; 4, pons varolii and medulla.

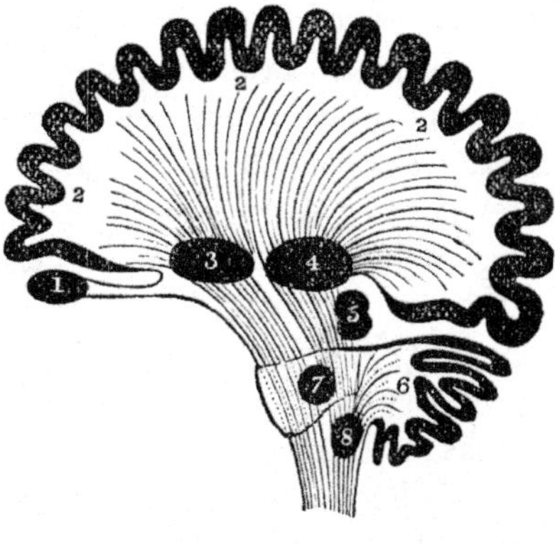

Fig. 11.—*Diagram of a vertical section of the Brain* (after Dalton). 1, Olfactory ganglion; 2, cerebral hemisphere; 3, corpus striatum; 4, thalamus; 5, corpora quadrigemina; 6, cerebellum; 7, ganglion of the pons varolii; 8, olivary body.

7. In man the Cerebrum is to the Cerebellum as 9 to 1. In the lower vertebrates the preponderance is still greater. The cerebrum is in our artificial systems commonly divided into three lobes. The frontal lobe is that portion which lies in front of the deep fissure named after Rolando; between

that fissure and the "internal perpendicular fissure" lies the parietal lobe; behind this we have the occipital lobe; and, below the fissure of Sylvius, the tempero-sphenoidal lobe. Each lobe is again subdivided according to its convolutions.

The disposition of the fibres in the brain is far too complex to be accurately followed. All that we can say is, that there are strands which connect one convolution with another, strands which connect one hemisphere with another, strands which connect cerebrum with cerebellum, and strands which connect the cerebrum with the lower ganglia. It is important to conceive this distinctly; for we shall hereafter see that the function of the Brain (by brain is here meant both Cerebrum and Cerebellum) is not that of *innervation*, but of *incitation and regulation*. To speak metaphorically, it is the coachman who holds in his hands the reins, and guides the team. One cardinal fact should arrest attention, namely, that not a single nerve in the body has its origin or centre of innervation in the cerebrum and cerebellum. The olfactory and optic nerves do indeed *seem* to issue from the cerebrum; and are commonly described as cerebral nerves. But the facts of Development, minute Anatomy, and Experiment prove this to be inexact. Although I shall continue to speak of the olfactory and optic nerves in accordance with universal usage, not wishing to burden the reader with unnecessary innovations, I must at the outset express my opinion that these nerves cannot be brought under the same general type as the other sensory nerves. Embryology and Anatomy suggest that they have no more claim to the title than the *crura cerebri*. Of this hereafter. Setting these aside, no one now refuses to acknowledge that Cerebrum and Cerebellum, although centres of Incitation and Association, are not the centres of direct Innervation: the organic mechanism in all its *physiological* processes will act independently of them (so far as such artificial distinctions are admissible at all). This does not throw a doubt on their *physiological* functions, nor on their participation in the normal execution of physiological processes.

8. From this rapid survey two important points may be

selected for special attention. First, the continuity of the neural axis throughout; secondly, the fundamental similarity of its *structure,* underlying great variations in its form and connections. This, which is the anatomical expression of the Unity of the nervous system, will become more evident after we have expounded what Embryology and Microscopic Anatomy teach. We may therefore digress here awhile to consider

THE EARLY FORMS OF NERVE CENTRES.

9. In the outermost layer of the germinal membrane of the embryo a groove appears, which deepens as its sides grow upwards, and finally close over and form a canal. This canal is composed of cells all alike. Its foremost extremity soon bulges into three well-marked enlargements, which are then called the *primitive cerebral vesicles.* The cavities of these vesicles are continuous. Except in position and size, there are no discernible differences in these vesicles, which are known as the Fore-brain, Middle-brain, and Hind-brain.

10. The *Fore-brain* soon buds off from each side a small vesicle. This is the optic vesicle, the first rudiment of what subsequently becomes optic nerve and retina. At this period it is simply a vesicle with a hollow stem, the cavity being continuous with the cavity of the cerebral vesicle, and the walls continuous with the cerebral wall.

It thus appears that the retina and optic "nerve" are primitive portions of the brain—a detached segment of the general centre, identical in structure with the cerebral vesicle, and not unlike in form. A cup-like depression quickly forms the optic vesicle into an inner and an outer fold. The inner or concave fold becomes the retina, and the outer or convex fold (that nearest to the brain) becomes its choroid membrane. On the fourth day of incubation the retina of the chick is composed of spindle-shaped cells, all alike. On the seventh day there is a differentiation into layers, one of which on the eighth day is granular; on the tenth two are granular; and on the thirteenth ganglionic cells appear. Some of the cells have elongated into radial fibres (known as Müller's fibres); and with the appearance of rods and cones the normal retinal elements are complete.

11. The researches of Foster and Balfour * confirm the statement that all the different parts of the retina (whether nervous or connective) are derived from one and the same layer of embryonic cells, which originally formed a portion of the first cerebral vesicle.

12. Meanwhile the hollow stem of this optic vesicle begins to develop fibres amidst the nuclei of its walls. The "optic nerve" arises: it is still hollow; and in birds remains so through life. The fibres as they are developed *grow forwards towards the retina,* and spread over its internal surface. *They also grow forwards towards the brain,* and spread over its substance; but it is *not,* as might be supposed, and is generally believed, with the cerebral hemispheres (or that portion of the Fore-brain from which these are derived), but with the Middle-brain (which becomes the *corpora quadrigemina*), that the optic fibres are in connection.†

13. This will be understood when the further development is traced. The Fore-brain after budding off the optic vesicles, buds off two larger vesicles—the future cerebral hemispheres. This is noticeable on the second day of incubation, and by the third day each vesicle is as large as the whole of the original Fore-brain. Their development is essentially like that of the optic vesicles; both as to the cellular and the fibrous elements.

The *convolutions, corpus callosum, nucleus lentiformis,* and *corpora striata* are then indicated. Meanwhile, that which originally was the Fore-brain, has lapsed into the secondary rank as Intermediate-brain (*Zwischenhirn*), and becomes the parts surrounding the third ventricle, namely, the *thalami, corpora candicantia, infundibulum,* and what is called the "posterior perforated substance."

* FOSTER and BALFOUR: *Elements of Embryology,* part i., 1874; Comp. SCHWALBE, Art. *Die Retina,* in the *Handbuch der Augenheilkunde* of GRAEFE *und* SÄMISCH, 1874, i. 363.

† The development of the olfactory lobe and bulb is similar; it need not be followed here.

14. The *Middle-brain*, or Second Vesicle, develops the *corpora quadrigemina* from the roof of its cavity, and the *crura cerebri* from its floor.

The *Hind-brain*, or Third Vesicle, divides into two, like the First Vesicle; it buds off the hemispheres of the cerebellum; its cavity forms the fourth ventricle; its walls the *medulla oblongata.*

15. It thus appears that the primitive membrane forms into a canal, which enlarges at one part into three vesicles, and from these are developed the encephalic structures. The continuity of the walls and cavities of these vesicles is never obliterated throughout the subsequent changes. It is also traceable throughout the medulla spinalis. And microscopic investigation reveals that underneath all the morphological changes the walls of the whole cerebro-spinal axis are composed of similar elements on a similar plan.*

16. Two conclusions directly follow from this exposition:—first, that *since the structure of the great axis is everywhere similar, the properties must be similar;* secondly, that *since there is structural continuity, no one part can be called into activity without at the same time more or less exciting that of all the rest.*

THE PERIPHERAL SYSTEM.

17. Following the analytical division, we now come to the Peripheral System of nerves and ganglia. The separation, I must often repeat, is purely artificial; but the artifice has conveniences. We separate in the same way the heart from veins and arteries, and the capillary circulation from the arterial.

* German anatomists divide this axis into trunk and crown (*Hirnstamm* and *Hirnmantel*). There is convenience in this division. If we remove all the grey matter of the cerebrum, with all the white matter radiating from it, until we again come upon grey matter—and if we then cut the cerebellum from its descending strands of white matter—we shall have removed the *crown*, and leave the *trunk* remaining. This trunk is constituted by the corpora striata, nucleus lentiformis, optic thalami, corpora quadrigemina, crura cerebri, pons, medulla oblongata, and medulla spinalis. From this trunk all the organs of the body are directly innervated (except those innervated from the sympathetic ?).

Each nerve has its direct connection with a particular centre, and indirectly with the whole system. It has its circumscribed territory, and individual office. Except in a few cases of anastomosis, the action of one nerve does not involve that of another: only one muscle or one group of muscles is moved, without exciting motion in a neighbour. It is through the centres that these individual territories are united; and a wave of excitation always passes throughout the central substance. Thus the centres are not simply organs of association, consequently of regulation, but are the nexus whereby the diversity of the actions is integrated into the unity of consensus.

18. Nothing further need at present be stated respecting the nerves; but it is needful to give precision to the ideas of

GANGLIA AND CENTRES,

usually spoken of as if they were convertible terms. That this is inexact may be readily shown, and that it is misleading appears in its causing physiologists to credit every ganglion, wherever found, with central functions; and, by an almost inevitable extension of the error, has led to the assignment of central functions to a single ganglionic cell! This is but part of that "superstition of the cell" against which I shall have to protest. I will not here raise the doubt which presses from various sides respecting the central functions of the ganglia in the heart and intestines, because the reader perhaps shares the general opinion on that point; but let me simply ask what central function can possibly be assigned to the ganglia on each of the spinal sensory nerves? above all to those grouped and scattered ganglionic cells which are found at the peripheral termination of some nerves, and in the very trunks of others? There may, indeed, be imagined a central function for the ganglia in the mesentery, and even in the choroid coat of the retina, on the hypothesis (quite gratuitous, I think) of their regulating the circulation; but even this explanation cannot be adopted with respect to the ganglionic cells which appear in the course of the nerve.*

The meaning of a physiological centre is, that it is a point *to* which stimulations proceed, and *from* which they are reflected. The meaning of a ganglion is, that it is a group of nerve cells dispersed among, or in continuation with, nerve fibres: it may be a centre of reflexion, or it may not; and in the latter case its physiological office is at present undetermined. A ganglion is no more a centre in virtue of its cell-group, than a muscle is a limb. All function depends on connection; and central function demands a connection of afferent and efferent parts.

19. The ganglia found in the ventral cord of the Invertebrate (see Fig. 1) are centres each of which has considerable independence, each regulating a single segment of the body, or a group of similar segments. As the scale of animal complexity ascends, these separated centres tend more and more to coalesce; and with this coalescence comes an increasing *combination* of movements.† Observe the caterpillar slowly

* "Ou s'est préoccupé du rôle spécial que pouvaient jouer les ganglions périphériques situés dans le voisinage de certaines organes ; et on a prétendu que les nerfs ne jouissaient de leur propriété d'agir sur ces organes qu'après avoir traversé ces ganglions. On avait admis que l'excitation portée sur le filet nerveux avant son entré dans le ganglion restait sans effet ; que pour obtenir l'action excitatrice des fonctions de l'organe il fallait exciter le nerf entre lui et le ganglion voisin."—CLAUDE BERNARD : *Système Nerveux*, ii. 169. But on proceeding to verify these statements by experiment, BERNARD is led to the conclusion, "que le ganglion n'a pas d'influence propre sur le mode de l'excitation transmise à l'organe."

I was delighted to find my opposition to the current teaching respecting the central functions of ganglionic cells thoroughly borne out by the elaborate researches of SIGMUND MAYER (*Archiv für Psychiatrie*, Bd. vi. Heft 2). Having artificially produced such cells, he pertinently asks, How can we attribute central functions to cells which appear in the process of regeneration of a divided nerve? The error has its origin in the confusion of functions with properties.

† It is often, though incorrectly, stated that every segment of an annulose animal has its separate ganglion. The fact is, that while the ganglia are usually fewer than the segments, they are sometimes more numerous.

crawling over a leaf; each segment of its body moves in succession; but when this caterpillar becomes a butterfly the body moves rapidly, and all at once. Open the caterpillar, and you find its nervous centres are thirteen separate ganglia, each presiding over a distinct part of the body, and each capable of independent action. Open the butterfly, and you find the thirteen ganglia greatly changed: the second and third are fused into one; the fourth, fifth, and sixth into another; the eleventh and twelfth into another; the only trace of the original separation is in a slight constriction of the surface. The movements of the caterpillar were few, simple, slow, and those of the butterfly are many, varied, and rapid.

20. In the Vertebrates the coalescence of ganglia is such that the spinal axis is one great centre. We do indeed anatomically and physiologically subdivide it into several centres, because several portions directly innervate separate organs; but its importance lies in the intimate blending of all parts, so that *fluctuating combinations* of its elements may arise, and varied movements result. Each centre combines various muscles; the axis is a combination of centres. The brainless frog, for instance, has still the spinal cord, and therefore the power not only of moving either of his limbs, but also of combining their separate movements: if grasped, he struggles and escapes; if pricked, he hops away. But these actions, although complex, are much less complex and varied than the actions of the normal frog.

There is not only a coalescence of ganglia, but a greater and greater concentration of the substance in the upper portions of the axis. In the inferior vertebrates, and in the mammalian embryo, the spinal cord occupies the whole length of the vertebral canal from the head to the tip of the tail; and here the centres of reflexion correspond with the several segments. But as the cranial mass develops there is a withdrawal of neural substance from the lower parts, and the centres of reflexion are then some way removed from the segments they innervate. In the animal development there is even a greater and greater predominance of the upper portions, so that the brain and medulla oblongata are of infinitely more importance than the spinal cord.

21. Besides the central group of elements which belong to fixed and definite actions, we must conceive these elements capable of variable combinations, like the pieces of coloured glass in a kaleidoscope, which fall into new groups, each group having its definite though temporary form. The elements constitute really a continuous net-work of variable forms. It is to such combinations, and not to fixed circumscribed ganglia, that we must refer the subordinate centres of the axis. We speak of a centre for Respiration, a centre for Laughing, a centre for Crying, a centre for Coughing, and so on, with as much propriety as we speak of a centre for Swallowing or for Walking. Not that in these cases there is a circumscribed mass of central substance set apart for the innervation of the several muscles employed in these actions, and for no other purpose. Each action demands a definite group of neural elements, as each geometric form in the kaleidoscope demands a definite group of pieces of glass; but these same pieces of glass will readily enter into other combinations; and in like manner the muscles active in Respiration are also active in Laughing, Coughing, &c., though differently innervated and co-ordinated.

22. The physiological rank of a centre is therefore the expression of its power of fluctuating combination. The medulla oblongata is higher than the medulla spinalis, because of its more varied combinations; the cerebrum is higher than all, because it has no fixed and limited combinations. It is the centre of centres, and as such the supreme organ.

CHAPTER II.

THE FUNCTIONAL RELATIONS OF THE NERVOUS SYSTEM.

23. The distinguishable parts of this system are the central axis, the cranial nerves, and the spinal nerves, with the chain of ganglia and nerves composing the Sympathetic. Let us briefly set down what is known of their special offices.

Men very early discovered that the nerves were in some way ministrant to Sensation and Movement; a divided nerve always being accompanied by insensibility and immobility in the limb. Galen, observing that paralysis of movement sometimes occurred without insensibility, suggested that there were two kinds of nerve; but no one was able to furnish satisfactory evidence in support of this suggestion

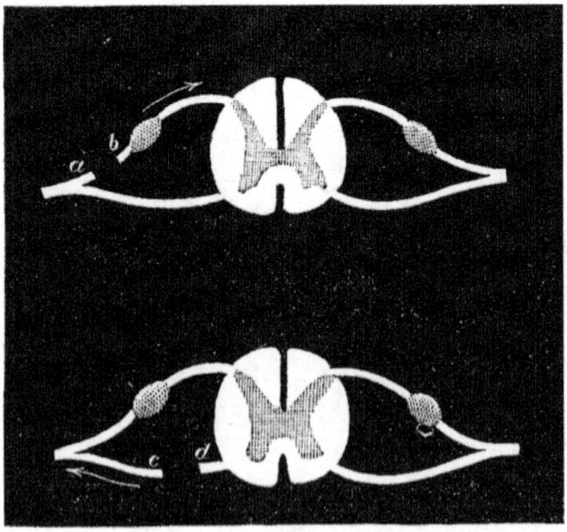

Fig. 12 —*Transverse sections of spinal cord (dorsal region).*

until early in the present century, when the experiments of Charles Bell, perfected by those of Majendie and Müller, placed the suggestion beyond dispute.

24. Fig. 12 is a *diagram* (not a drawing of the actual aspect, which would be hardly intelligible to readers unversed in such matters) representing two transverse sections of the spinal cord just where the nerve roots issue. The grey substance is somewhat in the form of a rude H, in the dorsal region, and of the expanded wings of a butterfly in the lumbar enlargements (figs. 4–6); the extremities of this grey substance are the *anterior and posterior horns.* We have already said that from the anterior horns of each half issue the roots of the motor nerves, which pass to the muscles. From the posterior horns issue the sensory nerves, which, soon after leaving the cord, enter the ganglia before joining the motor nerves, and then pass to the skin, in the same sheath with their companions, separating again as they reach the muscles and surfaces where they are to be distributed. When this mixed nerve is cut through, or tied, all sensation and movement disappear from the parts innervated. But if only one of the roots be cut through, above the ganglion, there will then be only a loss of movement, or a loss of sensation. Thus suppose the section be made at *a, b,* A: we have then divided a sensory nerve, and no pinching or pricking of the part innervated by that nerve will be felt; but movement will take place if the under nerve be irritated, or if a sensation *elsewhere* be excited. Now reverse the experiment, as at B, *c, d.* Then, pricking of the skin will be felt, but no movement will respond. The nerve which enters the cord at the upper (posterior) part is therefore a sensory nerve; that which enters at the under (anterior) part is motor. The direction is in each case indicated by the arrow. The central end *b* if irritated will produce sensation; whereas the peripheral end *a* produces neither sensation, nor movement. The central end *d* produces neither sensation nor movement; the peripheral end *c* produces movement.

25. Two facts are proved by these experiments. First, that the co-operation of the centre is necessary for Sensation, but not for Movement. Although normally all the muscles of the trunk are moved only when their centre has been excited, yet any irritation applied directly to the muscle nerve, even when separated from its centre, produces a movement. And to this we may add that a slighter stimulus will move the muscle by direct irritation of the nerve, than by indirect irritation through the centre; a slighter stimulus also will suffice when applied to the nerve, than when applied to the muscle itself.

26. The second fact proved is known as *Bell's Law*, that the sensory and motor channels are respectively the posterior and anterior nerves. The fact is indisputable, but its theoretic interpretation can no longer be accepted in its original form. Bell supposed the two nerves to be different in kind, endowed with different specific energies, the one sensitive, the other motor. The majority of writers still express themselves as if they adopted this view. We shall, however, presently see reason for replacing it by the more consistent interpretation which assigns one and the same property to both nerves, marking their distinction by the terms afferent and efferent; the one set being anatomically so disposed that it conveys stimuli from the surfaces to the centre, and the other set conveying stimuli from the centre to the muscles, glands, and other cells.*

27. Bell's discovery was rapidly generalised. The principle of localisation was extended to all nerves, and of course to the posterior and anterior columns of the spinal cord, which indeed were assumed to be continuations of the nerves. Bell, who was greater as an anatomist than as a philosopher, always maintained that anatomical deduction was superior to experiment. But this was to misunderstand the reach of deduction, which is only valid to the extent of its premisses.† In the present case, the premisses assumed that the posterior columns were continuations of the posterior roots, and carried

* It has been proved that the cells of the cornea and the pigment cells of the skin contract under nervous excitation. We cannot suppose that although these are the only cells which have hitherto been brought under experimental observation they are the only cells subject to nerve-influence. We may safely assume that wherever a nerve fibre terminates, its action will be transformed into an excitation of the part. Habitually, however, motor-nerves are spoken of as muscle-nerves.

† On Deduction, see *Problems: First Series*, vol. ii. p. 170.

impressions to the brain, the anterior columns carrying back from the brain the "mandates of the will." Experiment has, however, decisively shown that it is *not* through the posterior columns that sensory impressions travel to the brain, but through the central grey substance.

28. The spinal cord with its central grey substance is at each point a centre of reflexion. Connected as it is with different organs, we artificially consider it as a chain of different centres, and try to detect the functional relations of its parts. The inquiry is important, but we must bear in mind the cardinal principle that diversity of Function depends on the organs innervated, and not on a diversity of Property in the nervous tissue. Although all nerves have a common structure and common property, yet we distinguish them as sensory and motor; and the sensory we subdivide into those of Special Sensation and those of Systemic Sensation. The motor we divide into muscular, vasomotor, and glandular. The hypothesis of specific energies must be relinquished (§ 63).

In like manner all centres have a common structure and a common property, with a great diversity of functional relations. Here also the hypothesis of specific energies has been generally adopted, owing to a mistaken conception of the biological principle just mentioned. The cerebral hemispheres are credited with the properties of sensation, thought, and volition; the cerebellum with the property of muscular co-ordination; the spinal cord with the property of reflexion.

29. No attempt to assign the true functional relations of the centres will be made at the present stage of our exposition. We must learn more of the processes in Sensation, Thought, and Volition, before we can unravel the complex physiological web on which they depend. But here, provisionally, may be set down what observation and experiment have disclosed respecting the part played by certain centres. We know, for example, that when the cerebral hemispheres are carefully removed from a reptile or a bird, all the essentially *vital* functions go on pretty much as before, but a great disturbance in some of the *psychical* functions is observed.

The brainless bird eats, drinks, sleeps, moves its limbs separately and in combination, manifests sensibility to light, sound, and touch, performs such instinctive actions as pruning its feathers, or thrusting the head under the wing while roosting. Throw it into the air and it will fly. In its flight it will avoid obstacles, and will alight upon a ledge, or your shoulder. But it will not fly unless thrown into the air; it will not escape through the open door or window; it will avoid objects, but will show no fear of them—alighting on your head, for example, without hesitation. It is sensitive to light, and may in a certain sense be said to *see;* but it fails to *perceive* what is *seen.* It will eat and drink, if food and water be administered, but it will starve near a heap of grain and never peck it, not even if the beak be thrust into the heap. A grain, or strip of meat, may be thrust inside the beak; there it will remain unswallowed, unless it touches the back of the mouth, then swallowing at once follows the stimulus. The bird *with* its brain will fly away if you turn the finger, or stick, on which it is perching; *without* its brain, it makes no attempt to fly, but flutters its wings, and balances itself. If you open the mouth of a cat, or rabbit, and drop in some bitter fluid, the animal closes its mouth firmly, and resists your efforts to repeat the act; without its brain, the animal shows the same disgust at the taste, but never resists the preliminaries of the repetition.

30. These, and analogous facts, have been noted by various experimenters. They are very far from proving what is usually concluded; but they prove the important negative position that the cerebrum is not the centre of innervation for any of the organs on which the observed actions depend. Thus, the cerebrum is not necessary to sight; *ergo* it does not innervate the eye. It is not necessary to hearing: *ergo* it does not innervate the ear.* It is not necessary to breathing

* I do not here touch upon the question as to whether these actions of the senses are *sensations*, because that question demands that we should first settle what is Sensation. I may at once, however, say that what is ordinarily understood as a sensation of *colour*, or a sensation of *sound*, is, in my opinion, not possible without the cerebrum. But the sensibility of the eye and ear is manifestly preserved.

swallowing, flying, &c.: *ergo* it does not innervate the organs of these functions.

What then is lost? We have only to remember that the cerebrum is continuous with the thalami and corpora striata, and, through its crura, with the medulla oblongata and medulla spinalis, to foresee that its removal must more or less affect the whole neural axis, and consequently disturb the actions of the whole organism; this disturbance will often have the appearances which would be due to the removal of a central apparatus, so that we shall be apt to attribute the cessation of a function to the loss of its organ, when in fact the cessation is due simply to an arrest of the organ by irritation. Thus the cessation of consciousness, or of any particular movements, when the cerebrum is removed, is no decisive proof that the cerebrum is the organ of consciousness, or of the movement in question. This point will be duly considered hereafter. What we have now to consider is the facts observed after removal of the cerebrum.

First, we observe a loss of that power of combining present states with past states, present feelings with feelings formerly excited in conjunction with them, the power which enables the animal to adjust its actions to certain sensations *now unfelt* but which *will be* felt in consequence of the adjustment. Secondly, we observe a loss of Spontaneity: the bird, naturally mobile and alert, now sits moveless for hours in a sort of stupor, occasionally preening its feathers, but rarely quitting its resting-place. All the most conspicuous phenomena which we assign to Intelligence, and Will seem absent. The sensations are altered and diminished. Many Instincts have disappeared, but some remain. The sexual feeling is preserved, although the bird has lost all power of directing its actions so as to gratify the desire. But these effects are only observed when the whole of both hemispheres have been removed. If a small portion remain the bird retains most of its faculties, though with less energy. In frogs and fishes there is little discernible effect observed when a large portion of the cerebrum is removed.

31. Now take away from this mutilated bird its cere-

bellum: all the functions continue as before except that *some* combined movements can no longer be effected; flight is impossible; walking is a mere stagger. Remove only the lateral lobes, and though flight is still possible great *incoherence* of the wings is observed, whereas walking is not much affected. If only the cerebellum be removed, the cerebrum being intact, the phenomena are very different. All the perceptions and almost all the emotions, all the spontaneity and vivacity are retained; but the sexual instinct, which was manifested when the cerebrum was removed, is now quite gone. What we call Intelligence seems unaffected. The bird hears, and understands the meaning of the sounds, sees and perceives, sees and fears, sees and adjusts its movements with a mental vision of unseen consequences.*

32. Are we from these facts to conclude that the cerebrum is the "organ of the mind"? that it is "the seat" of sensation, thought, emotion, volition; and that the cerebellum is the "seat" of the sexual instinct, and muscular co-ordination? Such conclusions have found acceptance, even from physiologists who would have been startled had any one ventured to affirm that the medulla oblongata was the "organ" of Respiration, because Respiration ceases when this centre is destroyed. I shall have to combat this notion at various stages of my exposition. Here let me simply say that it is irreconcilable with any clear conception of organ and function; and is plainly irreconcilable with any survey of psychical phenomena in animals in whom the cerebrum does not exist, and in animals from whom it has been removed.

What the facts indisputably prove is that the cerebrum has an important part in the mechanism by which the most complex psychical combinations are effected, and that the cerebellum has an important part in the mechanism by which the most complex muscular combinations are effected. The supreme importance of the cerebrum may be inferred from its

* It has been observed that removal of the cerebellum affects the pigment cells of the skin. No doubt other parts are also affected, but the changes have hitherto escaped observation.

dominating all the other centres, and from its preponderance in size. In man it stands to all the other cranial centres together in the relation of 11 to 3. It is about five times as heavy as the spinal cord—that is to say from 1100 to 1400 grammes, compared with 27 to 30 grammes. The quantity of blood circulating through it is immense. Haller estimated the cranial circulation as one-fifth of the whole circulation. If, therefore, the Nervous Centres are agents in the production of Sensation and Intelligence, by far the largest share must be allotted to the cranial centres, and of these the largest to the Cerebrum.

33. It is, however, one thing to recognise the Cerebrum as having an important part in the production of psychical phenomena, another thing to localise all the phenomena in it as their organ and seat—a localisation which soon becomes even more absurd, when of all the cerebral structure the multipolar cells alone are admitted as the active agents!

As was said just now, we recognise in the Medulla Oblongata the nervous centre of Respiration, but we do not suppose that Respiration has its *seat* there, nor that this centre is absolutely indispensable for the essential part of the process. We respire by our skin, as well as by our lungs; many animals respire who have nothing like a medulla oblongata; as many animals feel, and manifest will, who have nothing like a cerebrum. The destruction of centres is of course a disturbance of the mechanisms which they regulate. But even the observed results of a destruction require very close examination, and are liable to erroneous interpretations. The disappearance of a function following the destruction, or disease of a particular part, is not to be accepted as a proof that this part is the organ of the lost function; because precisely the same phenomena may often be observed following the destruction of a totally different part.* But one result may always be relied

* OWSJANNIKOW describes the results of removing carefully the cranial ganglia of the crayfish; and these effects MEYER observes to be identical with those which follow removal of the large claw of the crayfish! A. B. MEYER: *Das Hemmungsnerven-system des Herzens*, 1869, p. 23. Let me add that the phenomena described by M. FAIVRE as

on, and that is the *persistence* of a function after removal of a particular part. Thus there is a certain spot of the cerebral convolutions from which movements of the limbs are excited when the electrodes are applied to it; removal of the substance is immediately followed by paralysis of the limbs. Are we to conclude that this spot is the organ of the function? It is true that the function is called into action by a stimulus applied to this spot: true that the function suddenly vanishes when the substance of this spot is destroyed. Nevertheless, what seems a loss of function is only a disturbance. In two or three days the paralysis begins to disappear, and at the end of a week the limbs are moved nearly in the normal manner. And the same is true when the spot in question is destroyed on both sides. The recovery of the function shows that the absent part was not its organ. There is a paradoxical experiment recorded by M. Paul Bert which may be cited here. He removed the right cerebral hemisphere from a chameleon, and found that the limbs on the left side were paralysed; but on his then removing the left cerebral hemisphere the limbs of the left side recovered their activity. A similar result was obtained by Lussana and Lemoigne by extirpation of the thalami. When we find combined movements persisting after the cerebellum has been destroyed, we may be sure that the cerebellum is not the organ by which such combinations take place; and when we find sensation and volition manifested after the cerebrum has been removed, we may be sure that the cerebrum is not the organ for these sensations and volitions.

34. And this we do find. Physiologists, indeed, for the most part, deny it; or rather, while they admit the observed facts, they refuse to admit the only consistent interpretation, biassed as they are by the traditional conception of the brain. After having for many years persistently denied Sensibility to any centre except the cerebrum, they are now generally agreed in including the medulla oblongata within

following the destruction of one subœsophageal ganglion in the *Dytiscus*, are so little to be referred to the mere absence of the ganglion, that I find them not to occur when the whole head is removed.

the privileged region; but they still exclude the medulla spinalis.

35. If all the cranial centres as far as the medulla oblongata are removed from young rabbits, dogs, or cats, there are unmistakable evidences of Sensibility in their *cries* when their tails are pinched, their *moving jaws* (as in mastication) when bitters are placed in their mouths, and their *raised paws rubbing their noses*, when irritating vapours are applied. It is said indeed that the cries are not signs of *pain;* and this is probable; but they are assuredly signs of Sensibility.

36. The frog thus mutilated has lost indeed all its special senses, except Touch, but it still breathes, struggles when grasped, thrusts aside the pincers which irritate it, or wipes away acid dropped on its skin. If the eye be lightly touched, the eyelid closes; if the touch be repeated three or four times, the foreleg is raised to push the irritant away; if still repeated, the head is turned aside; but however prolonged the irritation, the frog neither hops, nor crawls away, as he does when the cerebellum remains. Place the brainless frog on his back, and if the medulla oblongata remains he will at once regain the normal position; but if that part is absent he will lie helpless on his back. The power of preserving equilibrium in difficult positions—which of course implies a nice co-ordination of muscles—resides in the so-called *optic lobes* of the frog (what in mammals are called the *corpora quadrigemina*).

37. With the destruction of each part of the central mass there will necessarily be some disturbance of the mechanism; but difficult as may be the task of detecting by experiment what is the normal action of any one part, there ought to be no hesitation in recognising the persistence of functions after certain parts are destroyed. The spinal cord is anatomically known to be the centre from which the limbs, trunk, and genito-urinary organs are innervated. So long as the mechanism of the actions involving such organs is intact, no removal of other parts will prevent this mechanism from exhibiting its normal action. There may indeed arise, and there has arisen, the doubt whether Sensibility is involved in

the action of any nerve centre below the medulla oblongata. But this doubt is founded on the traditional hypothesis respecting the seat of Sensation, and is flagrantly at variance with the logical conclusions of Anatomy and Experiment.

38. Anatomy shows that the structure of the spinal cord is in all essential characters the same as that of the medulla oblongata; and indeed that the whole central axis has one continuous tissue, somewhat variously arranged, and in relation with various organs.

Abundant Experiment has shown that the spinal cord, apart from the encephalon, is capable of acting as a sensorial and volitional centre. The striking facts advanced by Pflüger, Auerbach, and myself, have not been impugned;* but their interpretation has been generally rejected. We showed that a brainless frog responded to stimulation in actions which bore so close a resemblance to actions admitted to be sensorial and volitional—showed the frog *adapting* itself to new conditions, and *acquiring* dexterity in executing actions which at first were impossible or difficult, *devising* combinations to effect a purpose which never by any possibility could have formed part of its habits—manifesting, in a word, such signs of Sensibility, that no one witnessing the experiments could hesitate as to the interpretation, had he not been biassed by the traditions of the schools.

39. Our opponents argued that in spite of all appearances there were profound differences between the actions of the normal and the brainless animal, and that the latter were due simply to Reflex Action. I also insist on profound differences; but underlying these there are fundamental identities. As to the Reflex Action, two points will hereafter be brought forward: 1°, that *all* central action is re-

* PFLÜGER : *Die Sensorischen Funktionen des Rückenmarks*, 1853.
AUERBACH : *Günzburg's Zeitschrift*. Jahrgang iv. p. 486.
LEWES : *Leeds Meeting of British Association*, 1858, and *Physiology of Common Life*, 1860.

This recognition of sensation, and even of volition, in spinal actions may be found in the writings of WHYTT, UNZER, PROCHASKA, LEGALLOIS, and MAYO; but the establishment of the Reflex Theory had displaced it, and its revival dates from PFLÜGER.

flex, the cerebral no less than the spinal; 2°, that the hypothesis of Reflex Action being purely *mechanical,* and distinguished from Voluntary Action in not involving Sensibility, is an hypothesis which must be relinquished.

40. Postponing, however, all discussion of these points, let me here say that the doctrine maintained in these pages is that the whole cerebro-spinal axis is a centre of Reflexion, its various segments taking part in the performance of different kinds of combined action. It has one common property, Sensibility; and different parts of it minister to different functions—the optic centre being different from the auditory, the cerebral from the spinal; and so on. To make this intelligible, however, we must first learn what is known respecting the properties of nerve-tissue.

CHAPTER III.

NEURILITY.

41. Observation having found that the activity of a nerve was always followed by a sensation when the nerve ended in a centre, and by a movement when the nerve ended in a muscle, Theory was called upon to disclose the nature of this peculiar property of nerves. That a peculiar and mysterious power did act in the nerves no one doubted; the only doubt was as to its nature. The ancient hypothesis of Animal Spirits seemed all that was needed. The spirits coursed along the nerves, and obeyed the mandates of the Soul. When this hypothesis fell into discredit, its place was successively taken by the hypotheses of Nervous Fluid, Electricity, and Nerve Force. The Fluid, though never manifested to Sense, was firmly believed in, even so late as the days of Cuvier;* but when the so-called electrical currents were detected in nerves, and the nervous phenomena were shown to resemble electrical phenomena, there was a general agreement in adopting the electrical hypothesis. The brain then took the place of a galvanic battery; the nerves were its electrodes.

42. Closer comparison of the phenomena detected various irreconcilable differences, which, if they proved nothing else, proved that nerve-action took place under conditions so special as to demand a special designation. Electricity itself is so little understood, that until its nature is more precisely known, we cannot confidently say more than that nerve-action resembles electrical-action; meanwhile the speciality

* Friedländer (*Versuch über die innern Sinne*, 1826, i. 77) declares it to be a rational necessity: "Die Annahme eines Nervenfluidums ist Nothwendigkeit der Vernunft."

of neural conditions renders all deduction illusory which is based on electrical-action as observed under *other* conditions. In presence of these difficulties, cautious physiologists content themselves with assigning the observed phenomena to the observed and inferred conditions, condensing these in the convenient symbol "nerve-force," without pretending to any specification of the nature of that force. It may be a wave of molecular movement dependent on isomeric change or on metamorphic change. It may be the liberation of molecular tension resembling electricity; it may be electricity itself. But whatever the nature of the change, it is an activity of the tissue, and as such comes under the general dynamic conception of Force or Energy.

43. In this sense the term has nothing equivocal or obscure. It is a shorthand expression symbolising certain well-defined observations. Nevertheless, it is a term which we shall do well to avoid when possible, and to replace by another having less danger of misinterpretation; the reason being that Force has become a sort of shibboleth, and a will-o'-wisp to speculative minds. All that we *know* of Force is Motion. But this is too meagre for metempirical thinkers, who disdain the familiar experiences expressed in the term Motion, and demand a transcendent cause "to account" for what is observed. They seek an entity to account for the fact. Motion is a very definite conception, expressing precise experiences: we know what it means; and know that the laws of moving bodies admit of the nicest calculation. A similar precision belongs to Force when understood as "mass acceleration," or $M V^2$. But this does not content those metaphysicians who understand by Force "the unknown reality behind the phenomena"—the *cause* of Motion. This cause they refuse to recognise in some antecedent motion (what I have termed a "differential pressure") but demand for it a physical or metaphysical *agent:* the physical agent being a subtle fluid of the nature of Ether, or a nerve atmosphere surrounding the molecules; the metaphysical agent being a Spirit or aggregate of Soul-atoms. The second alternative we may decline here to discuss. The first alternative is not only a pure fiction, but one which is inconsistent with the demonstrable velocity of the neural process, which is not greater than the pace of a greyhound, whereas the velocities of light and electricity are enormously beyond this. It is inconsistent also with the observation that a much feebler current of electricity is requisite for the stimulation of a muscle through its nerve than when directly applied to the muscle: a proof that the nerve does not act solely by transmission of electricity—unless we gratuitously assume that the nerve is a multiplicator.

When it is said that the living nerve is incessantly liberating Force which can be communicated to other tissues, the statement is acceptable only if we reject the metaphysical conceptions it will too generally suggest—the conceptions of Force as an entity, and of its being passed from one object to another like an arrow shot from a bow. The physical interpretation simply says that the molecules of the nerve are incessantly vibrating, and with varying sweep; these vibrations, when of a certain energy, will set going vibrations in another substance by disturbing the tension of its molecules, as the vibrations of heat will disturb the tension of the gunpowder molecules, and set them sweeping with greater energy: this is the *communication* of the force. Just as we say that a magnet communicates magnetic force to a bit of iron, though all we mean is that the magnet has so altered the molecular condition of the iron as to have given it the movements called magnetism—in short has excited in the iron the dormant property of becoming magnetic—so we say the nerve communicates its force to the muscle, exciting in the muscle its dormant property of contraction. But in truth nothing has passed from magnet to iron, or from nerve to muscle.

44. Do what we will, however, there is always, in the present condition of philosophical chaos the danger of being misunderstood when we employ the term Nerve-force; and I have proposed the term Neurility as an escape from the misleading suggestions. It is a symbol expressing the general property of nerve-tissue. For reasons presently to be stated, I restrict Neurility to the peripheral system, employing Sensibility for the central system. The excited muscle manifests its special property of Contractility; the excited nerve manifests its special property of Neurility; the excited centre manifests its special property of Sensibility.* The terms are simply descriptive, and carry with them no hypothesis as to *what* Neurility is in its hidden process, nor *how* Sensibility arises in a nerve centre, and not elsewhere. We know that a stimulated muscle contracts, and we express the fact by assigning to muscular tissue the property of Contractility. We know that a stimulated nerve translates an impulse from one point to another, and excites the muscle to contract; and we express the fact by assigning to nerve-tissue the property of transmitting stimulation, which is further specified, as unlike other transmissions, by the term Neurility.

45. What is the meaning attached to the term Property, and how it is distinguished from Function, has been already expounded in Problem I, §§ 81-6. There also was laid down

* These terms and the conception they embody were proposed by me in 1859 in a paper "On the necessity of a reform in Nerve-physiology," read at the Aberdeen meeting of the British Association, and were reproduced in the *Physiology of Common Life.* (Prof. OWEN, probably in forgetfulness of my suggestion, proposed "neuricity." *Lectures on the Comp. Anat. of Vertebrates*, 1866, i. p. 318.) The terms were fortunate enough to meet with acceptance from some physiologists both in England and France; and the conception has been more widely accepted than the terms. The most distinguished approver was Prof. VULPIAN. "Faute d'une meilleure détermination on peut, avec M. Lewes, donner à la propriété physiologique des fibres nerveuses le nom de *neurilité*; c'est là ce qui correspondra à la contractilité des fibres musculaires." *Leçons sur la physiologie du système nerveux*, 1866, p. 220. He also adopted my suggestion (since modified) of Sensibility as the property of ganglionic cells. Compare also GAVARRET: *Phénomènes physiques de la Vie*, 1869, pp. 213 and 222. TAULE: *Notions sur la nature de la matière orgranisée*, 1866, p. 131. CHARLES ROBIN: *Anatomie et physiologie cellulaires*, 1873, p. 166.

By these channels, and by the German, Italian, Russian, Polish, and Hungarian translations of my work, the suggestions were carried over Europe, crept into scientific journals, and became known to writers who never heard of me. I only mention these facts lest the reader should suppose that my views had been anticipated by certain continental writers.

the principle of *identity of structure implying identity of property.* Inasmuch as observation reveals a fundamental similarity in the structure of the nervous tissue throughout the animal kingdom, we must conclude the existence of a fundamental similarity in the property of that tissue: a conclusion confirmed by observation. There is a corresponding agreement in the organs and functions; so that, within certain limits, the experiments performed on an insect may be verified on a mammal. Everywhere nerve tissue has certain characters in common, accompanied by variations in the degree and mode of manifestation corresponding with variations in structure and connexion. Obvious as the fact is, we must emphasise the great variety which accompanies the underlying uniformity, for this is recognisable both in the individual organism and in the animal kingdom at large. Even such seemingly individual terms as nerve-cell and nerve-fibre are in truth generic; and the description which accurately represents one cell or fibre needs modifying for others.

Properties are generalised expressions; they result from the *composition,* the *structure,* and the *texture* of a substance. Thus one bar of iron may differ from another of equal bulk in being more or less crystalline in structure, though having the same composition, and the same texture. This difference will modify the mode of manifestation of the iron-properties. Cast-iron pillars, for example, will support, as a roof, a weight which would break them if suspended; wrought-iron pillars of similar bulk will bear a weight suspended which would crush them as a roof. Yet both cast and wrought iron pillars have the same properties, because they have the *same* composition and *similar* structure; the variation of structure only producing a difference in the modes. Texture may also vary. The bar of iron may be beaten into a plate, rolled into a cylinder, or split into wire-work, without any change in its properties, but with marked differences in its modes of manifestation, and in the *uses* to which it may be applied. These uses are of course dependent on the connexions established between the iron and other things. In Physiology, *uses* are called *functions.*

46. Nerve tissue must be understood as having everywhere the same general Property. In one animal and in another, in one part and in another, Neurility is the same in kind, but not everywhere manifesting the same degree, nor applied to the same Function. The *composition* of nerve tissue varies, but not more than the composition of all other organised substances; the *structure* is variable, but only within a small range; the *texture* also; while the *connexions* are very various. Hence, whatever the variations in composition or structure, the nerve-fibre has everywhere one fundamental property, which in connection with a muscle has the functional activity of exciting contraction; in connection with a gland of exciting secretion; and in connection with a centre of exciting reflexion.*

47. Had a clear idea of Function as dependent on connexion been present to their minds certain physiologists would hardly have raised the mirage of "Nerve-force," a mysterious entity endowed with "specific energies," and capable of producing vital and psychical phenomena by an occult process; nor would others have been led to the monstrous hypothesis of particular nerve-cells being endowed with thought, instinct, and volition. They would have sought an explanation of functions in the combined properties of the co-operant organs and tissues. They would not have endowed one nerve with Sensibility, and another nerve of identical structure with Motility; † one nerve with a motor property, and another with the opposite property of inhibition.

* "La force nerveuse n'existe pas comme puissance independant des propriétés de tissu. Elle consiste en l'action des parties excitée, sur les parties excitables, l'état de l'excitation des premières agissant comme impression ou stimulation sur les secondes." LANDRY: *Traité des Paralysies*, 1859, i. 142.

† "Le système nerveux est tout à la fois l'origine des sensations et l'origine des mouvements. Mais est—ce par une propriété unique, ou par deux propriétés diverses qu'il détermine deux phénomènes aussi distincts?" FLOURENS: *Recherches sur les propriétés et les fonctions du Système Nerveux*, 1824, p. 1. He concludes that "la puissance nerveuse n'est pas unique; il n'y a pas une seule propriété, il y en a deux," p. 24. In this he has been generally followed.

They would have seen that all nerves have the same *property*, but different *uses* when in different connexions.

48. Throughout the animal kingdom we see movement following on stimulation. Stimulation may be defined the change of molecular equilibrium. The stimulation of a muscle is produced indirectly through a change in the nerve, or directly through a change in the muscle itself. In the simplest organisms there is no trace of nerve tissue; but their substance manifests Irritability (or as it is often called Sensibility); and a stimulus to one part is propagated throughout—the whole body moves when touched. Even in Polypes, where there is the beginning of a differentiation, the motion is slowly propagated from one part to the rest. A single tentacle retracts when touched; but the movement rarely ends there; it is slowly communicated from one tentacle to the other, and from them to the whole mass. Touching the body, however, will not, if the touch be slight, cause the tentacles to move; so that we see here a beginning of that principle of specialisation which is so manifest in the higher organisms: the tentacles have become the specially sensitive parts. Ascending higher in the scale of organisms we find those which habitually move particular parts without at the same time necessarily moving the rest; and this independence of parts, accompanying a more perfect consensus, we find to be developed *pari passu* with a nervous system. An immense variety of part-movements, with varying combinations of such movements, is the physiological expression of the more complex nervous system.

48*a*. Deferring what has to be said of Sensibility till the next chapter, we may here touch on its relation to Irritability, which is often used as its synonym. *Objectively* it cannot be distinguished from Irritability, nor indeed from the most general phenomenon of reaction under stimulation; in this it is an universal property. But *subjectively* it is distinguishable as a peculiar mode of reaction, only known in nerve tissues. While all tissues are irritable, and react on being stimulated, each tissue has its special mode of reaction. The secreting-cell reacts differently from the muscle-cell.

The reaction of the nerve is the innervation of a centre or a muscle; the reaction of an innervated centre is sensation; of a muscle, contraction. There are three aspects of neural reaction: excitation, propagation of the disturbance, and innervation. The first is expressed by irritability, the second by conductibility, the third by sensibility; but these are only artificial distinctions in the general phenomenon of transmitted excitation. The nerve substance is specially distinguished by its instability of molecular equilibrium; it undergoes chemical change with a readiness comparable to that of explosive substances. Hence its facility of propagation of disturbance. There is irritability and propagation of disturbance in muscular tissue, notably evident in the continuous tissue of the heart, intestines, and ureter; but the propagation is slow and diffusive; whereas in the nerve it is rapid, and restricted along a definite path. By this rapidity and restriction the force of the impact is increased; and thus a slight stimulus applied to the nerve is capable of disturbing the state of the muscle.

49. Thus while molecular movement is a fundamental condition of Vitality, and is incessant throughout organised substance, the massive movements of the organism, and the movements of particular parts, are the *directed quantities* of this molecular agitation. They are due to stimulation. We distinguish this from mechanical impulsion. It is a vital process involving molecular change; it is not simply the *communication* of motion from without, but the *excitation* of motion within. It is not like the blow which merely displaces an object, but like the blow which disturbs its molecular equilibrium. The effect, therefore, depends on this molecular condition: the blow which scatters a heap of gunpowder will explode a fulminating salt, and this, in exploding, will excite the gunpowder to explode. The stimulus which is too feeble to excite contraction in a muscle will be powerful enough to excite the neurility of a nerve, and *that* will excite the contractility of the muscle. The nerve-force is simply neural stimulus. It acts upon the other tissues as the nitrogeneous salt upon the gunpowder.

Although it is now common to speak of nerves as transmitting waves of molecular motion, and to regard nerves as the passive medium for the "transference of force," whereby the force is thus made an abstract entity, we must always remember that such phrases are metaphors, and that the truer expression will be not "transference of force," but the "propagation of excitation." I mean that it is not the *force* of the impact nor its *energy* which a nerve transmits, it is the vibratory change produced in the nerve by the impact, which excites another change in the organ to which the nerve goes. We know by accurate measurements that the excitation of a nerve lasts much longer than the *stimulus*, a momentary impact producing an enduring agitation. We know also that the excitation of a centre lasts longer than the muscular contraction it has initiated. We know, moreover, that a nerve may be totally incapable of conducting an external stimulus, yet quite capable of conducting a central stimulus; were it a passive conductor like a wire this would not be so.*

50. The nerve is essentially an exciter of change, and thereby a regulator. A muscle in action does not appreciably determine action in any other (except in the comparatively rare cases of anastomosing muscles); a secreting cell does not propagate its excitation to others. The nerve, on the contrary, not only propagates its excitation, and awakens the activity of the muscle or gland with which it is connected, but through the centre affects the whole organism—

"Ein Schlag tausend Verbindungen schlägt."

Thus it is that stimulation which in the simpler organisms was diffused throughout the protoplasm, has in the complex organisms become the specialised property of a particular tissue.

51. Two general facts of supreme importance must now be stated: One is the law of stimulation—*every excitation*

* "I have raised and stretched the thick orbital nerve of horses on the handle of a scalpel, like a string on the bridge of a violin, without exciting the least sensation; but as soon as mechanical or chemical irritation had given rise to inflammation of the nerve a gentle touch caused violent pain."—ROMBERG: *Nervous Diseases* (translated for the Sydenham Society), i. 10.

pursues the path of least resistance. The second is the condition of stimulation—*unlike mechanical impulsion, it acts only at insensible distances.*

52. This means that although a nerve may be excited by any stimulus external to it which changes its molecular condition, no propagation of that change (*i.e.*, no stimulation through the nerve) is possible except through continuity of substance. Mere physical contact suffices to excite the nerve; but if there be an interruption of continuity in the nerve itself, no stimulus-wave passes across that line. Cut a nerve, and bring the divided surfaces once more into close contact, there will still be such a solution of continuity as to arrest the stimulus-wave, mere physical contact not sufficing for the propagation. Whereas across the cut ends of a divided nerve, even visibly separated, the electric current easily passes. This necessity for the vital continuity of tissue in the propagation of stimulation must always be borne in mind. The presence of a membrane, however delicate; or of any tissue having a different molecular constitution, suffices to arrest or divert the wave. I conceive, therefore, that it is absolutely indispensable that a nerve should terminate in and *blend* with a muscle or a centre, otherwise no stimulation of muscle or centre will take place through the nerve.

53. The difference between excitation from contact and stimulation from continuity may be thus illustrated. In fig. 13 we see the legs of a frog attached to the spine by the lumbar nerves (*l*), and lying on the muscles (*m*) of one leg is the nerve (*c*) of another frog's leg. Applying the electrodes to (*l*), the muscles (*m*) are violently contracted; not only so, but their contraction excites the other nerve (*c*), and the leg attached to this nerve is thereby thrown into contraction. This "secondary contraction," as Dubois Reymond calls it, might be supposed to be due to a diffusion of the electrical current; but that it is due to a change in the muscles (*m*) is proved by delicate experiments showing that the movements in the detached leg are of precisely the same kind as those in the legs directly stimulated. If there is only a muscular shock in the one case, there is only a muscular shock in the other;

if there is tetanus in the one, there is tetanus in the other; if the muscles of the first leg are fatigued and respond slowly and feebly, the response of the second is slow and feeble.

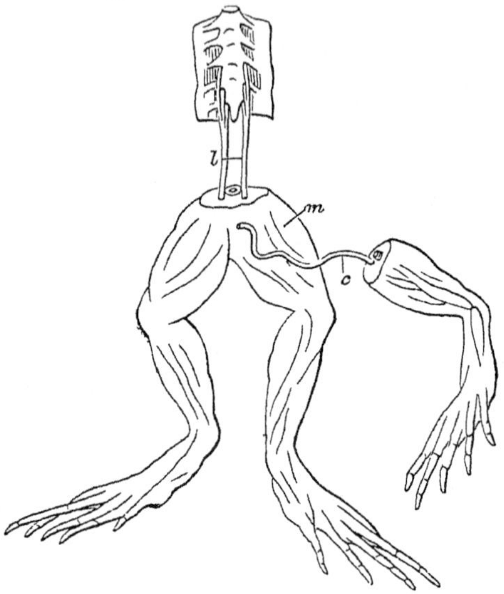

Fig. 13.

Moreover, the secondary contraction may be produced by chemical or mechanical stimulus, as well as by the electrical.

54. Although the contraction of a muscle is thus seen to be capable of exciting a nerve in contact with it, the reverse is not true: we can produce no contraction in a muscle by exciting a nerve simply in contact with the muscle, and not penetrating its tissue and terminating there. Accordingly we always find a nerve when about to enter a muscle or a centre losing its *protecting* envelopes; it gradually becomes identified as a protoplasmic thread with the protoplasm of the muscle or the centre.

55. Neurility, then, is the propagation of molecular change. Two offices are subserved by the nervous system, which may respectively be called Excitation—the disturbance of molecular *tension* in tissues, and consequent liberation of their energies; and Co-ordination—the direction of these several energies into combined actions. Thus, when the muscle is in a given state of molecular tension, the stimulation of its nerve will change that state, causing it to contract if it be in

repose. But this stimulation, which will thus cause a contraction, will be arrested, if at the same time a more powerful stimulation reaches the antagonist muscle, or some distant centre: then the muscle only *tends* to contract.

ORIGIN OF NERVE-FORCE.

56. After this brief account of Neurility we may pass to the consideration of its origin. Are we to understand that this property belongs to the nerves themselves in the sense in which Contractility belongs to the muscles? or are we to accept the teaching which assigns the origin of "nerve-force" to the ganglia, and regards the nerves simply as passive conductors of a force developed in the cells?

57. It is now many years since I ventured to criticise the reigning doctrine, and to urge the necessity of consistently carrying out the distinction between Property and Function. I called attention to the positive evidence which contradicted the idea of passive conduction; and pointed out the illusory nature of the favourite analogy, in which ganglia were likened to batteries, and nerves to the conducting wires. But the old image still exerts its empire; and writers are still found speaking of the brain as a telegraphic bureau, the ganglia as stations, and the nerves as wires. In the cells of the grey substance they place a constantly-renewing reservoir of nerve-force. There the force is elaborated, stored up, and from thence directed along the nerves. The sensory nerve "transmits an impression to the brain"—as the wire transmits a message to the bureau. The motor nerve, in turn, "transmits the mandates of the will"—and all is clear! Clear, until we come to translate metaphors into visible facts, or try to conjure up some mental image of the process. For myself, I can only conceive nerve-force as the activity of the nerve, and not of something *else*. This becomes still more evident when I find that the activity is equally manifest after its imaginary source has been removed. Transmitting impressions, or messages, implies as a preliminary that there should be an impressible agent, or a *message-sender*, at the periphery. No one supposes that simply touching one end of a wire would send an "impression" or a "message" to the battery; or that without the battery this touch would evolve a current. The battery is indispensable; in *it* is evolved the current which the wire transmits. Not so the ganglion, or brain. Remove the wire from its connection with the battery, and it is a bit of wire, nothing more. But remove a nerve from its connection with a ganglion, and it is still active as nerve, still displays its Neurility when excited, still moves the muscle as before. The amputated limb will move when its nerves are stimulated, just as when a reflex from its centre moved it. Every one knew the fact; it was staring them in the face, yet they disregarded it. Even the old anatomist, Willis, had recorded experiments which ought to have opened their eyes. He tied the phrenic nerve, and found that when he irritated it below the ligature, the diaphragm moved; but when he irritated it above the ligature, no movement followed. Since his days, thousands of experiments have shown that the presence of a ganglion is not necessary to the action of a nerve.*

58. Of course an explanation was ready. The nerve was said to have been "endowed with force" from its ganglion during their vital connection; and this force, stored up in the nerve, was disposable for some time after separation from the ganglion. We need not pause to criticise this misty conception of one part "endowing" another with force; the plain facts afford the best answer. There seemed, indeed, a confirmation of the hypothesis in the fact that although the nerve separated from its ganglion was capable of excitation, yet after a few excitations it was exhausted, and ceased to stimulate the muscle. It seemed like the piece of magnetised iron which would act as a temporary magnet, though quickly losing this borrowed power. But the whole fabric

* The experiments of HALLER: *Sur la nature sensible et irritable des parties*, i. 245; and the remarks of PROCHASKA: *De Functionibus Systematis Nervosi* (translated by LAYCOCK in the volume published by the *Sydenham Society*, p. 396), ought to have sufficed. See further on, Chap. V.

fell—or ought to have fallen—when extended observation discovered that this exhausted nerve would, if left in repose, *recover* its lost power. A nerve preserves its excitability as long as it preserves its structural integrity, and recovers its power in recovering that integrity. The length of time varies. Gratiolet found the muscles in the leg of a tortoise, which had been amputated a week before, contract when the nerves were irritated; and Schiff found the divided nerve of a winter frog excitable at the end of three weeks. Even after all excitability has disappeared, it will reappear if arterial blood be injected; just as muscles which have already begun to assume cadaveric rigidity recover their contractility after transfusion. Nor is this all. The separated nerve finally degenerates, and loses all its structural characters and physiological properties; yet under favourable conditions it will regenerate—recover its structures and properties; and this even apart from a centre, as Vulpian showed. Very noticeable is the fact that the force said to be produced in the centre, and only "conveyed" by the nerve, vanishes gradually from the centre to the periphery, and recovers from the periphery to the centre—the part of the nerve which is farthest from the centre being excitable when the part nearest the centre is still inexcitable. Again, when a nerve is pinched, contraction in the muscle follows; but the pinch has for a time so disturbed the structural integrity of the nerve (at that spot) that no irritant applied to the spot, or *between* it and the centre, will be followed by contraction, whereas *below* the spot an irritation takes effect. This is another form of the experiment of Willis. Even in its normal state, the nerve has different degrees of excitability in different parts of its course, a fact discovered by Pflüger which is quite irreconcilable with the hypothesis of passive conduction. Doubts have been thrown on Pflüger's interpretation,† namely, that there is an avalanche-like accumula-

* In mammals about three days, in birds four days, in frogs fourteen to twenty days.

† RUTHERFORD: in *Journal of Anatomy*, 1873, No. viii. p. 331. (FLEISCHL denies that the nerve *in situ* has different degrees of reaction: *Sitzungsberichte der Wiener Akad.*, December 1876.)

tion of energy proportionate to the length of the stimulated portion; but the fact remains, that one and the same irritant applied successively to two different points of a nerve does not irritate the muscle in the same degree. Munk also finds the velocity of transmission in a motor nerve increases as it approaches its termination in the muscle.*

59. Nothing can be more unlike the conduction of an electric current than this excitation of Neurility; nothing more accordant with the idea of it as a vital property of the tissue. The notion of its being derived from a centre is on a par with the notion first successfully combated by Haller,† that the muscle derived its Contractility from the nerves; or the analogous notion that the electric organ in fishes derived its property from the brain. Indeed it was in support of the hypothesis that the brain was a battery, and nerves the conductors, that the phenomena observed in electrical fishes were frequently cited. The electric organ was seen to be connected with the brain; its discharges were under the control of the animal; and were destroyed on one side when the brain on the corresponding side was destroyed. But Charles Robin long ago suggested, what indeed ought never to have been doubted, that the brain was not the source of the electricity; but that the tissue of the electric organ itself had this special property, which the nerve merely called into activity. The suggestion has been experimentally verified by M. Moreau, who divided all the nerves supplying the electric organ on one side, and having thus cut off all communication with the brain, produced electrical discharges by irritating the nerves; precisely as the muscles are made to contract when the divided nerves are irritated. Had the experiment ceased here, it might have been interpreted on the old hypothesis: the electric organ might be supposed to have a certain amount of electric force condensed in it, stored up there; as it is said to be in the nerves; and discharged when the organ is irritated. But experiment has decided this point also. Electric fishes notoriously exhaust their power by a

* MUNK: in the *Archiv für Anat.*, 1860, p. 798.

† HALLER: *Mémoires sur la nature sensible et irritable des parties.*

few discharges, and recover it after repose. When M. Moreau had exhausted his mutilated fishes, he replaced them in the water, and allowed them repose. On again irritating the divided nerves, the discharges were again produced.*

60. On all sides the idea of nerves deriving their power from another source than their own substance is seen to be untenable. *A priori* this might have been concluded. Neurility is the vital property of nerve-tissue. "Nerve-force" is nerve-action — molecular changes in the nerve itself, not in some remote substance. That nerve and centre are vitally connected is true; and what their physiological relations are will hereafter be examined; but we must dismiss the idea of nerves having the relation to centres that electrodes have to batteries.

61. In proposing the term Neurility, I not only wished to get rid of the ambiguities which hovered round "nerve-force" and "nerve-current," but to recall the physiological principle that properties are dependent on structures; and therefore that the special property of nerve-tissue is conditioned by its structure. Neurility is, of course, an abstraction; but so is *the* nerve an abstraction. The concrete manifestations are the several nerve-actions. These we classify and specify. One class we call sensory, another class motor; not because the nerve-action itself is different, but because it is in each class in a different functional relation to other parts. In classing men as governors and governed, employers and employed, we do not suppose anthropological distinctions, but only differences in their social functions.

62. This is the modification of the Law of Bell to which reference was made in § 26. It replaces the idea of two different kinds of nerve, sensory and motor, by that of two different anatomical connections. I need not reproduce here the argument with which I formerly criticised the supposed distinction between sensory and motor nerves; because the old idea is rapidly falling into discredit, and physiologists so eminent as Vulpian and Wundt have explicitly announced

* *Comptes Rendus*, 1862, liv. p. 965.

their adhesion to the principle of identity, a principle which, as Vulpian truly remarks, dominates the whole physiology of the nervous system.*

THE HYPOTHESIS OF SPECIFIC ENERGIES.

63. One development of the theory of Bell, respecting the different kinds of nerve, has been the still accredited hypothesis that each nerve has a "specific energy," or quality, in virtue of which it acts and reacts only in one way. The optic nerve, no matter how stimulated, only responds by a sensation of colour, the auditory nerve only by a sensation of sound; and so on. This hypothesis, which (as I learn from a correspondent †) was originally propounded by Bell himself, was developed and made an European doctrine by Johannes Müller, first in his remarkable treatise, *Über die phantastischen Gesichtserscheinungen* (1826), and afterwards in his *Physiology*. Like all good hypotheses, it has been fruitful; and Helmholtz still holds it to be of extraordinary importance for the theory of perception. Although combated by a few physiologists, it has kept its place firm in the general acceptance; no doubt because it forms a ready explanation of the facts. But, as I often have to remark, *explanation* is not *demonstration*.‡

64. The first criticism to be made on the hypothesis is that it commits the error of confounding function with property, assigning as a specific quality of the nerve the reaction of the organ innervated. Thus Müller speaks of the specific energy as "the essential condition of the nerves in virtue of which they see light and hear

* J'espère vous convaincre que tous les éléments anatomiques des nerfs sensitifs, moteurs, vasomoteurs, et autres, ont les mêmes propriétés, et ne sont distincts que par leurs fonctions. Cette question est de la plus haute importance pour la physiologie générale. C'est celle qui domine toute la physiologie des fibres nerveuses."—VULPIAN: *Leçons sur la Physiologie du Système Nerveux*, p. 11.

† Mr. JAMES ANDREWS.

‡ In the second number of *La Revue Philosophique*, Paris, 1876, I have treated this question of specific energies more at length than I could find space for in the present volume.

sound." But the optic nerve no more *sees*, than the liver-nerve *secretes* bile. That the optic nerve is one element in the mechanism on which vision depends, is all that we can say. Müller declares that it is not sufficient to assume each nerve to be so constituted that it has a susceptibility to certain stimuli rather than to others; but that "with Aristotle we must ascribe to each a peculiar energy as its vital quality. Sensation," he adds, "consists in the sensorium receiving through the medium of the nerves a *knowledge of certain qualities*,—a condition, not of the external bodies, but of the nerves themselves,"—and these qualities are different in different nerves. In other words, he assumes a special substance for each special energy. The sensation of colour depends on the special Visual substance (*Sehsinnsubstanz*); the sensation of sound on the Auditory substance (*Hörsinnsubstanz*); and so on.

65. We have here an hypothesis analogous to that of Innate Ideas, or *a priori* Forms of Thought. It is, in fact, only a reproduction of that conception carried into the sphere of Sense. No one thinks of assigning specific energies to the several muscles, yet a movement of prehension is as different from a movement of extension, a peristaltic movement is as different from a movement of occlusion, as a sensation of sound is from a sensation of colour. If movement is common to both of the one class, feeling is common to both of the other: the forms and mechanism are different and specific. Muscles have the common property of contracting under stimulation; whatever be the nature of the stimulus, each muscle has its own particular response, or mode of reaction: the flexor always bending, never extending the limb; the sphincter always closing, never opening the orifice. The movements of the heart are not the same as those of the eye; both are unlike the movements of the intestine. There are muscles which respond to some stimuli, and not to others. Those of the eye, or of the vocal chords, respond to impulses which would leave the masseter or biceps unstirred. According to Marey, the hyoglossus of a frog will become tetanic under a stimulus of only ten pulses in a second; whereas the gastrocnemius of

that same frog resists a stimulus of less than twenty in a second. We find the retina responding to ethereal pulses which leave the auditorius unaffected; we find the muscles of a gnat's wing so exquisitely susceptible that the wing beats eight thousand times in a second—a delicacy in comparison with which even our muscles of the eye are coarse.

66. The facts which the hypothesis of specific energies is called on to explain are more consistently interpreted on the admission of a common property in nerve-tissue, manifesting different degrees of excitability, and entering into different mechanisms, so that the functional results differ. A nerve which may be stimulated from the skin will not respond at all, or not in the same way, if the stimulus be applied under the skin. Are we to suppose that the specific energy resides in one part of the nerve, and not in another? * That the optic nerve responds to stimuli which will not sensibly excite a motor nerve, depends on the terminal structures through which the stimulation is excited; for the optic nerve itself, apart from the retinal expansion, is as insensible to light as the motor nerve is. And the specific sensation, or movement, which *results* from stimulation of a nerve depends not on the nerve, but on the mechanism of which the nerve is one element. Sensations of touch, temperature, and pain

* In 1859 I mentioned that if the nerves of a frog's back be exposed by raising the skin, they may be pricked or even cut without sensible effect, although a slight prick on the skin will excite the nerves, and cause a reflex action. In 1870 Prof. FICK expressed his astonishment at finding that after he had cut out a piece of the skin, leaving it attached to the body by a single nerve, electrical stimulation of this excised skin caused the frog to make the reflex movement of rubbing the irritated surface; whereas electrical stimulation of the nerve-trunk itself produced no reflex effect, only a twitching of a muscle. *Pflüger's Archiv*, 1870, p. 327. BROWN SÉQUARD tries to establish a distinct species of nerves as *conductors* of sensitive impressions, from those which are *impressionable*. The facts on which he founds these two properties simply show that nerves are so disposed that the stimulus which excites them in one place fails in another. He could hardly maintain that a skin nerve contained impressionable fibres at its periphery, and only conducting fibres in its trunk? See his communication to the Royal Society: *Proceedings*, 1856; and *Lectures* in the *Lancet*, 10th July 1858.

are assuredly specific; they are as unlike each other as a sensation of taste is unlike a sensation of smell. Yet the same nerves, variously stimulated, produce all three sensations.

67. We conclude, therefore, that the phrase specific energy is an elliptical expression for the particular office of a nerve. In this meaning there is no obscurity. The optic nerve is not a vasomotor nerve, the skin nerve is not a muscle nerve; the auditory nerve is a nerve of special sensation, the vagus is a nerve of systemic sensation; and so on. Neither movement nor sensation belongs to the nerves themselves.

CHAPTER IV.

SENSIBILITY.

68. THE principles laid down in the preceding chapter are equally applicable to the central system. But here greater difficulties await us. We cannot expect traditional views to be easily displaced, when they have taken such hold on the mind, as is the case with regard to Sensibility. To admit that all nerves have a common property, and that their functional relations depend on the organs which they innervate, demands small relinquishment of cherished opinions. But to admit that all nerve-centres have a common property, and that their functional relations depend on their anatomical connections, is to sweep away at once a mass of theoretic interpretations which from long familiarity have acquired an almost axiomatic force. That the brain, and the brain only, is the source and seat of Sensibility is the postulate of modern Physiology.

69. The question is one of extreme complexity, but may be greatly simplified, if we can manage to reduce it to purely physiological terms, and consider the phenomena in their objective aspect. In dealing with nerves and their actions this was comparatively easy; we had for the most part only physiological processes to unravel. It is otherwise in dealing with nerve-centres—the subjective or psychological aspect of the phenomena inevitably thrusts itself on our attention; and all the mysteries of Feeling and Thought cloud our vision of the neural process. Do what we will, we cannot altogether divest Sensibility of its psychological connotations, cannot help interpreting it in terms of Consciousness; so that even when treating of sensitive phenomena observed in molluscs and insects, we always imagine these more or less suffused with Feeling, as this is known in our own conscious states.

70. Feeling is recognised as in some way or other bound up with neural processes; but Physiology proper has only to concern itself with the processes; and the question whether these can, and do, go on unaccompanied by Feeling, is strictly speaking one which belongs to Psychology. It demands as a preliminary that the term Feeling be defined; and the answer will depend upon that definition, namely, whether Feeling be interpreted as synonymous with Consciousness in the restricted sense, or synonymous with the more general term Sentience. If the former, then since there are unquestionably neural processes of which we are not conscious, we must specify the particular groups which subserve Feeling; as we specify the particular groups which subserve the sensations of Sight, Hearing, Taste, &c.; and localise the separate functions in separate organs. If the latter, then, since all neural processes have a common character, we have only to localise the particular variations of its manifestation, and distinguish sensitive phenomena as we distinguish motor phenomena.

71. It is absolutely certain that the Feeling we attribute to a mollusc is different from that which we attribute to a man; if only because the organisms of the two are so widely different, and have been under such different conditions of excitation. If every feeling is the functional result of special organic activities, varying with the co-operant elements, we can have no more warrant for assuming the existence of the same *particular* forms of Feeling in organisms that are unlike, than for assuming the 47th proposition of Euclid to be presented by any three straight lines. The lines are the necessary basis for the construction, but they are not the triangle, except when in a special configuration. This is not denying that animals *feel* (in the general sense of that term), it is only asserting that their feelings must be very *unlike* our own. Even in our own race we see marked differences—some modes of feeling being absolutely denied to individuals only slightly differing from their fellows. If, however, we admit that different animals must have different modes of Feeling, we must also admit that the neuro-muscular activities are generically alike in all, because of the fundamental similarity in the structures. Whether we shall assign Feeling to the mollusc or not will depend on the meaning of the term; but, at all events, we require some term general enough to include the phenomena manifested by the mollusc, and those manifested by all other animals. Sensibility is the least objectionable term. Unless we adopt some such general designation, physiological and psychological interpretations become contradictory and obscure. The current doctrine which assigns Sensibility to the brain, denying it to all other centres, is seriously defective, inasmuch as it implies that tissues similar in kind have utterly diverse properties; in other words, that the same nerve-tissue which manifests Sensibility in the brain has no such property in the spinal cord.

72. How is this tenable? No one acquainted at first hand with the facts denies that the objective phenomena exhibited by the brainless animal have the same general character as those of the animal possessing a brain: the actions of the two are identical in all cases which admit of comparison. That is to say, the objective appearances are the same; differing only in so far as the mechanisms are made different by the presence or absence of certain parts. The brain not being a necessary part of the mechanical adjustments in swimming, or pushing aside an irritating object, the brainless frog swims and defends itself in the same way as the normal frog. But no sooner do we pass from the objective interpretation, and introduce the subjective element of Feeling among the series of factors necessary to the product—no sooner do we ask whether the brainless frog *feels* the irritation against which it struggles, or *wills* the movements by which it swims—than the question has shifted its ground, and has passed from Physiology to Psychology. The appeal is no longer made to Observation, but to Interpretation. Observation tells us here nothing directly of Feeling. What it does tell us, however, is the identity of the objective phenomena; and Physiology demands that a common term be employed to designate the character common to the varied phenomena. Sensibility is such a term. But most modern physiologists, under the bias of tradition, refuse to extend Sensibility to the spinal cord, in spite of the evidences of the spinal cord possessing that property in common with the brain. They prefer to invoke a new property; they assign spinal action to a Reflex Mechanism which has nothing of the character of Sensibility, because they have identified Sensibility with Consciousness, and have restricted Consciousness to a special group of sensitive phenomena.

73. Nor is it to be denied that on this ground they have a firm basis. Every one could testify to the fact that many processes normally go on without being accompanied by consciousness, in the special meaning of the term. Reflex actions,—such as winking, breathing, swallowing,—notoriously produced by stimulation of sensitive surfaces, take place without our "feeling" them, or being "conscious" of them. Hence it is concluded that the Reflex mechanism suffices without the intervention of Sensibility. I altogether dispute the conclusion; and in a future Problem will endeavour to show that Sensibility is necessary to Reflex Action. But without awaiting that exposition we may at once confront the evidence, by adducing the familiar fact that "unconscious" processes go on in the brain as well as in the spinal cord; and this not simply in the sphere of Volition, but also in the sphere of Thought.* We act and think "automatically" at times, and are quite "unconscious" of what we are doing, or of the data we are logically grouping. We often think as unconsciously as we breathe; although from time to time we become conscious of both processes.

* In consequence of this observation some physiologists have maintained that Feeling or Consciousness never arises in cerebral activity, unless the thalami and the connected tracts are at the same time in action. I go further, and maintain that there is no Consciousness (in the restricted meaning of the term) *unless the whole organism is involved.* Cerebral or spinal activity will be activity of Sensibility; but this is only the basis of Consciousness.

Yet who will assert that these unconscious processes were independent of Sensibility? Who will maintain that because cerebral processes are sometimes unaccompanied by that peculiar state named Consciousness, therefore all its processes are unaccompanied by Feeling? And if here we admit that the Reflex mechanism in the brain is a *sensitive* mechanism, surely we must equally admit that the similar Reflex mechanism in the spinal cord is sensitive?

74. Let it be understood that Sensibility is the common property of nerve-centres, and physiological interpretations will become clear and consistent. Consciousness, as understood by psychologists, is not a property of tissue, it is a function of the organism, dependent indeed on Sensibility, but not convertible with it. There is a greater distinction between the two than between Sensation, the reaction of a sensory organ, and Perception, the combined result of sensory and cerebral reactions; or than that between Contractility, the property of the muscles, and Flying, the function of a particular group of muscles. It is not possible to have Consciousness without Sensibility; but perfectly possible to have Sensations without Consciousness. This will perhaps seem as inconceivable to the reader as it seemed to Schröder van der Kolk.*

75. Let us illustrate it by the analogy of Pain. There is a vast amount of sensation normally excited which is totally unaccompanied by the feelings classed as painful. The action of the special senses may be exaggerated to an intolerable degree, but the exaggeration never passes into pain: the retina may be blinded with excess of light, and the ear stunned with sound—the optic nerve may be pricked or cut—but no pain results. The systemic sensations also are habitually painless, though they pass into pain in abnormal states. Clearly, then, Pain is not the necessary consequence of Sensibility; and this is true not only of certain sensitive parts, but

* "An unconscious sensation, which Lewes distinguishes from perception, is to me an inconceivable (ist für mich ein Unding)." —SCHRÖDER VAN DER KOLK: *Die Pathologie des Geistes-Krankheiten*, p. 22.

of all; as is proved in the well-known facts of Analgesia, in which complete insensibility of the skin as regards Pain co-exists with vivid sensibility as regards Touch and Temperature. Hence the majority of physiologists refuse to acknowledge that the struggles and cries of an animal, after removal of the brain, are evidences of pain; maintaining that they are "simply reflex actions." This is probable; the more so as we know the struggles and cries which tickling will produce, yet no pain accompanies tickling. But if the struggles and cries are not evidence of pain, they are surely evidence of Sensibility.

76. Now for the term Pain in the foregoing paragraph substitute the term Consciousness, and you will perhaps allow that while it may be justifiable to interpret the actions of a brainless animal as due to a mechanism which is unaccompanied by the *specially conditioned forms* of Sensibility classed under Consciousness — just as it is unaccompanied by the specially conditioned forms of Perception and Emotion—there is no justification for assuming the mechanism not to have been a *sensitive* mechanism. The wingless bird cannot manifest any of the phenomena of flight; but we do not therefore deny that its *other* movements depend on Contractility.

77. Difficult as it must be to keep the physiological question apart from the psychological when treating of Sensibility, we shall never succeed in our analysis unless the two questions are separately treated. The physiologist considers organisms and their actions from their objective side, and tries to detect the mechanism of the observed phenomena. These he has to interpret in terms of Matter and Motion. The psychologist interprets them in terms of Feeling. The actions which we *see* in others we cannot *feel*, except as visual sensations; the changes which we feel in ourselves we cannot see in others, except as bodily movements. The reaction of a sensory organ is by the physiologist called a sensation,—borrowing the term from the psychologist; he explains it as due to the stimulus which changes the molecular condition of the organ; and this changed condition, besides being seen to be followed by a muscular movement, is *inferred* to be accompanied by a change of Feeling. The psychologist has direct knowledge only of the change of Feeling which follows on some other change; he infers that it is originated by the action of some external cause, and infers that a neural process precedes, or accompanies, the feeling. Obviously there are two distinct questions here, involving distinct methods. The physiologist is compelled to complete his objective observations by subjective suggestions; compelled to add Feeling to the terms of Matter and Motion, in spite of the radical diversity of their aspects. The psychologist also is compelled to complete his subjective observations by objective interpretations, linking the internal changes to the external changes. A complete theory must harmonise the two procedures.

78. In a subsequent Problem we shall have to examine the nature of Sensation in its psychological aspect; here we have first to describe its physiological aspect. To the psychologist, a sensation is simply a fact of Consciousness; he has nothing whatever to do with the neural process, which the physiologist considers to be the physical basis of this fact; and he therefore regards the physiologists as talking nonsense when they talk of "unconscious sensations," the phrase being to him equivalent to "unfelt feelings," or "invisible light." It is quite otherwise with the physiologist, who viewing a sensation solely as a neural process, the reaction of a sensory organ, can lawfully speak of unconscious sensations, as the physicist can speak of invisible rays of light,—meaning those rays which are of a different order of undulation from the visible rays, and which may become visible when the susceptibility of the retina is exalted. He knows that there are different modes, and different complexities of neural process; to one class he assigns consciousness, to the other unconsciousness. If he would be severely precise, he would never speak of sensation at all, but only of sensory re-action. But such precision would be pedantic and idle. He wants the conotatians of the term sensation, and therefore uses it.

79. The functional activity of a gland is stimulated by a

neural process reflected from a centre; by a similar process a muscle is called into action. No one supposes that the neural process is in the one case secretory, in the other motory: in both it is the same process in the nerve; and our investigation of it would be greatly hampered if we did not disengage it from all the suggestions hovering around the ideas of secretion and muscular action. In like manner we must disengage the neural process of a sensory reaction from all the suggestions hovering around the idea of Consciousness, when that term designates a complex of many reactions. In Problem III. we shall enter more particularly into the distinction between Sensibility and Consciousness; for the present it must suffice to say that great ambiguity exists in the current usage of these terms. Sometimes Consciousness stands as the equivalent of Sensibility; sometimes as a particular *mode* of Sensibility known as Reflection, Attention, and Thought. The former meaning is an extension of the term similar to that given to the word Rose, which originally meaning Red came to be restricted to a particular red flower; and after other flowers of the same kind were discovered which had yellow and white petals, instead of red, the term rose still adhered even to these. "Yellow Rose" is therefore as great a verbal solecism as unconscious sensation. We have separated the redness from the rose, and can then say that the colour is one thing, the flower another. By a similar process of abstraction we separate Consciousness from Sensation, and we can then say that there are sensations without consciousness. In consequence of this, psychologists often maintain that to have a sensation and be conscious of it are two different states. We are said to hear a sound, and yet not to be conscious of hearing it. The sound excites a movement, but it does not excite our consciousness. Now although it is true that there are roses which are not red, it is not true that there are roses which have no colour at all. Although it is true that there are sensations which are not of the particular mode of Sensibility which psychologists specially designate as Consciousness, it is not true that there are sensations which are not modes of Sensibility.

80. And what is Sensibility which, on its subjective side, is Sentience? In one sense it may be answered that we do not know. In another sense it is that which we know most clearly and positively: Sentience forms the substance of all knowledge. Being the ultimate of knowledge, every effort must be vain which attempts to explain it by reduction to simpler elements. The human mind, impatient of ultimates, is always striving to pierce beyond the fundamental mysteries; and this impatience leads to the attempts so often made to explain Sensibility by reducing it to terms of Matter and Motion. But inasmuch as a clear analysis of Matter and Motion displays that our knowledge of these is simply a knowledge of modes of Feeling, the reduction of Sentience or Sensibility to Matter and Motion is simply the reduction of Sensibility to some of its modes. This point gained, a clear conception of the advantages of introducing the ideas of Matter and Motion will result. It will then be the familiar and indispensable method of explaining the little known by the better known. The objective aspect of things is commonly represented in the visible and palpable; because what we can see we can also generally touch, and what we can touch we can taste and smell; but we cannot touch an odour nor a sound; we cannot see them; we can only connect the odorous and sonorous objects with visible or palpable conditions. Everywhere we find sensations referred to visible or palpable causes; and hence the desire to find this objective basis for every change in Sensibility. The sensation, or state of consciousness, is the ultimate fact; we can only *explain* it by describing its objective conditions.

81. Thus much on the philosophical side. Returning to our physiological point, we must say that a sensation is, objectively, the reaction of a sensory organ, or organism; subjectively, a change of feeling. Objectively it is a phenomenon of movement, but distinguishable from other phenomena by the speciality of its conditions. It is a vital phenomenon, not a purely mechanical phenomenon. Although the molecular movement conforms, of course, to mechanical principles, and may be viewed abstractly as a purely mechan-

ical result, yet, because it takes place under conditions never found in machines, it has characters which markedly separate it from the movements of machines. Among these differential characters may be cited that of *selective adaptation*,* which is most conspicuous in volition.

82. In the early stages of animal evolution there is no differentiation into muscle and nerve. The whole organism is equally sensitive (or irritable) in every part. Muscles appear, and then they are the most sensitive parts. Nerves appear, and the seat of Sensibility has been transferred to them; not that the muscles have lost theirs, but their irritability is now represented by their dominant character of Contractility, and the nerves have taken on the special office of Sensibility. That is to say, while both muscle and nerve form integral elements of the sensitive reaction, the process itself is analytically conceived as a combination of two distinct properties, resident in two distinct tissues.

83. Carrying further this analytical artifice, I propose to distinguish the central organs as the seat of Sensibility, con-

* By selective adaptation is meant the varying combination of motor impulses to suit the varying requirements of the effect to be produced. Physical mechanisms are limited to the performance of definite actions; sensitive mechanisms employ fluctuating combinations of elements in response to fluctuations of stimuli. The wheels, levers, springs, and valves of a machine cannot be differently combined according to varying degrees of the motor-force, as the nerves and muscles of an organism are differently combined by varying sensations. An automaton may be constructed to play on the violin; but it will only play the air to which it is *set*, it cannot vary the performance: cannot play a false note, or throw in a *crescendo* here, a *largo* there, according to a caprice of feeling. We must admit that a violinist has his delicate and changing movements guided by sensations, auditory and muscular; any interruption in the sensations would arrest the movements, which in truth *incorporate* them. And yet it is well known that the violinist may perform while completely "unconscious." I do not simply refer to the fact that his thoughts and attention may be elsewhere; I refer to such facts as are recorded in Pathology. TROUSSEAU, for example, had an epileptic patient who was occasionally seized with attacks of complete unconsciousness while he was performing in the orchestra; yet on re-awakening to consciousness, he found that he had continued to play, had kept proper time, and played the proper notes.

fining Neurility to the peripheral nerves. In physiological reality both systems, central and peripheral, are one; the separation is artificial. Strictly speaking, therefore, Neurility—or nerve-action—is the general property of nerve tissue, central and peripheral. But since Neurility may be manifested by nerves apart from centres, whereas Sensibility demands the co-operation of both, and since we have often to consider the central process in itself, without attending to the process in the nerves, it is well to have two characteristic terms. I shall therefore always use the term Sensibility for the reactions of the nervous centres—Sentience being its psychological equivalent; although the reader will understand that in point of fact there is no break, nor transformation, as the wave of change passes from sensory nerve to centre, and from centre to motor nerve: there is one continuous process of change. But just as we analytically distinguish the sensory from the motor element of this indissoluble process, so we may distinguish the ingoing and outgoing stages from the *combining* stage. Sensibility, then, represents the property of combining and grouping stimulations.

84. Fully aware of the misleading conotations of the term, and of the difficulty which will l e felt in disengaging it from these, especially in reference to Consciousness, I have long hesitated before adopting it. But the advantages greatly outweigh the disadvantages. Sensibility has long been admitted to express the peculiar modes of reaction in plants and animals low down in the scale. No one hesitates to speak of a sensitive plant, or a sensitive surface. The tentacles of a polype are said to be sensitive; though probably no one thereby means that the polype has what psychologists mean by Consciousness. By employing the general term Sensibility to designate the whole range of reactions peculiar to the nerve-centres, when these special organs exist, it will be possible to interpret all the physiological and psychological phenomena observed in animals and men on one uniform method. The observed variations will then be referable to varieties in organisms.

85. Suppose, for illustration, an organism like the human

except that it is wholly deficient in Sight, Hearing, Taste, and Smell. It has no sense but Touch—or the general reaction under contact with external objects. It will move on being stimulated, and will combine its movements differently under different stimulations. It will feel, and logically combine its feelings. But its mass of feeling will be made of far simpler elements than ours; its combinations fewer; and the contents of its Consciousness so very different from ours that we are unable to conceive what it will be like; we can only be sure that it will *not* be very like our own. This truncated organism will have its Sensibility; and we must assign this property to its central nerve-tissue, as we assign our own. If now we descend lower, and suppose an organism with no centres whatever, but which nevertheless displays evidence of Sensibility—feelings and combinations of movements—we must then conclude that the property specialised in a particular tissue of the highly differentiated organism, is here diffused throughout.

It is obvious that the sensations or feelings of these supposed organisms will have a common character with the feelings of more highly differentiated organisms, although the modes of manifestation are so various. If we recognise a common character in muscular movements so various as the rhythmic pulsation of the heart, the larger rhythm of inspiration and expiration, the restless movements of the eye and tongue, the complexities of manipulation, the consensus of movements in flying, swimming, walking, speaking, singing, &c., so may we recognise a common character in all the varieties of sensation. The special character of a movement depends on the moving organ. The special character of a sensation depends on the sensory organ. Contractility is the abstract term which expresses all possible varieties of contraction. Sensibility—or Sentience—is the abstract term which expresses all possible varieties of sensation.

86. The view here propounded may find a more ready acceptance when its application to all physiological questions has been tested, and it is seen to give coherence to many scattered and hitherto irreconcilable facts. Meanwhile let a glance be taken at the inconsistencies of the current doctrine. That doctrine declares one-half of the grey substance of the spinal cord to be capable only of *receiving* a sensitive stimulation, the other half capable only of *originating* a motor stimulation. We might with equal propriety declare that one-half of a muscle is capable only of receiving a contractile stimulation, and the other half of contracting. The ingoing nerve, passing from the surface to the posterior part of the spinal cord, excites the activity of the grey substance into which it penetrates; with the anterior part of this grey substance an outgoing nerve is connected, and through it the excitation is propagated to a muscle: contraction results. Such are the facts. In our analysis we separate the sensory from the motor aspect, and we then imagine that this ideal distinction represents a real separation. We suppose a phenomenon of Sensibility independent of a phenomenon of Contractility—suppose the one to be "transformed" into the other—and we then marvel "how during this passage the excitation changes its nature." *

87. Before exerting ingenuity in explaining a fact, it is always well to make sure that the fact itself is correctly stated. *Does* the neural excitation change its nature in passing from the posterior to the anterior grey substance? I can see no evidence of it. Indeed the statement seems to confound a neural process with a muscular process. The neural process is one continuous excitation along the whole line of ingoing nerve, centre, and outgoing nerve, which nowhere ceases or changes into another process, until the excitation of the muscle introduces a new factor. So long as the excitation keeps within the nerve-tissue, it is one and the same process of change; its issue in a contraction, a secretion, or a change in the conditions of consciousness, depends on the organs it stimulates.

88. I have already called attention to the artificial nature

* CLAUDE BERNARD: *Système Nerveux*, 1858, i. 349.

of all our distinctions, and the necessity of such artifices. They are products of that

> "Secondary power
> By which we multiply distinctions, then
> Deem that our puny boundaries are things
> That we perceive, and not that we have made." *

The distinction of Central and Peripheral systems is not simply anatomical, it has a physiological justification in this, that the Central System is the organ of connexion. Any one part of it directly excited by an ingoing nerve propagates that excitation throughout the whole central mass, and thus affects every part of the organism. Therefore we place Sensibility in it.

But this general Property subserves various Functions, according as the Central System is variously related to different organs. This fact has given rise to the idea that different portions of the cerebro-spinal axis have different properties—which is a serious error. What is certain is that the Cerebrum must have a different function from that of the Thalami, and the Cerebellum one different from the Medulla Oblongata; while that of the Medulla Spinalis is different from all. Precisely on the same grounds that a muscle-nerve has a different office from a skin-nerve, or the pneumogastric from the acoustic. But all nerves have one Neurility in common; all centres have one Sensibility in common.

* WORDSWORTH: *The Prelude.*

CHAPTER V.

ACTION WITHOUT NERVE-CENTRES.

89. It has long been one of the unquestioned postulates of Physiology that no nerve-action can take place without the intervention of a centre; and as a corollary, that all movement has its impulse—reflex or volitional—from a centre.* The postulate rests on the assumption that nerves derive their "force" from their centre. This assumption we have seen to be erroneous. Yet, in consequence of its acceptance, experimenters have failed to notice the many examples of nerve-action independent of centres. Indeed, except Schiff, Goltz, and Engelmann, I can name no one who has ventured to suggest that movements may be excited through nerves without the co-operation of centres; † nor have even they explicitly formulated the conclusion to which their observations point.

It is true that the majority of muscular movements are determined by a reflex from centres; and that any break in the triple process of the in-going nerve, centre, and out-going nerve, prevents such movements. It is true that the more conspicuous and harmoniously co-ordinated phenomena

* "On peut dire que toujours un phénomène de mouvement reconnait pour point de départ une impression sensitive."—Claude Bernard: i. 267.

† Since this was written Prof. Michael Foster and Mr. Dew Smith have published their very important researches on the motions of the heart, which establish beyond a doubt that, in the molluscs at least, there is no co-operation of either centre or nerve.—*Proceedings of the Royal Society*, 18th March 1875. (See also *Studies from the Physiological Laboratory of Cambridge*, Part II., 1876.) Mr. Foster knows that I had independently, and from a totally different line of research, arrived at the same conclusion respecting the heart's movement.

belong to this class. But it is also demonstrable that many nerve-actions *may*, and some *do*, take place by direct stimulation of the nerve, or direct stimulation of the muscle, without the intervention of a centre, without even the intervention of a ganglion. This must obviously be the case in animals which have no centres; and even in some which have well-developed nervous centres, there is every reason to believe that these centres often act rather in the way of co-ordinating than of directly stimulating actions.

90. I was first led to doubt the reigning doctrine by a surprising observation (frequently repeated) after I had removed the whole nervous centres from a garden snail (*Helix pomatia*). The muscular mass called "the foot" was thrown into slow but energetic contraction whenever the skin was pricked with the point of a scalpel, or touched with acid; nay, even when a glass rod dipped in the acid was brought close to, without absolutely touching, the skin, the foot curled up, and then slowly relaxed. The same effect was produced on the "mantle"—where there was of course no centre. But direct irritation of the muscles under the skin produced no such contraction; only through the skin could the stimulation take effect. In one case I observed this strange phenomenon five hours after removal of the centres. It was a great puzzle. At first I concluded that there must be minute ganglia in the skin, serving as reflex-centres. I searched for them in vain; and although a longer search on better methods might *possibly* have detected ganglionic cells, I soon relinquished the search, because I had other grounds for believing that even the presence of abundant ganglia would not suffice, until some better proof were afforded that such ganglia were reflex-centres.

91. That direct stimulation of the nerve suffices to move the muscles, is familiar to all experimenters. There is no centre, or ganglion, in the amputated leg of the frog, which nevertheless contracts whenever the sciatic nerve is stimulated. And after the nerve has been exhausted, and refuses to respond to any stimulus, the muscle itself may be directly stimulated. Inasmuch as the movement depends on the contractility of the muscles, a stimulation through centre, through motor-nerve, or through muscle, will be followed by contraction. Let us take a clear case of reflex action. The pupil of the eye contracts when a beam of light falls on it, and dilates when the beam is shut off. The path of the neural process is normally this: the light stimulates the optic nerve, which in turn stimulates the corpora quadrigemina; (here the nerves which move the eye are experimentally proved to be stimulated;) and it is through these that the pupil is caused to contract. If the optic nerve be divided, no such reflex takes place—proving that the contraction does not, at least normally, come from the ciliary ganglion.

But now it is matter of observation that the pupil will contract and dilate under the stimuli of light and darkness, when there is no such reflex pathway open. Removal of the eye from the body obliterates this path, cuts the eye off from all connection with the centre. Brown Séquard removed both eyes from a frog, placed one in a dark box, and left the other exposed to the light: the pupil of the former was found dilated, that of the latter contracted. On reversing the experiment, and placing the eye with contracted pupil in the dark box, he found it there dilate, while the dilated pupil exposed to the light contracted.* In frogs with very irritable tissues,

* *Comptes Rendus de la Société de Biologie*, 1847, i. 40. In 1856 he showed that not only were the muscles of the iris directly stimulated by light (and this not by its calorific or chemical rays), but that sixteen days after removal of the eye from the orbit, this effect was observable in the eel. Yet a very few days after extirpation of the eye the nerves are disintegrated.—*Proceedings of the Royal Society*, 1856, p. 234.

Donders has the following observations :—"The movements of the iris are of two kinds—reflex and voluntary. Reflex action is exhibited as constriction of the pupil in consequence of the stimulus of incident light upon the retina. Fontana has shown that the light falling upon the iris produces no remarkable contraction. We have confirmed this result by causing the image of a small distant light to fall, by means of a convex lens, upon the iris, whereby, during slight perception of light, a doubtful contraction occurred, which gave way to a strong contraction so soon as the light entering the pupil excited a vivid perception. Nevertheless, the experiments of Harless and Budge have shown that even after death, so long as irritability remains, the pupil still contracts upon the continued action of light. Of the correctness of this we have satisfied our-

I have found not only the pupil contracting, after the whole cranial cavity has been emptied, but even the eyelid close, on irritating the conjunctiva *—yet this is one of the typical reflex actions! I am disposed to think that even the action of swallowing may be faintly excited by stimulation of the pharynx of a brainless frog; but I have not observations sufficiently precise to enable me to speak confidently. Goltz has, however, shown that after removal of brain and spinal cord and heart, there is spontaneous and active movement in œsophagus and stomach.† This will no doubt be referred to the agency of the ganglionic plexus; but similar movements have been observed by Engelmann in the ureter, and in isolated fragments of the ureter in which not a ganglionic cell was present.‡

92. That nerves are stimulated by internal changes has long been recognised with reference to "subjective sensations." The divided nerve, in that portion which remains connected with the centre, will at times cause great pain. Obscure organic conditions, changes of temperature, states of the blood, excite the nerves, and the patient feels as if the surface of the amputated limb were irritated. It is all very well to call these "subjective sensations;" that does not alter the fact of the nerve being called into activity by other than the normal stimuli from the surface; in like manner muscular movements (which are not to be explained as "subjective movements") will be excited by organic stimuli

selves. In a dog killed by loss of blood the one eye was closed, the other opened and turned to the light: after the lapse of an hour, the pupil of the opened eye was perceptibly smaller than that of the closed eye. The latter now remained also exposed to the light, and on the following day the diameter of both eyes was equal. The upper jaw, along with the eyes, was taken out of some frogs; one eye was exposed to the light, while the other was covered with a closely-folded piece of black paper: after the lapse of half an hour the pupil turned to the light was narrow, the other wide. But the latter also contracted almost immediately after the removal of the paper."—DONDERS: *On the Anomalies of Accommodation and Refraction of the Eye.* Trans. of the New Sydenham Society, p. 572.

* The experiment often fails, but I have seen it several times succeed.

† *Pflüger's Archiv.*, 1872, p. 618.

‡ See his Researches in *Pflüger's Archiv. Bde.* ii. and iv.

when motor nerves are separated from their centres. In each case it has sufficed that the nerve should be excited; and when excited, no matter by what means, the effect is always similar.

93. Here are a few facts. Stimulation of the nerves which send filaments to the chromatophores of the skin in reptiles causes the skin to become paler, and even colourless: the colour-specks disappear under this contractile stimulus. This being known, Goltz deprived a frog of brain, spinal cord, and heart, thus eliminating all possible influence from them, slit up the skin of the back, and displayed the nerves which pass from each side of the spine to the skin; these nerves he then divided on the right side, and observed the skin on this side slowly become paler and paler, till finally it was as yellow as wax; the left side, having its nerves intact, retained its colour. Two conclusions seemed to him warranted by this experiment: First, that even in the dead frog the nerves separated from their centre were still active; secondly, that the irritation of the nerves resulting from their section was the cause of the colour-specks disappearing. This second conclusion was strengthened when he found that the irritation was increased when he cut the nerves bit by bit.

It is not at present, I believe, clearly made out that the colour-specks of the Cephalopoda are in direct connection with nerves; but it is tolerably certain that they are in some way under the influence of nervous stimulation, directly or indirectly. D'Orbigny, indeed, goes so far as to say they are dependent on the will of the animal.* This seems very lax language; but restricting ourselves to the fact of nervous influence, the experiments of Goltz receive further illustration in an observation I have elsewhere recorded.† I found that a strip of skin taken from the dead body of a calamary (*Loligo*) showed the colour-specks expanding and contracting with vigour.

94. The heart is well known to beat after death, if death be not the result of a gradual decay. Sometimes, indeed, its

* D'ORBIGNY: *Des Mollusques Vivants et fossils*, p. 113.
† *Seaside Studies*: 2d ed., p. 101.

muscular irritability is so active that the heart will beat for hours. E. Rousseau observed it beating in a woman twenty-seven hours after she had been guillotined.* Not only will it beat after death, but in many animals even after removal from the body: the heart of a young puppy, or kitten, will beat for three or four hours after its removal; that of a full-grown dog, or cat, not one hour; whereas the beating of that of a tortoise, or a frog, will, under proper precautions, be preserved for days—and even after it has stopped, it may be stimulated to fresh pulsations.

Physiologists explain this spontaneous movement of the heart as due to the ganglia in its substance. This explanation, which is founded on what I cannot but regard as a purely imaginary view of the functions of ganglionic cells, must stand or fall with that hypothesis. A long and arduous investigation has led me to doubt whether in *any* case the heart's movements are primarily due to its ganglia; at all events, the same spontaneous movements are observed in the hearts of molluscs and crustaceans, which are without even a trace of ganglia; and in the hearts of mammalian embryos long before ganglia or nerve fibres make their appearance. Not less certain is it that movements of contraction and dilatation are produced in the blood-vessels independently of all central influence. This has been decisively proved by the Italian physiologist, Mosso, when experimenting on an organ isolated from the organism; and although the vessels have their nerve cells and fibres, he justly doubts whether it is to these that the stimulation is due, because the phenomena are observed after the nervous vitality has disappeared. Goltz severed all the tissues in the leg of a rabbit, so that the only connection of the leg with the rest of the body was through the crural vein and artery, which kept up the circulation; yet although the nerves of the skin were thus separated from their centre, so that no sensation could be produced by stimulating the skin of the leg, consequently no reflex from the centre on the vessels, Goltz found that a marked reddening of the skin from congestion of the capillaries followed the

*Cited by BROWN SÉQUARD: *Journal de la Physiologie*, 1858, p. 359.

application of mustard to the skin. Physiologists who believe that the constriction and dilatation of blood-vessels are due to the action of the ganglionic cells distributed over the walls of the vessels will explain Goltz's observation as a case of reflex action; but those who agree with me that such an hypothesis respecting the part played by the cells is untenable, will class the observation among other cases of direct stimulation.

95. But passing from these perhaps questionable cases, let us glance at other cases. The mobile iris of the bird displays movements after the nerves have been divided. Even the voluntary striped muscles are not altogether motionless. Schiff divided the hypoglossus on one side, and found, of course, the tongue paralysed on that side; but he also found that on the third day after the operation some of the muscles of that side were quivering: the agitation spread to others, till by the end of the fourth day all the fibres were *rhythmically* contracting. From this time onwards, the contractions were incessant; though they were never able to move the tongue, because the fibres did not contract simultaneously.

Schiff also observed that the hairs over the eyes and the "whiskers" of cats, rabbits, and guinea pigs were for months after section of their nerves in incessant rhythmical vibration. This was observed when the animals were asleep as when awake. Valentin records the spontaneous movements in the diaphragm of animals just killed; and this even after section of the phrenic nerve. The same movements may be seen in the operculum of fishes. Henle observed the spontaneous contractions of the intercostal muscles; which Schiff confirms, adding that the movements observed by him in cats and birds were not simply contractions of some fibres, but of all the muscles, so that three or four excised ribs rhythmically contracted and expanded.

I have performed a great many experiments with a view of determining this question, but the phenomena were so variable that I refrain from adducing any,* and merely state

* Dr. NORRIS has recorded some striking observations in his paper on "Muscular Irritability" in the *Journal of Anatomy*, 1867, No. II.

the general result as one in harmony with the foregoing examples. The great variability of the phenomena depends upon the variable conditions of muscular irritability and anatomical relations. When the heart of one woman is found beating twenty-seven hours after death, while in most men and women it ceases after a few minutes, we must be prepared to find different, and even contradictory phenomena under varying unknown conditions. There is, however, a general agreement among experimenters that muscular irritability increases after separation from nerve-centres, and then quickly decreases again.

96. Although the stimulation of muscles usually comes *through* a nerve-centre, yet since the muscles do not derive their Contractility from nerve-centres any stimulation will suffice. Now since we have abundant proof that sensory nerves are stimulated by certain organic changes, by poisons in the blood, excess of carbonic acid, &c., we are justified in concluding that motor nerves will be stimulated in like manner, and thus muscular movement be produced occasionally without the intervention of a centre. Pressure on a motor nerve, or the irritation which results from inflammation, will determine contraction, or secretion directly. Recently, Erb and Westphal have disclosed the fact that the leg will be suddenly jerked out if the patella be gently tapped; and they prove this not to be a reflex action, because it follows with the same certainty after the skin has been made insensible.*

There are doubtless many other phenomena which, though commonly assigned to reflex stimulation, are really due to direct stimulation. Research might profitably be turned to-

p. 217. Here is the only one I can find room for: "On taking up the *dead* frog and touching the limb (which during life had been paralysed by section of its nerve) with my finger, *it was suddenly shot out as if alive.* I placed the body down, and one or two *apparently spontaneous movements* of small extent afterwards occurred. On touching the skin gently with the point of a needle, by the slight pressure upon the muscle beneath, movements of the limb were also induced, but this high degree of exaltation very rapidly disappeared."

* See their papers in the *Archiv für Psychiatrie*, 1875, Bd. v. Heft 3.

wards the elucidation of this point. Since there is demonstrable evidence that a nerve when no longer in connection with its centre, or with ganglionic cells, may be excited by electricity, pressure, thermal and chemical stimuli, we must conclude that even when it is in connection with its centre, any local irritation from pressure, changes in the circulation, &c., will also excite it. But as such local excitations will have only local and isolated effects, they will rarely be conspicuous.

CHAPTER VI.

WHAT IS TAUGHT BY EMBRYOLOGY?

97. SUBJECT to the qualification expressed in the last chapter, stimulation of muscles and glands involves a neural process in ingoing nerve, centre, and outgoing nerve. These are the triple elements of the "nervous arc." If muscles were directly exposed to external influences, they would be stimulated without the intervention of a centre; but as a matter of fact they never are thus exposed, being always protected by the skin. Did the skin-nerves pass directly to the muscles underneath, they would move those muscles, without the intervention of a centre; but as a matter of fact the skin-nerves pass directly to a centre, so that it is only *through* a centre that they can act upon the muscles. Were muscles and glands directly connected with sensitive surfaces, their activity would indeed be awakened by direct stimulation; but unless the muscles were so connected the one with the other, by anastomosis of fibres or continuity of tissue, that the movement of one was the movement of all, there would need to be some other channel by which their separate energies should be combined and co-ordinated. In the higher organisms anastomosis of muscles is rare, and the combination is effected by means of the nerves.

98. Although analysis distinguishes the two elements of the neuro-muscular system, assigning separate properties to the separate tissues, an interpretation of the phenomena demands a synthesis, so that a movement is to be conceived as always involving Sensibility, and a sensation as always involving Motility.* In like manner, although analysis dis-

* This latter statement will be justified when I come to expound the Triple Process, which I have named the *Psychological Spectrum.*

tinguishes the various organs of the body, assigning separate functions to each, our interpretation demands their synthesis into an organism; and we have thus to explain how the *whole* has different *parts,* and how these different parts are brought into unity. Embryology helps us to complete the fragmentary indications of Anatomy and Physiology.

99. Take a newly-laid egg, weigh it carefully, then hatch it, and when the chick emerges, weigh both chick and shell: you will find that there has been no increase of weight. The semifluid contents have become transformed into bones, muscles, nerves, tendons, feathers, beak, and claws, all without increase of substance. There has been *differentiation* of structure, nothing else. Oxygen has passed into it from without; carbonic acid has passed out of it. The molecular agitation of heat has been required for the rearrangements of the substance. Without oxygen there would have been no development. Without heat there would have been none. Had the shell been varnished, so as to prevent the due exchange of oxygen and carbonic acid, no chick would have been evolved. Had only one part of the shell been varnished, the embryo would have been deformed.

99*a*. The patient labours of many observers (how patient only those can conceive who have made such observations !) have detected something of this wondrous history, and enabled the mind to picture some of the incessant separations and reunions, chemical and morphological. Each stage of evolution presents itself as the consequence of a preceding stage, at once an emergence and a continuance; so that no transposition of stages is possible; each has its appointed place in the series (PROBLEM I. § 107). For in truth each stage is a *process*—the sum of a variety of co-operant conditions. We, looking forward, can foresee in each what it will become, as we foresee the man in the lineaments of the infant; but in this prevision we always presuppose that the regular course of development will proceed unchecked through the regular succession of special conditions: the infant becomes a man only when this succession is uninterrupted. Obvious as this seems, it is often disregarded; and the old metaphysical conception of *potential* powers obscures the real significance of Epigenesis. The potentiality of the cells of the germinal membrane is simply their capability of reaching successive stages of development under a definite series of co-operant conditions. We foresee the result, and personify our prevision. But that result will not take place unless all the precise changes that are needful serially precede it. A slight pressure in one direction, insufficient to alter the chemical composition of the tissue, may so alter its structure as to disturb the regular succession of forms necessary to the perfect evolution.

100. The egg is at first a microscopic cell, the nucleus of which divides and subdivides as it grows. The egg becomes a hollow sphere, the boundary wall of which is a single layer of cells, all so similar that to any means of appreciation we now possess they are indistinguishable. They are all the progeny of the original nucleus and yolk, or cell contents. Very soon, however, they begin to show distinguishable differences, not perhaps in *kind*, but in *degree*. The wall of this hollow sphere is rapidly converted into the *germinal membrane*, out of which the embryo is formed. Kowalewsky (confirmed by Balfour) has pointed out how in the Amphioxus the hollow sphere first assumes an oval shape, and then, by an indentation of the under side, with corresponding curvature of the upper side, presents somewhat the shape of a bowl. The curvature increases, and the curved ends approaching each other, the original cavity is reduced to a thin line separating the upper from the under surface. The cavity of the body is formed by the curving downwards of this double layer of the germinal membrane.

101. This is not precisely the course observable in other vertebrates; but in all, the germinal membrane, which lies like a watch-glass on the surface of the yolk, is recognisable as two distinct layers of very similar cells. What do these represent? They are the starting-points of the two great systems: Instrumental and Alimental. The one yields the dermal surface; the other the mucous membrane. Each follows an independent though analogous career. The yolk fur-

nishes nutrient material to the germinal membrane, and so passes more or less directly into the tissues; but unlike the germinal membrane, it is not itself to any great extent the seat of generation by segmentation. There are two yolks: the yellow and the white (which must not be confounded with what is called the *white of egg*); and their disposition may be seen in this diagram copied from Foster and Balfour's work:

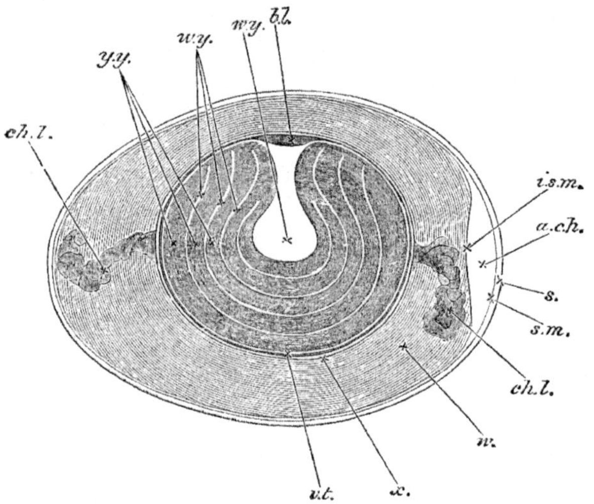

Fig. 14.—*Diagrammatic section of an unincubated hen's egg.* *bl*, blastoderm; *w y*, white yolk; *y y*, yellow yolk; *v t*, vitelline membrane; *x* and *w*, layers of albumen; *ch l*, chalaza; *a ch*, air-chamber; *i s m*, internal layer of shell membrane; *s m*, external layer; shell.

The importance of the white yolk is that it passes insensibly into a distinct layer of the germinal membrane, between the two primary layers.* Each of the three layers of the germinal membrane has its specific character assigned to it by embryologists, who, however, are not all in agreement. Some authorities regard the topmost layer as the origin of the nervous system, the epidermis, with hair, feathers, nails, horns, the cornea and lens of the eye, &c. To the middle layer are assigned the muscular and osseous systems, the sexual organs,

* FOSTER and BALFOUR: *Elements of Embryology*, 1874, part i. p. 52. HIS: *Untersuchungen über die erste Anlage des Wirbelthierleibes*, 1868, p. 197.

&c. To the innermost layer, the alimentary canal, with liver, pancreas, gastric and enteric glands. Other authorities are in favour of two primary layers: one for the nervous, muscular, osseous, and dermal systems; the other for the viscera and unstriped muscles. Between these two layers, a third gradually forms, which is specially characterised as the vascular.

102. Messrs. Foster and Balfour, avoiding the controverted designations of serous, vascular, and mucous layers, or of sensorial, motor germinative, and glandular layers, employ designations which are independent of theoretic interpretation, and simply describe the position of the layers, namely, *epiblast* for the upper, *mesoblast* for the middle, and *hypoblast* for the under layer. From the epiblast they derive the epidermis and central nervous system (or would even limit the latter to the central grey matter), together with some parts of the sense-organs. From the mesoblast, the muscles, nerves (and probably white matter of the centres), bones, connective tissue, and blood-vessels. From the hypoblast, the epithelial lining of the alimentary canal, trachea, bronchial tubes, as well as the liver, pancreas, &c.* Kölliker's suggestion is much to the same effect, namely, that the three layers may be viewed as two epithelial layers, between which subsequently arises a third, the origin of nerves, muscles, bones, connective tissue, and vessels.†

103. The way in which the history may be epitomised is briefly this: There are two germinal membranes, respectively representing the Instrumental and Alimental Systems. Each membrane differentiates, by different appropriations of the yolk substance, into three primary layers, *epithelial*, *neural*, and *muscular*. In the epiblast, or upper membrane,

* They state that the cells of the epiblast are the results of direct segmentation, whereas the cells of the other layers are formed at a subsequent period, and are only indirectly results of segmentation. But if the observations of KOWALEWSKY are exact, this is not the case with the hypoblast of the Amphioxus, which is from the first identical with the epiblast.

† KÖLLIKER: *Entwicklungsgeschichte des Menschen und der höheren Thiere*, 1861, p. 71.

these layers represent: 1°, the future epidermis with its derivatives—hair, feathers, nails, skin glands, and chromatophores; 2°, the future nervous tissue; 3°, the future muscular tissue.* (Bone, dermis, connective tissue, and blood-corpuscles are subsequent formations.)

The hypoblast, or under membrane, in an inverted order presents a similar arrangement: 1°, the unstriped muscular tissue of viscera and vessels; 2°, the nervous tissue of the sympathetic system; 3°, the epithelial lining of the alimentary canal with its glands.

Fundamentally alike as these two membranes are, they have specific differences; but in both we may represent to ourselves the *embryological unit* constituted by an epithelial cell, a nerve-cell, and a muscle-cell. All the other cells and tissues are adjuncts, necessary, indeed, to the working of the vital mechanism, but subordinated to the higher organites.

104. This conception may be compared with that of His in the division of Archiblast and Parablast assigned by him to the germ and accessory germ.† We can imagine, he says, the whole of the connective substances removed from the organism, and thus leave behind a scaffolding in which brain and spinal cord would be the axis, surrounded by muscles, glands, and epithelium, and nerves as connecting threads. All these parts stand in more or less direct relation to the nervous system. All are continuous. By a similar abstraction we can imagine this organic system removed, and leave behind the connected scaffolding which is formed from the accessory germ; but this latter has only *mechanical* significance; the truly vital functions belong to the other system.

105. The researches of modern histologists have all converged towards the conclusion that the organs of Sense are modifications of the surface, with epithelial cells which on the one side are connected with terminal hairs, or other elements adapted to the reception of stimuli, and are connected

* [According to BALFOUR's recent observations, a large part of the muscular tissue is derived from the layer of the mesoblast belonging to the hypoblast.]

† HIS: *Untersuchungen*, pp. 39, 40.

on the other side through nerve-fibres with the perceptive centres. It has been shown that nerve-fibres often terminate in (or among) epithelial cells—sensory fibres at the surface, and motor-fibres in the glands.* Whether the fibres actually penetrate the substance of the cell, or not, is still disputed. Enough for our present purpose to understand that there is a *physiological* connection between the two, and above all that sensory nerves are normally stimulated through some epithelial structure or other.

106. And this becomes clear when we go back to the earliest indications of development. Look at Fig. 15, representing a transverse section of the germinal membranes in a chick after eighteen hours' incubation. Here the three

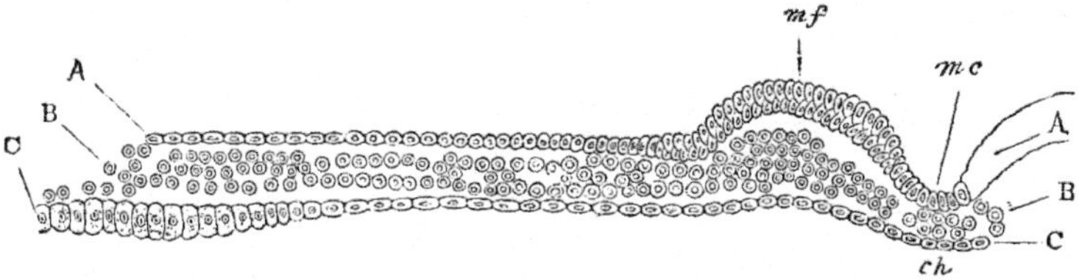

Fig. 15.—*Transverse section of a Blastoderm incubated for eighteen hours.* The section passes through the medullary groove, *m c.* A, epiblast. B, mesoblast. C, hypoblast. *m f*, medullary fold; *c h*, notochord.

layers, A, B, and C, have the aspect of simple cells very slightly differing among each other. Yet since each layer has ultimately a progeny which is characteristically distinguishable, we may speak of each not as what it now is, but what it will become. Although the most expert embryologist is often unable to distinguish the embryo of a reptile from that of a bird or of a mammal, at certain stages of evolution, so closely does the one resemble the other, yet inasmuch as the

* Quite recently OWSJANNIKOW has pointed out the termination of fibres in the phosphorescent cells of the *Lampyris Noctiluca.* See his paper in the *Mémoires de l'Acad. de St. Petersbourg*, 1868, xi. 17. These phosphorescent cells are said to be ganglion-cells by PANCERI: *Intorno della luce che emana dalle celleule nervose* (Rendiconto della Accad. delle Scienze, April 1872); and by EIMER: *Archiv für mikros. Anatomie*, 1872, p. 653. KÖLLIKER also calls the phosphorescent organ a nervous organ. This is not to be interpreted as meaning that neurility is phosphorescence, but simply that in some nerve cells there is phosphorescent matter, which is called into activity by stimulus of the nerves.

embryo of a reptile does not, cannot become a bird, nor that of a bird a mammal, he is justified in looking forward to what each will become, and in calling each embryo by its future name. On the same ground, although we cannot point to any such distinction between the layers of the blastoderm as I have indicated in the separation of Instrumental and Alimental Systems, nor specify any characters by which the cells can be recognised as epithelial, neural, and muscular, yet a forward glance prefigures these divisions. We know that the first result of the segmentation of the yolk is the formation of cells all alike, which in turn grow and subdivide into other cells. We know that these cells become variously modified both in composition and structure, and that by such differentiations the simple organism becomes a complex of organs.

107. But here it is needful to recall a consideration sometimes disregarded, especially by those who speak of Differentiation as if it were some magical Formative Principle, quite independent of the state of the organised substance which is formed. There is a luminous conception—first announced by Goethe, and subsequently developed by Milne Edwards—which regards the organism as increasing in power and complexity by a physiological "division of labour," very similar to that division of employments which characterises the developed social organism. But the metaphor has sometimes been misleading; it has been interpreted as indicating that Function creates Organ (see PROBLEM I. § 88), and as if Differentiation itself were something more than the expression of the changes resulting from the introduction of different elements. In the Social Organism a "division of labour" presupposes that labourers with their labour-materials are already existing; the change is one of re-arrangement: instead of each labourer employing his skill in doing many kinds of work, he restricts it to one kind, which he is then able to do with less loss of time and power. Thus is social power multiplied without increase of population; and the social organism becomes more complex by the differentiation of its organs. It is not precisely thus with the

Animal Organism during its evolution. Indeed to suppose that the differentiation of the germinal membrane into special tissues and organs takes place by any such division of employments, is to fall into the ancient error of assuming the organism to exist *preformed* in the ovum. The unequivocal teaching of Epigenesis is that each part is produced out of the elements furnished by previous parts; and for every differentiation there must be a difference in composition, structure, or texture—the first condition being more important than the second, the second more important than the third. The word protoplasm has almost as wide a generality as the word animal, and is often used in forgetfulness of its specific values: the protoplasm of a nerve-cell is not the *same* as that of a blood-cell, a muscle-cell, or a connective-tissue cell, any more than a bee is a butterfly, or a prawn a lobster. No sooner has the specific character been acquired, no sooner is one organite formed by differentiation, than there is an absolute barrier against any transformation of it into any other kind of organite. The nerve-cell, muscle-cell, and epithelial cell have a common starting-point, and a community of substance; but the one can no more be transformed into the other, than a mollusc can be transformed into a crustacean. In the homogeneous cellular mass which subsequently becomes the "vertebral plates," a group of cells is very early differentiated: this is the rudimentary spinal ganglion, which becomes enveloped in a membrane, and then pursues a widely different course from that of the other cells surrounding it, so that "the same cell which was formerly an element of the vertebral plate now becomes a nerve-cell, while its neighbours become cartilage-cells." * Indeed all the hypotheses of transformation of tissues by means of Differentiation are as unscientific as the hypotheses of the transformation of animals. In the organism, as in the Cosmos,

* BIDDER und KUPFFER: *Textur des Rückenmarks*, 1857, p. 108. [What is said in the text has been rendered doubtful by the recent researches of Mr. F. BALFOUR, *On the Development of the Spinal Nerves in Elasmobranch Fishes* (*Philos. Trans.*, vol. clxvi., part i.), which show that in these fishes the ganglion has its origin in the spinal cord.]

typical forms once attained are retained. There probably was a time in the history of the animal series when masses of protoplasm by appropriating different materials from the surrounding medium were differentiated into organisms more complex and more powerful than any which existed before. But it is obvious that from a common starting-point there could have been no variations in development without the introduction of new elements of composition: there might have been many modifications of structure, but unless these facilitated modifications of composition, there could never have resulted the striking differences observed in animal organisms.*

108. To return from this digression, we may liken the three primary layers of the germinal membranes to the scattered and slightly different masses of protoplasm out of which the animal kingdom was developed. In this early stage there are no individualised organites—no nerve-cells or muscle-cells. They are cells ready to receive modifications both of composition and structure, appropriating slightly different elements from the yolk, and according to such appropriation acquiring different properties. And this is necessarily so, since the different cells have not exactly the same relation to the yolk, nor are they in exactly the same relation to the incident forces which determine the molecular changes. The uppermost layer (epiblast) under such variations develops into epithelium and central nerve-tissue; the epithelial cell cannot develop into a nerve-cell, the two organites are markedly unlike, yet both spring from a common root. Another modification results in the development of muscle-cells from the inner layer.

109. Hence we can understand how the surface is sensitive even in organisms that are without nerve-tissue; and also how even in the highest organisms there is an intimate blending of epithelial with neural tissues. The same indication explains the existence of neuro-muscular cells in the *Hydra*, recorded by Kleinenberg, and of neuro-

* Comp. PROBLEM I. § 130, with the remarks of CHARLES ROBIN: *Anatomie et Physiologie Cellulaires*, 1873, p. 20.

muscular fibres in the *Beroë*, by Eimer.* In the simpler organisms the surface is at once protective, sensitive, and absorbent. It shuts off the animal from the external medium, and thus individualises it; at the same time it connects this individual with the medium; for it is the channel through which the medium acts, both as food and stimulus. The first morphological change is one whereby a part of the surface is bent inwards, and forms the lining of the body's cavity. Soon there follows such a modification of structure between the outer and inner surfaces (*ectoderm* and *endoderm*) that the one is mainly sensitive and protective, the other mainly protective and absorbent. The outer surface continues indeed to absorb, but its part in this function is insignificant compared with that of the inner surface, which not only absorbs but secretes fluids essential to assimilation. The inner surface although sensitive is subjected to less various stimulation, and its sensibility is more uniform.

110. The uppermost of the primary layers we have seen to be epithelial; and we know that the first lines of the central nervous system are laid there. A depression called the medullary groove is the first indication of the future cerebro-spinal axis. Some writers—Kölliker, for instance—regard this medullary groove as continuous with but different from the epithelial layer; others maintain that it lies underneath the epithelium, just as we see it in later stages, when the differentiation between epithelial and nerve-cell has taken place. Since no one disputes the fact that when the groove

* KLEINENBERG: *Hydra; Eine Anatomisch-Entwickelungs-Untersuchung*, 1872, p. 11. EIMER: *Zoologische Studien auf Capri*, 1873, p. 66.

A similar formation is described by Dr. ALLMAN in the *Myriothela;* he says, however, that he has never been able to trace a direct continuity of the caudal processes of the cells with muscular fibrils. He believes that the processes make their way to the muscular layer through undifferentiated protoplasm.—*Philos. Transactions*, vol. clxv. pt. ii. p. 554.

An intermediate stage between this neuro-muscular tissue and the two differentiated tissues seems presented in the Nematoid worms which have muscles that send off processes into which the nerves pass. GEGENBAUR declares his inability to decide whether these processes are muscles or nerves. BÜTSCHLI thinks the nerve process blends with the muscle process.—*Archiv für mikros. Anatomie*, 1873, p. 89.

becomes a closed canal its lining is epithelial, one of two conclusions is inevitable: either the cells of the primary layer develop in the two diverse directions, epithelial and neural; or else epithelial cells can be developed on the surface of neural cells and out of them. The latter conclusion is one which, involving the conception of transformation, would seem to be put out of court. I think, then, we must admit that the under side of the primary layer of cells becomes differentiated into nerve-cells; and this is in accordance with the observations of Messrs. Foster and Balfour.*

111. While there is this intimate morphological and physiological blending of epithelial and neural organites, there is an analogous relation between neural and muscular organites. As the neural layer lies under the epithelial, the muscular lies under the neural. The surface stimulation passes to the centre, and is reflected on the muscles. Embryology thus teaches why a stimulus from the external medium must be propagated to a nerve-centre before it reaches the muscles; and why a stimulus on one part of the surface may set all the organism in movement, by passing through a centre which co-ordinates all movements. This, of course, only applies to the higher organisms. In the simpler structures the sensitive surface is directly continuous with the motor organs.

It is unnecessary here to pursue this interesting branch of our subject; nor need we follow the analogous evolution of the second germinal membrane representing the Alimental System. Our attention must be given to what is known and inferred respecting the elementary structure of the nerves and centres, on which mainly the interest of the psychologist settles, since to him the whole of Physiology is merged in nerve actions.

* "The grey matter of the cord seems undoubtedly to be formed by a metamorphosis of the external cells of the epiblast of the neural tube, and is directly continuous with the epithelium; there being no strong line of demarcation between them."—*Op. cit.*, p. 185.

CHAPTER VII.

THE ELEMENTARY STRUCTURE OF THE NERVOUS SYSTEM.

112. THE progress of science involves an ever-increasing Analysis. Investigation is more and more directed towards the separated details of the phenomena previously studied as events: the observed facts are resolved into their component factors, complex wholes into their simpler elements, the organism into organs and tissues. But while the analytical process is thus indispensable, it is, as I have often to insist, beset with an attendant danger, namely, that in drawing the attention away from one group of factors to fix it exclusively on another, there is a tendency to forget this artifice, and instead of restoring the factors provisionally left out of account, we attempt a reconstruction in oblivion of these omitted factors. Hence, instead of studying the properties of a tissue in all the elements of that tissue, and the functions of an organ in the anatomical connections of that organ, a single element of the tissue is made to replace the whole, and very soon the function of the organ is assigned to this particular element. The "superstition of the nerve-cell" is a striking illustration. The cell has usurped the place of the tissue, and has come to be credited with central functions; so that wherever anatomists have detected ganglionic cells, physiologists have not hesitated to place central functions. By such interpretations the heart and intestines, the glands and blood-vessels, have, erroneously I think, their actions assigned to ganglionic cells.

It is unnecessary to point out the radical misconception which thus vitiates a great mass of anatomical exposition and physiological speculation. I only call the reader's attention to the point at the outset of the brief survey we have now to make of what is known respecting the elementary structure of the nervous system.

DIFFICULTIES OF THE INVESTIGATION.

113. So great and manifold are the difficulties of the search, that although hundreds of patient observers have during the last forty years been incessantly occupied with the elementary structure of the nervous system, very little has been finally established. Indeed we may still repeat Lotze's sarcasm, that "microscopic theories have an average of five years' duration." This need not damp our ardour, though it ought to check a too precipitate confidence. Nothing at the present moment needs more recognition by the student than that the statements confidently repeated in text-books and monographs are very often for the most part only ingenious guesses, in which Observation is to Imagination what the bread was to the sack in Falstaff's tavern bill. Medical men and psychologists ought to be warned against founding theories of disease, or of mental processes, on such very insecure bases; and physiological students will do well to remember the large admixture of Hypothesis which every description of the nervous system now contains. Not that the potent aid of Hypothesis is to be undervalued; but its limits must be defined. It may be used as a finger-post, not as a foundation. It may suggest a direction in which truth may be sought; it cannot take the place of Observation. It may link together scattered facts, it must not take the place of a fact. We are glad of corks until we have learned to swim. We are glad of a suggestion which will for the nonce fill up the gaps left by observation, and hold the facts intelligibly together. And both as suggestion and colligation, Hypothesis is indispensable. Indeed every *discovery* is a verified hypothesis; and there is no discovery until verification has been gained: up to this point it was a guess, which might have been erroneous—a torchbearer sent out to look for a missing child in one direction, while the child was wandering in another; only when he finds the child can we acknowledge that the torchbearer pursued the right path. Hypothesis satisfies the intellectual need of an explanation, but we must be wary lest we accept this fulfilment of a need as equivalent to an enlargement of knowledge; we must not accept explanation as demonstration, and suppose that because we can form a mental picture of the possible stages of an event, therefore this picture represents the actual stages. Let us be alert, forewarned against the tendency to seek evidence in support of a conclusion, instead of seeking to unfold the conclusion step by step from the evidence. To seek for evidence in support of a *guess* is very different from seeking it in support of a *conclusion;* which latter practice is like that of people asking advice, and only following it when it chimes in with their desires.

114. Is not the warning needed, when we find anatomists guided by certain "physiological postulates," and consequently *seeing* only what these postulates demand? For example, there is the postulate of "isolated conduction," which is said to require that every nerve-fibre should pursue its course singly from centre to periphery. Accordingly the fibres are described as unbranched. Whatever may be the demand of the postulate, or the felt necessity of the deduction, the fact is that nerve-fibres do branch off during their course at various points; nay, it is doubtful whether any lengthy fibre is unbranched. Other postulates demand what fact plainly denies. It is said to be "necessary" that every cell should have at least two fibres, and that sensory and motor nerves should be directly connected through their respective cells. These things cannot be seen, but they are described with unhesitating precision. Diagrams are published in which the sensory fibres pass into the cells of the posterior horn of the spinal cord, and these cells send off prolongations to the cells of the anterior horn, and thence the motor fibres pass out to the muscles: an absolutely impossible arrangement, according to our present data! Again, the postulate that nerve-force originates in the cells, and that nerve-functions depend on cells, required that the cells should be most abundant where the function was most energetic. Of course they were found most abundant in the required places —no notice whatever being taken of the facts which directly contradicted the deduction.

115. Among the serious obstacles to research we must reckon this tendency to substitute Imaginary Anatomy for Objective Anatomy. I am conscious of the tendency in myself, as I note it in others; and have constantly to struggle against it, though not perhaps always aware of it. Many a time have I had to relinquish plausible explanations, which would have supported my speculations could I but have believed that they represented the facts; but being unable to believe this, I had to remember that hypotheses and explanations appear and disappear—only the solid fact lives. If there is one lesson emphatically taught by Philosophy, it is the unwisdom of founding our conclusions on our desires rather than on the objective facts.

116. In the following pages a constantly critical attitude is preserved: this is simply to keep active the sense of how much is still needed to be done before a satisfactory theory of the nervous system can be worked out. The objective difficulties are greater than in any other department of Anatomy. The problem is to form a precise picture of what the organites are, and of how they are arranged in the living tissue; yet our present means of investigation involve as a preliminary that we should *alter* that arrangement, *removing* some elements of the tissue, and *changing* the state of others, without knowing what were their precise state and arrangement before the change. Place a piece of nerve-tissue under the microscope, without having subjected it to various mechanical and chemical operations, and you can see next to nothing of its structure. You must tear the parts asunder, and remove the fat and nerve-sap (plasmode) before you can see anything; you must coagulate the albumen, and otherwise chemically alter the substances before a thin section can be made; you must get rid of the tissues in which it is embedded, without knowing what are the connections thus destroyed. Living neurine has no greater consistence than cream, often no greater than oil. How, then, can thin sections be made until this viscid substance has been hardened by alcohol or acids? But substances thus acted on lose their constituent water, which can no more be removed without alteration of their structure, than it can be removed from certain salts without destruction of their special properties. Losing their water alone, they become deformed. They lose much more. Sometimes the loss can be estimated, as in the case of the hyaline substance investing the nucleus during the process of segmentation in embryonic cells, which may be seen to disappear when a weak solution of acid is applied.* At other times we are unable to say what has disappeared. Under different modes of preparation very different appearances are observed, and anatomists are accordingly at variance. Yet unless some hardening method be adopted little can be seen! Stilling, who has given his life to the study, declares that no results are reliable which are obtained from the unprepared tissue, because the mechanical isolation of the elements destroys the textural arrangement.† There is one method of hardening, and only one, which we can be certain does not chemically alter the structure, and that is the freezing method. The experiments of Dr. Weir Mitchell and Dr. Richardson prove this, because they prove that the brain of the living animal may be frozen and frozen again and again, yet recover its vital activity when thawed. Professor Rutherford has invented an admirable instrument for making sections of the frozen tissue, of any delicacy that may be required; but with the thinnest section there will still be certain difficulties of observation, unless the tissue has undergone a staining process. Whatever is seen, however, in the frozen tissue is to be accepted as normal.

117. Two points must be determined before reliance can be placed on observations of tissues chemically acted on:

* Robin: *Anat. et Physiol. Cellulaires*, p. 332.

† Stilling: *Bau der Nervenprimitiv-Fasern*, 1856, p. 16.

First, we must prove that the forms now visible existed before the preparation—the chemical action merely unveiling them; secondly, we must estimate the part played by the elements which have been removed in order to make the rest visible. We know, for example, that the nucleus often exists in the cell, though an acid may be needed to make it visible. We also know that cells which during life are quite free from visible granules are distinctly granulated after death, even without external chemical action. Imagine the explanation of a steam-engine to be attempted by first taking it to pieces, and examining these pieces, with no account of the coals and steam which had previously been *removed* in order to facilitate the examination. When we know the part played by coals and steam, we may disregard these items of the active machine. So when we know the part played by water, fat, amorphous substance, and plasmode, we may describe nerve-tissue without taking these into account.

118. "You have convinced me," said Rasselas to Imlac, "that it is impossible to be a poet." My readers may, perhaps, infer from this enumeration of the difficulties that a knowledge of the minute anatomy of the nervous system is impossible. Not so; but a knowledge of these difficulties should impress us with the necessity for a vigilant scepticism, and the search after new methods. If the difficulties are fairly faced, they may be finally overcome. What we must resign ourselves to at present is the conviction that our knowledge is not sufficiently accurate to be employed as a basis of deduction in the explanation of physiological and psychological processes.*

119. Having said so much, let me add that there are some positive materials, and these yearly receive additions. The

* "There was a time," says KÖLLIKER, "when I confidently believed that an hypothetical explanation of the arrangement of elements in the spinal cord could be grounded on a basis of fact; but the deeper my insight into the minute anatomy, the less my confidence became; and now I am persuaded that the time is not yet come to frame such an hypothesis."—*Gewebelehre*, 5te Auf. 1867.

organites are described with a general agreement as to their composition and structure—although there is much that is hypothetical even here. Neurine is known under two aspects: the amorphous and the figured. The figured, which is the better known, comprises cells of different kinds, fibres and fibrils. The amorphous, more generally called *Neuroglia*, or nerve-cement, is less understood, and is indeed by many authorities excluded altogether from the nerve-tissue proper, and relegated to the class of connective tissues.

THE NERVE-CELL.

120. It is unfortunate that the term nerve-cell is applied to organites of very variable structure. Nerve-cell is a generic term of which the species are many; under it are designated organites in different stages—as infancy, childhood, and manhood are all included under Man. Most commonly by nerve-cell is understood the ganglionic corpuscle, conspicuous in its size and its prolongations, such as it appears in the great centres, and in ganglia. It also designates smaller different organites, sometimes called "nuclei" (*Kerne*), sometimes grains (*Körner*). There would be advantage in designating the earlier stages as *neuroblasts*, reserving the word *cells* for the more developed forms. Such a distinction would facilitate the discussion of whether nerve-fibres had or had not their origin in cells; because while I, for one, see very coercive evidence against the accepted notion that all the fibres have their origin in the processes of ganglionic corpuscles, I see no reason to doubt that both fibres and corpuscles have their origin in neuroblasts. Of this anon.

The cell is a composite organite, the primary element being a microscopic mass of protoplasm, or what may more conveniently be termed *neuroplasm*. It appears as finely granulated and striated or fibrillated substance on a hyaline ground, with water, fat, and diffused pigment in varying quantities. The cell contains a nucleus, and nucleolus—

sometimes two. Like other animal cells, it sometimes has a distinct cell-wall, sometimes not. Its size and shape are variable: sometimes distinctly visible to the naked eye, generally visible only under the microscope.* It is round,

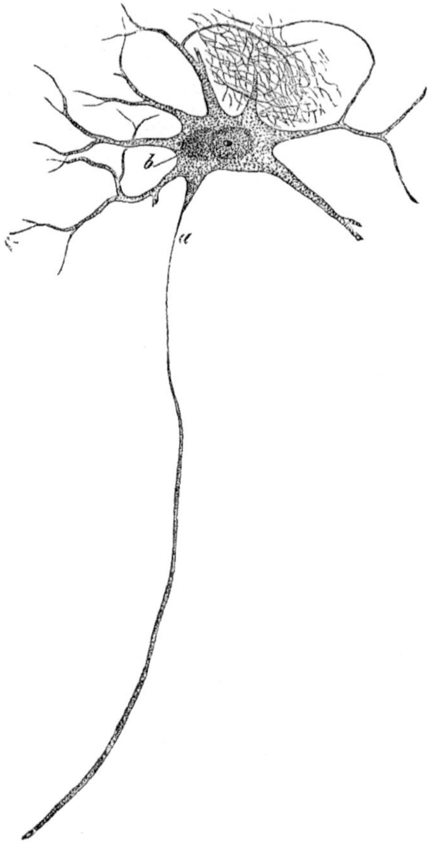

Fig. 16.—*Nerve-cell from anterior horn of spinal cord (man), magnified* 150 *diameters.* *a*, cell process unbranched passing into or joining an axis cylinder, the other processes are branched; *b*, pigment. The nucleus and nucleolus are visible.

oval, pyramidal, club-shaped, pear-shaped, or many-cornered. It has one, two, three, or many outgrowths called "processes,"

* In the Gasteropoda the cells range from 220 μ to 3 μ (μ=0,001 millimètre).

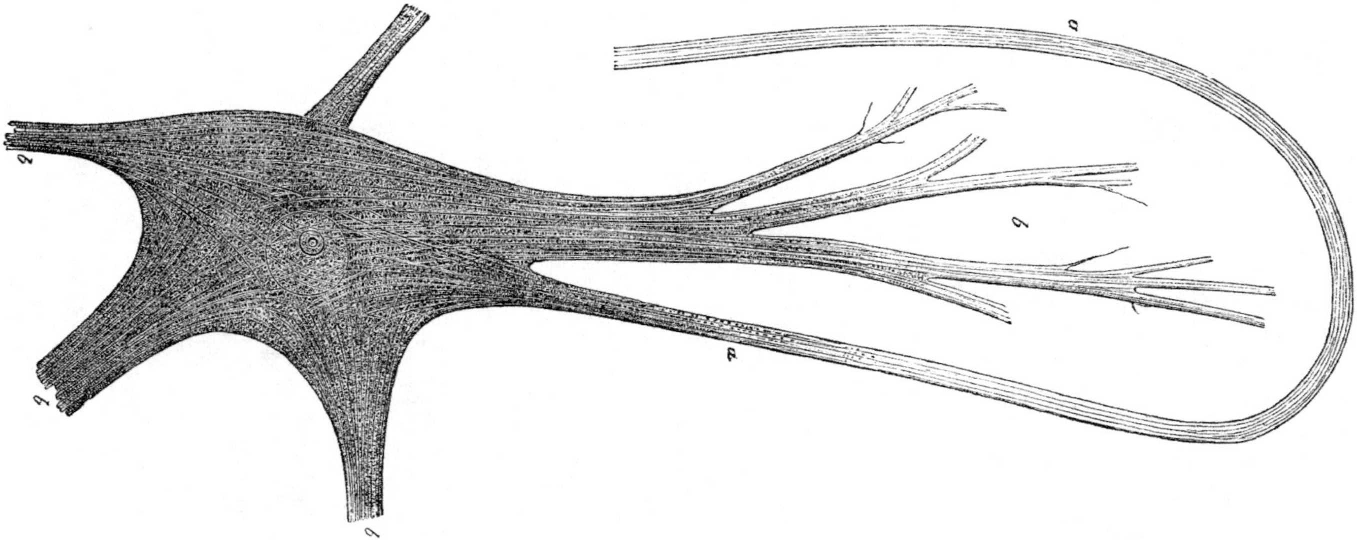

Fig. 17.—*Nerve-cell from the anterior grey substance of the spinal cord of a calf, magnified 600.* *a*, the axis cylinder; *b*, the branched processes. The neuroplasm is represented as distinctly fibrillated, with granular substance interspersed. Nucleus and nucleolus very distinct

and according to the processes it is known as unipolar, bipolar, and multipolar. When there are no processes the cell is called apolar. Some idea of these processes may be formed if they are likened to the pseudopodia of Amœbæ and Foraminifera. Compare fig. 16, a nerve-cell, figured by Gerlach, with fig. 17,' one highly magnified, in which Max Schultze's hypothesis is represented.

121. Such is a general description of the nerve-cell as it is seen in various places, and under various modes of preparation. How much is due to preparation we cannot positively say. While we always discover fibrine in the blood after it is withdrawn from the vessels, we know that fibrine as such does not exist in the circulating blood. And if neurine is a semi-liquid substance, we may doubt whether in the living cell it is fibrillated. Doubts have been thrown even on the normal existence of the granular substance, which has been attributed to coagulation. Thus we know that the nucleus of the white blood-corpuscle appears perfectly homogeneous until subjected to heat, yet at a certain temperature (86° F.) it assumes the aspect of a fine network. Haeckel observed the hyaline substance of the neurine in crayfish become troubled and changed directly any fluid except its own blood-serum came in contact with it. Leydig noticed the transparent ganglion of a living Daphnia become darker and darker as the animal died; and I saw something like this, after prolonged struggles of a Daphnia to escape from a thread in which its leg was entangled. Charles Robin, indeed, asserts that the passage from the hyaline to the finely-granulated state is a characteristic of the dying cell.*

* HAECKEL : *Muller's Archiv*, 1857. LEYDIG : *Vom Bau des thierischen Körpers*, 1864, i. 84. ROBIN : *Anat. et Physiol. Cellulaires*, p. 89. Should the observations of HEITZMANN be confirmed, there would be ground for believing that neurine is normally fibrillated. He says that the living protoplasm in the Amœba, white blood-corpuscle, &c., is an excessively fine network, which condenses into granules at each contraction. (Cited in the *Jahresberichte über Anat. und Physiol.*, 1873, Bd. ii.) WALTHER, who examined frozen brains, describes the cells as quite transparent at first, with very rare granules, but gradually while under obser-

On the other hand, it should be noted that Max Schultze describes a fibrillated appearance in cells just removed from the living animal, and placed in serum.

When, therefore, one observer describes the neuroplasm as being clear as water, another as finely granular, and a third as fibrillated, we must conclude that the observations refer to cells, 1°, under different states of vitalisation, or, 2°, under different modes of preparation. On the first head we note that some nerve-cells are so perishable that Trinchese declares he could find no cells in the ganglia of a cuttlefish which had been dead twenty-four hours, although they were abundant in one recently killed.* On the second head we note that the changes wrought by modes of preparation cannot be left out of consideration. Auerbach notices that the cells and fibres apparent in the *plexus myentericus* after an acid has been applied, cannot be detected before that application —nothing is visible but a pale gelatinous network, with here and there knots of a paler hue; and I remember my surprise on examining the fresh spinal cord of a duck-embryo, and finding no trace of cells such as I had that very morning seen in the cord of a chick of earlier date, but which had been soaked in weak bichromate of potash. Now we have excellent grounds for believing that in both cases these organites were present, and that it was the reagent which disclosed their presence in the chick; and so in other cases we must ask whether the forms which appear under a given mode of preparation are simply *unmasked*, or are in truth *produced* by the reagent? This question we can rarely answer.

If one of the very large cells be taken from the ganglion of a living mollusc, and be gently pressed till it bursts, the

vation the granules became more numerous: *Centralblatt*, 1868, p. 459. According to MAUTHNER: *Beiträge zur Kenntniss der morphologischen Elemente des Nervensystems*, 1862, p. 41, neurine has three cardinal forms—transparent, finely granular, and coarsely granular.

* TRINCHESE: *Struttura del sistema nervoso dei Cefalopodi*, Florence, 1868, p. 7.

discharged contents will be seen to be of a hyaline viscid substance, with fine granules but no trace of fibres. Yet we must not rashly generalise from this, and declare that in the vertebrate cells the substance is not also fibrillated. As a good deal of speculation rests on the assumption of the fibrillated cell-contents, I have thought it worth while to note the uncertainty which hovers round it.

122. Among the uncertainties must be reckoned the question as to the cell-processes. The existence of apolar and unipolar cells is flatly denied by many writers, who assert that the appearances are due to the fragility of the processes. Fragile the processes are, and evidence of their having been broken off meet us in every preparation; but the denial of apolar and unipolar cells seems to me only an example of the tendency to substitute hypothesis for observation (§ 114). The "postulate" which some seem to regard as a "necessity of thought" that every nerve-cell shall have at least two fibres, one ingoing, the other outgoing, is allowed to override the plain evidence.* It originated in the fact first noticed by Wagner and Charles Robin that certain cells in the spinal ganglia of fishes are bipolar. The fact was rapidly generalised, in spite of its not being verified in *other* places; the generalisation was accepted because (by a strange process of reasoning running counter to all physiological knowledge) it was thought to furnish an elementary illustration of the reflex process. As the centre had its ingoing and outgoing nerve, so the cell was held to be a centre "writ small," and required its two fibres. No one paused to ask, how a cell placed in the *track* of an ingoing nerve could fulfil this office of a reflex centre; no one supposed that the portion of the sensory fibre which continued its course, after the interruption of the cell, was a motor fibre.

What does Observation teach? It teaches that at first all

* An eminent friend of mine was one day insisting to me that the physiological postulate made it *impossible* for a nerve-cell to be without its ingoing and outgoing fibres; and he was not a little astounded when I replied, "Come into my workroom and I will show you a thousand."

nerve-cells are apolar. Even in the cortex of the cerebrum, where (unless we include the nuclei and grain-like corpuscles under cells) all the cells are finally multipolar, there is not one which has a process, up to the seventh or eighth day of incubation (in the chick); from that day, and onwards, cells with one process appear; later on, cells with two, and later still, with three. By this time all the apolar cells have disappeared. They may therefore be regarded as cells in their infancy. However that may be, we must accept the fact that apolar cells exist; whether they can co-operate in neural functions, is a question which must be decided after the mode of operation of cells is placed beyond a doubt.

123. If apolar cells are embryonic forms of cells which afterwards become multipolar, this interpretation will not suffice for the unipolar cells. They are not only abundant, but are mature forms in some organs, and in some animals; though in some organs they may truly be regarded as embryonic. Thus in the human embryo up to the fourth month all the cells of the spinal cord are said to be unipolar,* later on they become multipolar. But in birds, rabbits, dogs, and even man, the cells in the spinal ganglia are mainly (if not wholly) unipolar; † nor is there any difficulty in observing the same fact in the œsophageal ganglia of molluscs (see fig. 22).

* EICHHORST in *Virchow's Archiv*, 1875, lxiv. p. 432.

† AUERBACH (*Ueber einen Plexus Myentericus*, 1862) describes the ganglia as filled with apolar cells, among which only a few are unipolar. STIEDA (*Centralnervensystem der Vögel*, 1868) finds both apolar and unipolar cells in the spinal ganglia of birds. AXMANN (*De Gangliorum Systematis Structura penitiori*, 1847) says the spinal cells are all unipolar. SCHWALBE (*Archiv für mikros. Anat.*, 1868) and COURVOISIER (*ibid.*, 1869) say the same. So also RANVIER: *Comptes Rendus*, 1875. KÖLLIKER (*Gewebelehre*) speaks decidedly in favour of both apolar and unipolar cells, but thinks the apolar are embryonic. PAGLIANI (*Saggio sullo Stato attuale delle Cognizioni della Fisiologia intorno al Sistema nervoso*, 1873), who represents the views of MOLESCHOTT, admits the existence of apolar and unipolar cells. The authors just cited are those I happen to have before me during the rewriting of this chapter, and

Such are the observations. They have indeed been forced into agreement with the bipolar postulate, by the assumption that the single process branches into two, one afferent, the other efferent.* But before making observation thus pliant to suit hypothesis, it would be well to look more closely into the evidence for the hypothesis itself. For my own part, I fail to see the justification of the postulate; whereas the existence of unipolar cells is an observation which has been amply verified.

124. Bipolar cells abound; multipolar cells are still more abundant; and these are the cells found in the grey substance of the neural axis. Deiters, in his epoch-making work,† propounded an hypothetic *schema* which has been widely accepted. Finding that the large cells in the anterior horn of the spinal cord gave off processes of different kinds, one branched, the other unbranched, he held that the latter process was the origin of the axis cylinder of a nerve-fibre, whereas the branched process was protoplasm which divided and subdivided, and formed the connection between one cell and another. Gerlach has modified this by supposing that the minute fibrils of the branching process reunite and form an axis cylinder (fig. 18). There is no doubt that some processes terminate in a fine network; and there is a probability (not more) that the unbranched process is always continuous with the axis cylinder of a motor nerve, as we know it sometimes is with that of a dark-bordered fibre in the white substances. This, though probable, is, however, very far from having been de-

the list might easily be extended if needful. AUERBACH, BIDDER, and SCHWEIGGER-SEIDEL describe unipolar cells which in some places present the aspect of bipolar cells simply because two cells lie together, their single poles having opposite directions. I will add that the bipolar cells do not really render the physiological interpretation a whit more easy than the unipolar, for they are simply cells which form enlargements in the course of the nerve-fibres.

* When Dr. BEALE says "that it is probable no nerve-cell exists which has only *one single fibre* connected with it" (*Bioplasm*, p. 186), he has no doubt this in his mind; since he would not, I presume, deny that there are cells each with a single *process*.

† DEITERS: *Untersuchungen über Gehirn und Rückenmark*, 1865.

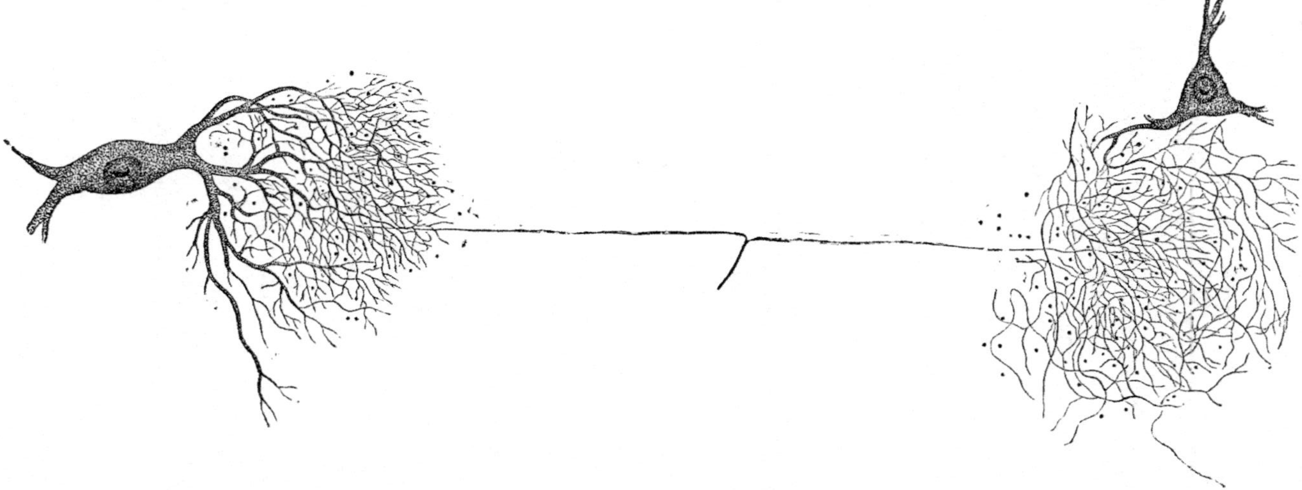

Fig. 18.—*Supposed union of two nerve-cells and a fibre.* The processes subdivide into a minute network, in which the fibre also loses itself.

monstrated. Once or twice Kölliker, Max Schultze, and Gerlach have followed this unbranched process as far as the *root* of a motor nerve; and they infer that although it could not be traced further, yet it did really join an axis cylinder there. In support of this inference came the observations of Koschennikoff,* that in the cerebrum and cerebellum, processes were twice seen continuous with dark-bordered nerve-fibres. But the extreme rarity of such observations amid thousands of cells is itself a ground for hesitation in accepting a generalised interpretation, the more so since we have Henle's observation of the similar entrance of a *branched* process into the root.† Now it must be remembered that the branched process is by no anatomist at present regarded as the origin of the axis cylinder; so that if it can enter the root without being the origin of a nerve-fibre, we are not entitled to assume that the entrance of the unbranched process has any other significance (on this head compare § 145), especially when we reflect that no trustworthy observer now professes to have followed a nerve-fibre of the posterior root right into a multipolar cell. Figures, indeed, have been published which show this, and much else; but such figures are diagrams, not copies of what is seen. They belong to Imaginary Anatomy.‡ The relation of the cell-process to the nerve-fibre will be discussed anon.

125. A word in passing on the contradictory assertions respecting the anastomosis of nerve-cells. That the grey substance forms a *continuum* of some kind is certain from the continuity of propagation of a stimulus. But it is by no

* *Archiv für mikros. Anat.*, 1869, p. 217. Compare also Butzke: *Archiv für Psychiatrie*, 1872, p. 584.

† Henle: *Nervenlehre*, 1871, p. 58, fig. 21.

‡ When men of such experience and skill as Kölliker, Bidder, Goll, and Lockhart Clarke declare that they have never seen a cell-process pass directly into a dark-bordered fibre in the anterior root, what are we to say to such figures and descriptions as those given in the works of Schröder van der Kolk, Gratiolet, and Luys? Even did such arrangements exist, no transverse nor longitudinal section could display them, owing to the different planes at which the fibres enter, and the length and irregularity of their course.

means certain that one cell is directly united to its neighbour by a cell-process. Eminent authorities assert that such direct union never takes place; others, that it is a rare and insignificant fact; others, that it is constant, and "demanded by physiological postulates." I will not, in the presence of distinct affirmations, venture to deny that such appearances as are presented in fig. 19 may occasionally be observed;

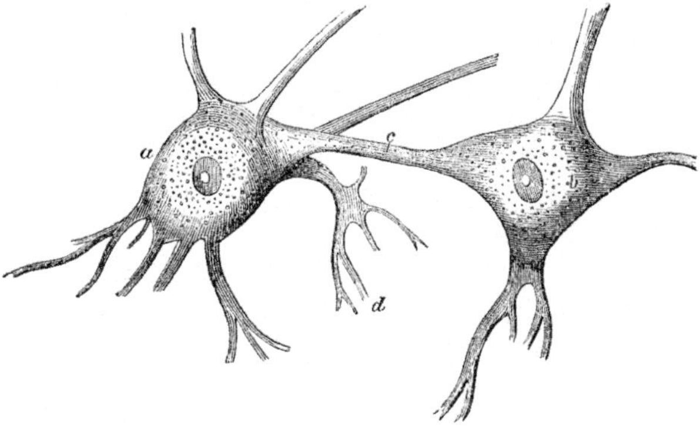

Fig. 19.—*Anastomosing nerve-cells* (after Gratiolet). *a*, body of the cell; *c*, process of uniting two cells; *d*, branching process.

the more so as I have myself seen perhaps half-a-dozen somewhat similar cases; but it is the opinion of Deiters and Kölliker that all such appearances are illusory.* Granting that such connections occur, we cannot grant this to be the normal mode; especially now the more probable supposition is that the connection is normally established by means of the delicate ramifications of the branching processes.

Imaginary Anatomy has not been content with the cells of the anterior horn being thus united together, to admit of united action, but has gone further, and supposed that the cells of the posterior horn, besides being thus united, send off processes which unite them with the cells of the anterior horn —and thus a pathway is formed for the transmission of a sensory impression, and its conversion into a motor impulse.

* Long after the text was written, WILLIGK published in *Virchow's Archiv*, 1875, lxiv. p. 163, observations of anastomoses which even KÖLLIKER admitted to be undeniable. Yet out of sixty-four preparations, amid hundreds of cells, he could only reckon seven cases of conjunction.

What will the reader say when informed that not only has no eye ever beheld such a pathway, but that the first step—the direct union of the sensory nerve-fibre with a cell in the *posterior* horn—is confessedly not visible?

126. The foregoing criticisms will perhaps disturb the reader who has been accustomed to theorise on the data given in text-books; but he may henceforward be more cautious in accepting such data as premisses for deduction; and will look with suspicion on the many theories which have arisen on so unstable a basis. When we reflect how completely the modern views of the nervous system, and the physiological, pathological, and psychological explanations based on these views, are dominated by the current notions of the nerve-cell, it is of the last importance that we should fairly face the fact that at present our knowledge even of the structure of the nerve-cell is extremely imperfect; and our knowledge of the part it plays—its anatomical relations and its functional relations—is little more than guesswork!

THE NERVES.

127. We now pass to the second order of organites; and here our exposition will be less troubled by hesitations, for although there is still much to be learned about the structure and connections of the nerve-fibres, there is also a solid foundation of accurate knowledge.

A nerve is a bundle of fibres within a membranous envelope supplied with blood-vessels. Each fibre has also its separate sheath, having annular constrictions at various intervals. It is more correctly named by many French anatomists a nerve-*tube* rather than a nerve-*fibre;* but if we continue to use the term *fibre,* we must reserve it for those organites which have a membranous sheath, and thereby distinguish it from the more delicate *fibril* which has none.

The nerve tube or fibre is thus constituted: within the sheath lies a central band of neuroplasm identical with the neuroplasm of nerve-cells, and known as the *axis cylinder;* surrounding this band is an envelope of whitish substance, variously styled *myeline, medullary sheath,* and *white substance of Schwann:* it is closely similar to the chief constituent of the yolk of egg; and to its presence is due the whitish colour of the fibres, which in its absence are greyish. The axis cylinder must be understood as the primary and essential element, because not only are there nerve-fibrils destitute both of sheath and myeline yet fulfilling the office of Neurility, but at their terminations, both in centres and in muscles, the nerve-fibres always lose sheath and myeline, to preserve only the neuroplasmic threads of which the axis cylinder is said to be composed. In the lowest fishes, in the invertebrates, and in the so-called sympathetic fibres of vertebrates, there is either no myeline, or it is not separated from the neuroplasm.

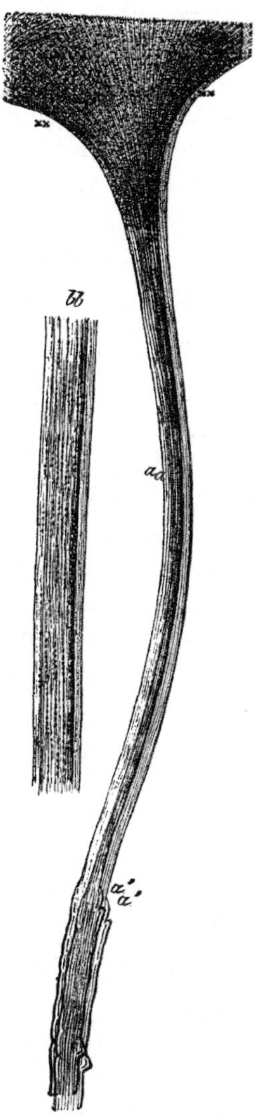

Fig. 20.—*a*, axis cylinder formed by the fibrils of the cell contents, and at *a′* assuming the medullary sheath; *b*, naked axis cylinder from spinal cord.

128. Nerve-fibres are of two kinds —1°. The *dark-bordered* or *medullary* fibres, which have both sheath and myeline, as in the peripheral system; or only myeline, without the sheath, as in the central system. 2°. The *non-medullary* fibres, which have the sheath, without appreciable myeline—such are the fibres of the olfactory, and the pale fibres of the sympathetic.

Nerve-fibrils are neuroplasmic threads of extreme delicacy, visible only under high magnifying powers (700 – 800), which abound in the centres, where they form networks. The fibrils also form the terminations of the fibres. Many fibrils are supposed to be condensed in one axis cylinder. This is represented by Max Schultze in figs. 17 and 20.

129. As may readily be imagined, the semi-liquid nature of the neuroplasm throws almost insuperable difficulties in the way of accurately determining whether the axis cylinder in the living nerve is fibrillated or not; whether, indeed, any of the aspects it presents in our preparations are normal. Authorities are not even agreed as to whether it is a pre-existent solid band of homogeneous substance, or a bundle of primitive fibrils, or a product of coagulation.* Rudanowsky's observations on frozen nerves convinced him that the cylinder is a tubule with liquid contents.† My own investigations of the nerves of insects and molluscs incline me to the view of Dr. Schmidt of New Orleans, namely, that the cylinder axis consists of minute granules arranged in rows and united by a homogeneous inter-fibrillar substance, thus forming a bundle of granular fibrils enclosed in a delicate sheath ‡—in other words, a streak of neuroplasm which has a fibrillar disposition of its granules. We ought to expect great varieties in such streaks of neuroplasm; and it is quite conceivable that in the Rays and the Torpedo there are axis cylinders which are single fibrils, and others which are bundles, with finely-granulated inter-fibrillar substance.§

The fibres often present a varicose aspect, as represented in fig. 21. It is, however, so rarely observed in the fresh tissue, that many writers regard it (as well as the double contour) as the product of preparation.‖ It is, indeed, always visible after the application of water.

* See the history given in STILLING's learned work, *Ueber den Bau der Nervenprimitiv-Faser*, p. 34; and compare MAX SCHULTZE, *De Retinæ Structura*, p. 8, and *Bau der Nasenschleimhaut*, p. 66; WALDEYER, in the *Zeitschrift für rat. Med.*, 1863; LISTER and TURNER: *Observations on the Structure of Nerve-Fibres*, in *Quarterly Micros. Journal*, 1859; RANVIER, in the *Archives de Physiologie*, 1872.

† *Virchow's Archiv*, Bd. lxxii. p. 193.

‡ *Monthly Journal of Micros. Science*, 1874, xi. p. 214.

§ BABUCHIN: *Centralblatt*, 1868, p. 756.

‖ Even so eminent an authority as W. KRAUSE holds this both with regard to the varicose aspect and the double contour: *Handbuch der menschlichen Anatomie*, 1876, i. 367. BUTSCHLI, however, describes

We need say no more at present respecting the structure of nerve-fibres, except to point out that we have here an organite not less complex than the cell.

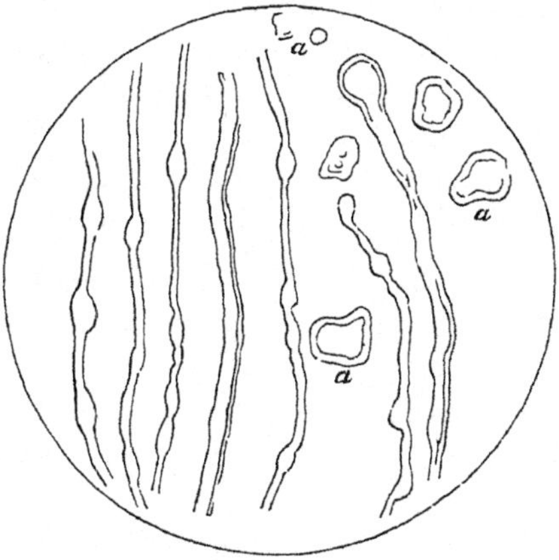

Fig. 21.—*Nerve-fibres from the white substance of the cerebrum. a, a, a,* the medullar contents pressed out of the tube as irregular drops.

THE NEUROGLIA.

130. Besides cells and fibres, there is the *amorphous substance*, which constitutes a great part of the central tissue, and also enters largely into the peripheral tissue. It consists of finely granular substance, and a network of excessively delicate fibrils, with nuclei interspersed. Its character is at present *sub judice.* Some writers hold it to be nervous, the majority hold it to be simply one of the many forms of connective tissue: hence its name neuroglia, or nerve-cement.

In the convolutions of the frozen brain Walther finds the cells and fibres embedded in a structureless semi-fluid substance wholly free from granules; the granules only appear there when cells have been crushed. It is to this substance he attributes the fluctuation of the living brain under the

the nerves in a living Nematode as varicose: *Archiv für Anat.*, 1873, p. 78; and I have somewhere met with an observation of the double contour being visible in the living animal.

touch, like that of a mature abscess; the solidity which is felt after death is due to the coagulation of this substance. Unhappily we have no means of determining whether the network visible under other modes of investigation is present, although invisible, in this substance. The neuroglia, as it appears in hardened tissues, must therefore be described with this doubt in our minds.

If we examine a bit of central grey substance where the cells and fibres are sparse, we see, under a low power, a network of fibrils in the meshes of which lie nerve-cells. Under very high powers we see outside these cells another network of excessively fine fibrils embedded in a granular ground substance, having somewhat the aspect of hoar-frost, according to Boll. It is supposed that the first network is formed by the ultimate ramifications of the nerve-cell processes, and that the second is formed by ramifications of the processes of *connective* cells. In this granular, gelatinous, fibrillar substance nuclei appear, together with small multipolar cells not distinguishable from nerve-cells except in being so much smaller. These nuclei are more abundant in the tissue of young animals, and more abundant in the cerebellum than in the cerebrum. The granular aspect predominates the fresher the specimen, though there is always a network of fibrils; so that some regard the granules as the result of a resolution of the fibrils, others regard the fibrils as the linear crystallisation (so to speak) of the granules.*

131. Such is the aspect of the neuroglia. I dare not venture to formulate an opinion on the histological question whether this amorphous substance is neural, or partly neural and partly connective (a substance which is potentially both, according to Deiters and Henle), or wholly connective. The

* BUTZKE: *Archiv für Psychiatrie*, 1872, p. 594, states that the granular substance has the chemical composition of myeline. If this be so, we may suppose the "fibrils of crystallisation" to represent the coagulation of the substance which is in solution amid the myeline granules, and corresponds with the axis cylinder of a fibre. I may remark that in almost every good preparation nerve-cells will be found in which while one process is distinctly granular, another is striated or even fibrillated.

question is not at present to be answered decisively, because what is known as connective tissue has also the three forms of multipolar cells, fibrils, and amorphous substance; nor is there any decisive mark by which these elements in the one can be distinguished from elements in the other. The physical and chemical composition of Neuroglia and Neuroplasm are as closely allied as their morphological structure. And although in the later stages of development the two tissues are markedly distinguishable, in the early stages every effort has failed to furnish a decisive indication.* Connective tissue is dissolved by solutions which leave nerve-tissue intact. Can we employ this as a decisive test? No, for if we soak a section of the spinal cord in one of these solutions, the *pia mater* and the membranous septa which ramify from it between the cells and fibres, disappear, leaving all the rest unaltered. This proves that Neuroglia is at any rate chemically different from ordinary connective tissue, and more allied to the nervous. As to the *staining* process, so much relied on, nothing requires greater caution in its employment. Stieda found that the same parts were sometimes stained and sometimes not; and Mauthner observed that in some cells both contents and nucleolus were stained, while the nucleus remained clear, in other cells the contents remained clear; and some of the axis cylinders were stained, the others not.† Lister found that the connective tissue between the fibres of the sciatic nerve, as well as the *pia mater*, were stained like the axis cylinders;‡ and in one of my notes there is the record of both (supposed) connective cells and nerve-cells being stained alike, while the nerve-fibres and the (supposed) connective fibres were unstained. Whence I conclude that the supposition as to the nature of the one group being different from that of the other was untenable, if the staining test is to be held decisive.

* BOLL: *Die Histiologie und Histiogenese der nervösen Centralorgane*, in the *Archiv für Psychiatrie*, 1873, p. 47.

† STIEDA: *Studien über das Centralnervensystem der Vögel*, 1868, p. 65. MAUTHNER: *Op. cit.*, p. 4.

‡ TURNER and LISTER: *Op. cit.*, p. 8.

132. The histological question is raised into undue importance because it is supposed to carry with it physiological consequences which would deprive the neuroglia of active co-operation in neural processes, reducing it to the insignificant position of a mechanical support. I cannot but regard this as due to the mistaken tendency of analytical interpretation, which somewhat arbitrarily fastens on one element in a complex of elements, and assigns that one as the sole agent. Whether we call the neuroglia connective or neural, it plays an essential part in all neural processes, probably a more important part than even the nerve-cells, which usurp exclusive attention! To overlook it, or to assign it a merely *mechanical* office, seems to me as unphysiological as to overlook blood-serum, and recognise the corpuscles as the only nutrient elements. The notion of the neuroglia being a mere vehicle of support for the blood-vessels arises from not distinguishing between the alimental and instrumental offices. In the function of a limb, bone is a co-operant. In the function of a centre, connective tissue is a co-operant; so that even if we acknowledge neuroglia to be a special form of connective tissue, it is an agent in neural processes; *what* its agency is, will be hereafter considered.

Following Bidder and Kupffer, the Dorpat school proclaimed the whole of the grey substance of the posterior half of the spinal cord to be connective tissue; and Blessig maintained that the whole of the retina, except the optic fibres, was connective tissue.* Even those anatomists who regarded this as exaggerated, admitted that connective tissue largely enters into the grey substance, especially if the granular ground substance be reckoned as connective, the nerve-cells being very sparse in the posterior region. Be it so. Let us admit that the grey matter of the frog's spinal cord is mainly composed of neuroglia, in which a very few multipolar nerve-cells are embedded. What must our conclusion be? Why, that since this spinal cord is proved to be a centre of energetic and manifold reflex actions—even to the extent of forcing many investigators to attribute sensation and voli-

* BLESSIG: *De Retinæ Structura*, 1857.

tion to it—this is proof that connective tissue does the work of nerve-tissue, and that the neuroglia is more important than nerve-cells!

Three hypotheses are maintainable—1°. The neuroglia is the amorphous ground-substance of undeveloped tissue (neuroplasm) out of which the cells and fibres of nerve-tissue and connective tissue are evolved. 2°. It is the product of dissolved nerve cells and fibres. 3°. It is the undeveloped stage of connective tissue. For physiological purposes we may adopt any one of these views, provided we keep firm hold of the fact that the neuroglia is an essential element, and in the centres a dominant element. To make this clear, however, we must inquire more closely into the relations of the three elements, nerve-cells, fibres, and neuroglia.

THE RELATIONS OF THE ORGANITES.

133. In enumerating among the obstacles to research the tendency to substitute hypothetic deductions in place of objective facts, I had specially in my mind the wide-reaching influence of the reigning theories of the nerve-cell. Had we a solidly-established theory of the cell, equivalent, say, to our theory of gas-pressure, we should still need caution in allowing it to override exact observation; but insecure as our data are, and hypothetical as are the inferences respecting the part played by the cell, the reliance placed on deductions from such premisses is nothing less than superstition. Science will take a new start when the whole question is reinvestigated on a preliminary setting aside of all that has been precipitately accepted respecting the office of the cell. This exercise of the imagination, even should the reigning theories subsequently be confirmed, would not fail to bring many neglected facts into their rightful place.

I am old enough to remember when the cell held a very subordinate position in Neurology, and now my meditations have led me to return, if not to the old views of the cell, at least to something like the old estimate of its relative importance. Its existence was first brought prominently forward by Ehrenberg in 1834, who described its presence in the sympathetic ganglia; and by Remak in 1837, who described it in the spinal ganglia. For some time afterwards the ganglia and centres were said to contain irregular masses of vesicular matter which were looked on as investing the fibres; what their office was, did not appear. But there rapidly arose the belief that the cells were minute batteries in which "nerve-force" was developed, the fibres serving merely as conductors. Once started on this track, Hypothesis had free way, and a sort of fetichistic deification of the cell invested it with miraculous powers. In many works of repute we meet with statements which may fitly take their place beside the equally grave statements made by savages respecting the hidden virtues of sticks and stones. We find the nerve-cells credited with "metabolic powers," which enable them to "spiritualise impressions, and materialise ideas," to *transform* sensations into movements, and *elaborate* sensations into thoughts; not only have they this "remarkable aptitude of metabolic local action," they can also "act at a distance." * The savage believes that one pebble will cure diseases, and another render him victorious in war; and there are physiologists who believe that one nerve-cell has sensibility, another motricity, a third instinct, a fourth emo-

* LUYS: *Recherches sur le Système nerveux*, 1865, p. 267. In a recent and remarkable treatise the student is informed that "plus une cellule est chargée d'un rôle purement mécanique plus elle est volumineuse; plus l'acte qu'elle produit tend à revêtir un caractère psychique plus elle est petite;" to move a limb the *agitation* of the cerebral cells must *materialise itself* more and more, "Il a besoin de passer par des cellules, de moins en moins spirituelles et de plus en plus matérielles. . . . De même pour les cellules sensitives. L'impression extérieure va en se modifiant, en se spiritualisant, de la périphérie au centre. . . . Un phénomène de l'ordre spirituel ne saurait devenir sans transition un phénomène d'ordre physique." And what is this marvellous transition between spiritual and physical? It is the action of medium-sized cells which "travaillent la vibration reçue, la modifient de façon à lui ôter de son spiritualisme et à la rapprocher davantage des ébranlements physiques." I will not name the estimable author, because he is simply restating what many others implicitly or explicitly teach; but I will only ask the reader to try and realise in thought the process thus described.

tion, a fifth reflexion: they do not say this in so many words, but they assign to cells which differ only in size and shape, specific qualities. They describe sensational, emotional, ideational, sympathetic, reflex, and motor-cells; nay, Schröder van der Kolk goes so far as to specify hunger-cells and thirst-cells.* With what grace can these writers laugh at Scholasticism?

134. The hypothesis of the nerve-cell as the fountain of nerve-force is supported by the gratuitous hypothesis of cell-substance having greater chemical tension and molecular instability than nerve-fibre. No evidence has been furnished for this; indeed the only experimental evidence bearing on this point, if it has any force, seems directly adverse to the hypothesis. I allude to the experiments of Wundt, which show that the faint stimulus capable of moving a muscle when applied directly to its nerve, must be increased if the excitation has to pass through the cells by stimulation of the sensory nerve.† Wundt interprets this as proving that the cells retard every impulse, whereby they are enabled to store up latent force. The cells have thus the office of locks in a canal, which cause the shallow stream to deepen at particular places. I do not regard this interpretation as satisfactory; but the fact at any rate seems to prove that so far from the cells manifesting greater instability than the fibres, they manifest less.

135. The hypothesis of nerve-force being developed in the ganglia, gradually assumed a more precise expression when the nerve-cells were regarded as the only important elements of a ganglion. It has become the foundation-stone of Neurology, therefore very particular care should be taken to make sure that this foundation rests on clear and indisputable evidence. Instead of that, there is absolutely no evidence on which it can rest; and there is much evidence decidedly

* SCHRÖDER VAN DER KOLK: *Pathologie der Geisteskrankheiten*, 1863, p. 69.

† WUNDT: *Physiologische Psychologie*, p. 261. In his *Mechanik der Nerven*, 2 *Abth.* (published just as this sheet is going to press), he shows that a stimulus is both retarded and weakened in its passage through a ganglion.

opposed to it. Neither structure nor experiment points out the cells as the chief agents in neural processes. Let us consider these.

Fig. 22 shows the contents of a molluscan ganglion which has been teased out with needles.

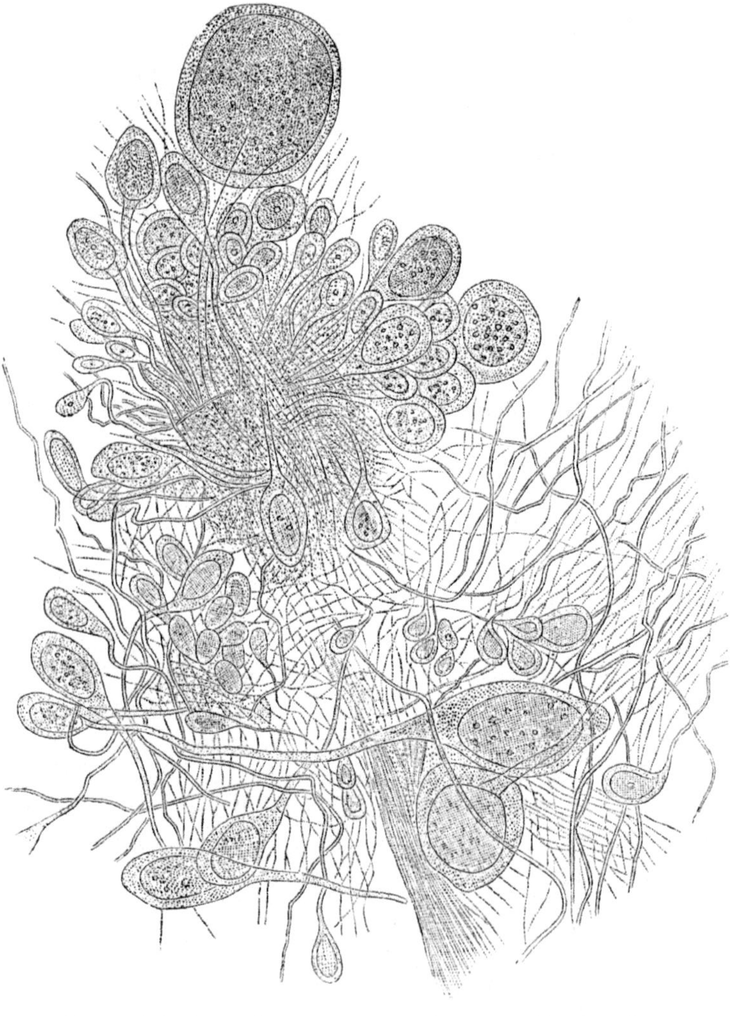

Fig. 22.—*Cells, fibres, and amorphous substance from the ganglion of a mollusc* (after Bucholtz).

The cells are seen to vary in size, but in all there is a rim of neuroplasm surrounding the large nucleus, and from this neuroplasm the fibre is seen to be a prolongation. The dotted substance in the centre is the neuroglia. Except in the possession of a nucleus, there is obviously here no essential difference in the structure of cell and fibre.

Now compare this with fig. 23, representing three fibres from the auditory nerve.

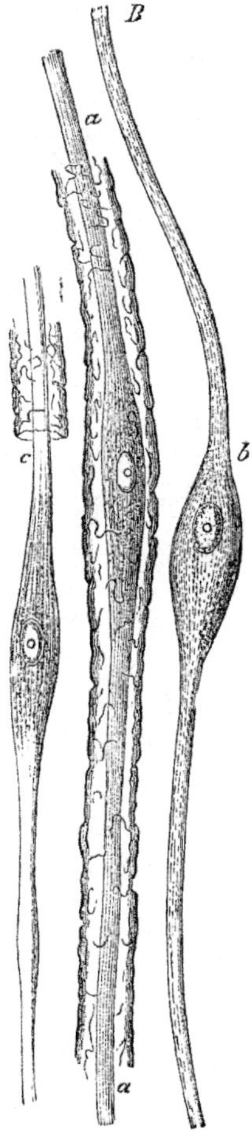

Fig. 23.—*Fibres from the auditory nerve.* *a*, the axis cylinder; *b*, the cellular enlargement; *c*, the medullary sheath.

Here the cell substance, as Max Schultze remarks, "is a continuation of the axis cylinder, and encloses the nucleus. The medulla commonly ceases at the point where the axis enters the cell, to reappear at its exit; but it sometimes stretches across the cell to enclose it also: so that such a ganglion cell is in truth simply the nucleated portion of the cylinder axis."* There are many places in which fibres are thus found with cells inserted in their course as swellings: in the spinal ganglia of fishes these are called bipolar cells; they are sometimes met with even in the cerebellum; but oftener in peripheral nerves, where they are mostly small masses of granular neuroplasm from which usually a branching of the fibre takes place. The point to which attention is called is that in some cases, if not in all, the nerve-fibre is structurally continuous with the cell contents.

* TRINCHESE also says that the fibres "provengono dalle cellule e *non son altro che i loro prolungamenti o poli.*"—*Op. cit.*, p. 13. An unequivocal example is seen in the *Torpedo*, where the large cells have each their prolongation continuing without interruption into the electrical organ. See the figure given by REICHENHEIM in the *Archiv für Anat.*, 1873, Heft vi.

The two organites—fibre and cell—differ only as regards the nucleus and pigment. Haeckel, who affirms that in the crayfish (*Astacus fluviatilis*) he never saw a cell which did not continue as a fibre, thinks there is always a marked separation of the granular substance from its "hyaline protoplasm," and that only this latter forms the axis cylinder. But although my observations agree with this as a general fact, I have seen even in crayfish the granular substance prolonged into the axis cylinder; and in other animals the granular substance is frequently discernible.

Indeed it may be said that anatomists are now tolerably unanimous as to the axis cylinder being identical with the protoplasmic cell substance. If this be so, we have only to recall the principle of identity of property accompanying identity of structure, to conclude that *whatever properties we assign to the cells* (unless we restrict these to the nucleus and pigment) *we must assign to the axis cylinders.* We can therefore no longer entertain the hypothesis of the cells being the fountains or reservoirs of Neurility; the less so when we reflect that cells do not form the hundredth part of nerve-tissue: for even the grey substance bears but a small proportion to the white; and of the grey substance, Henle estimates that one-half is fibrous, the rest is partly cellular, partly amorphous. Those who derive Neurility from the cells, forget that although the organism begins as a cell, and for some weeks consists mainly of cells, yet from this time onwards there is an ever-increasing preponderance of cell-derivatives—fibres, tubes, and amorphous substance—and corresponding with this is the ever-increasing power and complexity of the organism.

136. From another point of view we must reject the hypothesis. Not only does the evidence which points to the essential continuity in structure of nerve cell and fibre discredit the notion of their physiological diversity, but it is further supported by the fact that although the whole nervous system is structurally continuous, an immense mass of nerve-fibres have no *immediate* connection with ganglionic cells:—neither springing from nor terminating in such cells, their activity cannot be assigned to them. To many readers this statement will be startling. They have been so accustomed to hear that every fibre begins or terminates in a cell, that a doubt thrown on it will sound paradoxical. But there is an equivoque here which must be got rid of. When it is said that every fibre has its "origin" in a cell, this may be true if origin mean its *point of departure in evolution*, for "cells" are the early forms of all organites; but although every organite is at first a cell, and in this sense a nerve-fibre must be said to originate in a cell, we must guard against the equivoque which arises from calling the highly-differentiated organite, usually designated ganglionic cell, by the same name as its starting-point. On this ground I suggest the term neuroblast, in lieu of nerve-cell, for the earlier stages in the evolution of cell and fibre. Both Embryology and Anatomy seem to show that cell and fibre are organites differentiated from identical neuroblasts, with a somewhat varying history, so that in their final stages the cell and fibre have conspicuous differences in form with an underlying identity; just as a male and female organism starting from identical ova, and having essential characters in common, are yet in other characters conspicuously unlike. The multipolar cell is not necessarily the origin of a nerve-fibre, although it is probable that some short fibres have their origin in the prolongations of cells. Although the latter point has not, I think, been satisfactorily established, except in the invertebrata, I see no reason whatever to doubt its probability; what seems the least reconcilable with the evidence is the notion that all fibres arise as prolongations from ganglionic cells, instead of arising independently as differentiations from neuroblasts. The reader will observe that my objection to the current view is purely anatomical; for the current view would suit my physiological interpretations equally well, and would be equally irreconcilable with the hypothesis of the cell as the source of Neurility, so long as the identity of structure in the axis cylinder and cell contents is undisputed.

137. The evidence at present stands thus: There are numerous multipolar cells which have no traceable connection with nerve-fibres; and fibres which have no direct connection with multipolar cells. By the first I do not mean the disputed apolar cells, I mean cells in the grey substance of the centres which send off processes that subdivide and terminate as fibrils in the network of the Neuroglia (figs. 16, 18). It is indeed generally assumed that these have each one process—the axis-cylinder process—which is prolonged as a nerve-fibre; nor would it be prudent to assert that such is never the case; though it would be difficult to distinguish between a fibre which had united with a process and a fibre which was a prolongation of a process, in both cases the neuroplasm being identical. I only urge that the assumption is grounded not on anatomical evidence, but on a supposed necessary postulate. All that can be demonstrated is that some processes terminate in excessively fine fibrils; and occasionally in thousands of specimens processes have been traced into dark-bordered fibres. It is true that they often present appearances which have led to the inference that they did so terminate—appearances so deceptive that Golgi and Arndt independently record observations of unbranched processes having the aspect of axis cylinders being prolonged to a considerable distance (600 μ in one case), yet these were found to terminate *not* in a dark-bordered fibre, but in a network of fibrils.*

138. While it is thus doubtful whether dark-bordered fibres are always immediately connected with cells, it is demonstrable that multitudes of fibres have only an indirect connection with cells, being developed as outgrowths from other fibres. Dr. Beale considers that in each such outgrowths have their origin in small neuroplasmic masses (his "germinal matter"). That is another question. The fact

* GOLGI: *Sulla struttura della sostanza grizia del Cervello.* ARNDT: *Archiv für mikros. Anat.*, 1870, p. 176. RINDFLEISCH also traces these processes into the neuroglia (*ibid.*, 1872, p. 453). "Deiters, Boddaert, and other observers have stated that one dark-bordered nerve-fibre enters each cell. . . . My own observations lead me to conclude that *all* the fibres are composed of the same material, but that one fibre does not divide until it has passed some distance from the cell, while others give off branches much closer to it."—BEALE: *Bioplasm*, p. 189.

here to be insisted on is that we often find groups of cells with only two or three fibres, and groups of fibres where very few cells exist. Schröder van der Kolk says that in a sturgeon (*Accipenser sturio*) weighing 120 pounds he found the spinal cord scarcely thicker than that of a frog; the muscles of this fish are enormous, and its motor nerves abundant; yet these nerves entered the cord by roots no thicker than a pig's bristle; and in the very little grey matter of the cord there was only a cell here and there found after long search. Are we to suppose that these rare cells were the origins of all the motor and sensory nerves? A similar want of correspondence may be noticed elsewhere. Thus in the spinal cord of the Lamprey my preparations show very few cells in any of the sections, and numerous sections show none at all. Stieda counted only eight to ten cells in each horn of some osseous fishes, except at the places where the spinal roots emerged. In the eel and cod he found parts of the cord quite free from cells, and in other parts found two, three, never more than ten. In birds he counted from twenty-five to thirty. Particular attention is called to this fact of the eel's cord being thus deficient, because every one knows the energetic reflex action of that cord, each separate segment of which responds to peripheral stimulation.

It may indeed be urged that these few cells were the origin of all the fibres, the latter having multiplied by the well-known process of subdivision; and in support of this view the fact may be cited of the colossal fibres of the electric fishes, each of which divides into five-and-twenty fibres, and in the electric eel each fibre is said by Max Schultze to divide into a million of fibrils. But I interpret this fact otherwise. It seems to me to prove nothing more than that the neuroplasm has differentiated into few cells and many fibres. And my opinion is grounded on the evidence of Development, presently to be adduced. If we find (and this we do find) fibres making their appearance anywhere *before* multipolar cells appear, the question is settled.

139. Dr. Beale regards the large caudate cells of the centres as different organites from the oval and pyriform

cells, and thinks they are probably stations through which fibres having different origins merely pass, and change their directions; and Max Schultze says that no single fibril has been found to have a central origin; every fibril arises at the periphery, and passes through a cell, which is thus crossed by different fibrils.* (Comp. fig. 17.)

The teaching of Development is on this point of supreme importance. Unhappily there has not yet been a sufficient collection of systematic observations to enable us to speak very confidently as to the successive stages, but some negative evidence there is. The changes take place with great rapidity, and the earliest stages have hardly been observed at all. Although for several successive years I watched the development of tadpoles, the difficulties were so great, and the appearances so perplexing, that the only benefit I derived was that of being able the better to understand the more successful investigations of others. Four or five days after fecundation is the earliest period of which I have any recorded observation; at this period the cerebral substance appeared as a finely granular matter, having numerous lines of segmentation marking it off into somewhat spherical and oval masses, interspersed with large granules and fat globules. Here and there hyaline substance appeared between the segments. Similar observations have since been recorded by Charles Robin in the earliest stages of the Triton.† He says that when the external gills presented their first indications, nuclei appeared, each surrounded by a rim of hyaline substance, from which a pale filament was prolonged at one end, sometimes one at both ends, and this filament subdivided as it grew in length until it had all the appearance of an axis

* BEALE: *Bioplasm*, p. 177. MAX SCHULTZE, in *Stricker's Handbuch*, p. 134. Comp. STILLING: *Nervenprimitiv-Faser*, p. 133. ARNDT: *Archiv für mikros. Anat.*, 1868, p. 512; and 1869, p. 237.

Weighty as these authorities are, their view is questionable—firstly, because the forms of these cells are too constant and definite in particular places to result from the union of fibrils coming from various origins; but secondly, and mainly, because the teaching of Development is opposed to it.

† ROBIN: *Anat. et Physiol. Cellulaires*, p. 335.

cylinder. This, however, he says, is a striation, not a fibrillation; he refuses to admit that the axis cylinder is a bundle of fibrils. He further notices the simultaneous appearance of amorphous substance; and as this is several days before there is any trace of a *pia mater*, or proper connective tissue, he urges this among the many considerations which should prevent the identification of neuroglia with connective tissue.

In a very young embryo of a mole (I could not determine its age) the cortex of the hemispheres showed granular amorphous substance, in which were embedded spherical masses of somewhat paler colour, which had no nuclei, and were therefore not cells. Besides these, there were nucleated masses (apolar cells, therefore) and more developed cells, unipolar, bipolar, and tripolar. Not a trace of a nerve-fibre was visible. In agreement with this are the observations of Masius and Van Lair, who cut out a portion of the spinal cord in a frog, and observed the regenerated tissue after the lapse of a month. It contained apolar, bipolar, and multipolar cells, together with "corpuscles without processes, for the most part larger than the cells, and appearing to be mere agglomerations of granules"—these latter I suppose to have been what I describe as segmentations of the undeveloped substance. Grey fibres, with a few varicose fibres, also appeared.*

140. The admirable investigations of Franz Boll have given these observations a new significance. He finds in the cerebral substance of the chick on the third or fourth day of incubation a well-marked separation between the neuroglia and nerve-tissue proper. Fig. 24, A, represents three nerve-cells, each with its nucleus and nucleolus, and each surrounded with its layer of neuroplasm. The other four masses he regards as nuclei of connective tissue. Three days later the distinction between the two is more marked (fig. 24, B). Not only have the nerve-cells acquired an increase of neuroplasm, they also present indications of their future processes, which at the twelfth day are varicose

* *Archives de Physiologie*, 1872, p. 268.

(fig. 24, C). (All this while the connective corpuscles remain unchanged.) Although Boll was unable to trace one of these processes into nerve-fibres, he has little doubt that they do ultimately become (unite with?) axis cylinders.

It is difficult to reconcile such observations with the hypothesis of the cells being simply points of *reunion of fibrils.* We see here multipolar cells before any fibrils appear. Respecting the development of the white substance, *i.e.*, the nerve-fibres, Boll remarks that in the *corpus callosum* of the chick the first differentiation resembles that of the grey substance.

The polygonal and spindle-shaped cells represented in fig. 25, A, are respectively starting-points of connective and neural tissues. The spindle-shaped cells elongate, and rapidly become bipolar. This is supposed to result in the whole cell becoming transformed into a fibre, the nucleus and nucleolus vanishing; but the transformation is so rapid that he confesses that he was unable to trace its stages; all that can positively be asserted is that one or two days after the appearance presented in fig. 25, B, the aspect changes to that of fibrils. The columns of polygonal cells between which run these fibrils, he regards as the connective corpuscles described by several anatomists in the white substance both of brain and cord, and which are sometimes declared to be multipolar nerve-cells.*

141. Dr. Schmidt's observations on the human embryo were of course on tissue at a very much later stage. According to him, the fibrils of the axis cylinders are formed by the linear disposition and consolidation of elementary granules.

* The fact of the existence of cells in the white substance is one which is very difficult of interpretation on the current hypotheses. The cells are found in regular columns and irregularly scattered. Boll thinks that while in the white substance of both cerebrum and cerebellum there are true nerve-cells as well as connective corpuscles, in the cord there are only the latter. But hitherto there has been no decisive test by which a nerve-cell can be distinguished from a connective corpuscle.

The fibrils thus formed are separated by interfibrillar granules which in time become fibrils. Not earlier than three months and a half does the formation of individual axis cylinders begin by the aggregation of these fibrils into

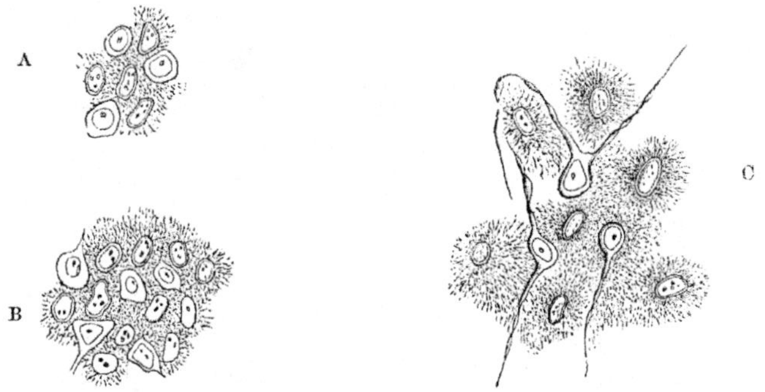

Fig. 24.—*Embryonic nerve-cells.*

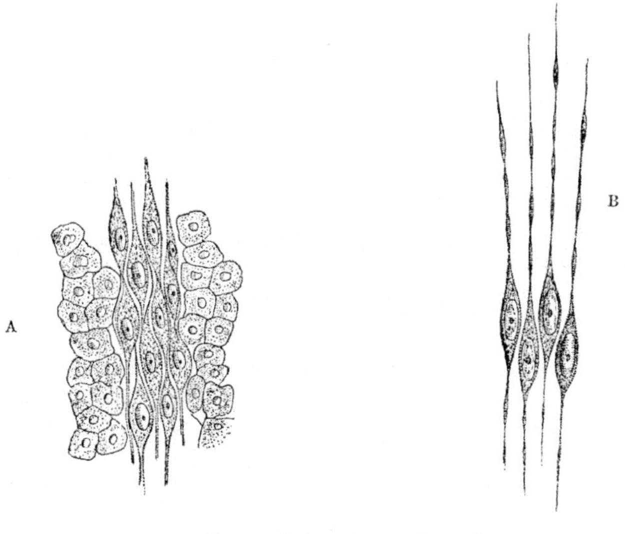

Fig. 25.—*Embryonic nerve-fibres.*

minute bundles, which are subsequently surrounded by a delicate sheath.*

142. With respect to the transition of the spindle-shaped cells into fibrils, since there is a gap in the observations of Boll, and since those of Schmidt are subsequent to the disappearance of the cells, and in both cases all trace of nucleus has disappeared, I suggest that we have here an analogy with what Weismann has recorded of the metamorphoses of insects. In the very remarkable memoir of that investigator † it is shown that the metamorphoses do not take place by a gradual modification of the existing organs and tissues, but by a *resolution* of these into their elements, and a *reconstruction* of their elements into tissues and organs. The muscles, nerves, tracheæ, and alimentary canal, undergo what may be called a fatty degeneration, and pass thence into a mere blastema. *It is out of these ruins of the old tissues that the new tissues are reconstructed.* On the fourth day the body of the pupa is filled with a fluid mass—a plasma composed of blood and dissolved tissues. The subsequent development is thus in all essential respects a repetition of that which originally took place in the ovum.‡

Two points are especially noticeable: First, that in this resolved mass of granules and fat globules there quickly appear

* *Monthly Journal of Micros. Science*, xi. 219. This accords with what KUPFFER says respecting the entire absence of cells in the earliest stages observed by him in the sheep. The white substance of the spinal cord he describes as soft, transparent, and gelatinous, in which dark points are visible; these dark points are seen in longitudinal sections to arise from the fibrillation of the substance.—BIDDER und KUPFFER: *Op. cit.*, p. 111.

† WEISMANN: *Die nachembryonale Entwick. der Musciden*, in the *Zeitschrift für Wissen. Zoologie*, 1864, Bd. xiv. Heft iii.

‡ The suggestion in the text has since received a striking confirmation in the observations of SIGMUND MAYER on the regeneration of nerves. The nerve when divided rapidly undergoes fatty degeneration, which is succeeded by a transformation of the myeline and axis cylinder into a homogeneous mass; in this resolved pulp new longitudinal lines of division appear, which subsequently become new fibres, and new nuclei are developed in the remains of the untransformed substance.—*Archiv für Psychiatrie*, Bd. vi. Heft ii.

large globular masses which develop a fine membrane, and subsequently nuclei. A glance at the figure 51 of Weismann's plates reveals the close resemblance to the earliest stages of nerve-cells; and the whole process recalls the regeneration of nerves and nerve-centres after their fatty degeneration.

Secondly, the nerves reappear in their proper places in the new muscles, and this at a time when the nerve-centres are still unformed; so that the *whole peripheral system is completely rebuilt in absolute independence of the central system.* The idea, therefore, that nerve-fibres are the products of ganglia must be relinquished. This idea is further discountenanced by Boll's observations, which show that the fibre-cells are from the first different from the ganglionic cells; and by the observations of Foster and Balfour, that "fibres are present in the white substance on the third day of incubation;" *whereas cell processes do not appear until the eighth day.* Foster and Balfour are inclined to believe "that even on the seventh day it is not possible to trace any connection between the cells and fibres." In the later stages, the connection is perhaps established.*

* Strong confirmation of various statements in the text, since they were written, has been furnished by the researches of EICHHORST, published in *Virchow's Archiv*, lxiv. Our knowledge of the development of nerve-tissue in human embryos is so scanty that these researches have a great value. EICHHORST describes the striation of the cells in the cord to begin only at the fourth month; up to this time they are, what I find most invertebrate cells to be, granular, not fibrillar. There is very slight branching of the cell processes until the ninth or tenth month, when the multipolar aspect first appears; the cells are unipolar up to the end of the fourth month. The connection between the white columns and the grey columns is very loose up to the fifth month; and the two are easily separated. Subsequently the union is closer. The substance of the white columns readily separates into bundles and fibres, but that of the grey columns falls into a granular detritus if attempted to be teased out with needles. But after the fifth month this is no longer so. Instead of a granular detritus there appears a network of fine fibres and fibrils. Although the white posterior columns are developed before the fifth month, not a single cell can be seen in the posterior grey columns until the second half of the ninth month. (Yet the fibres are imagined to arise in the cells !) The passage from the granu-

143. We may, I think, conclude from all this that in the higher vertebrates the white substance of brain and cord is not the direct product of the grey substance ; in other words, that here nerve-fibres, even if subsequently in connection with the ganglionic cells, have an independent origin. They may grow towards and blend with cell processes ; they are not prolongations of those processes. They may be identical in structure and property, as one muscle is identical with another, but one is not the parent of the other.

144. Sigmund Mayer emphatically declares that in no instance has he traced a cell process developed into a dark-bordered nerve-fibre. The process, he says, may often be traced for a certain distance alongside of a fibre ; but it then suddenly ceases, whereas the fibre is seen continuing its course unaltered. Still more conclusive is the evidence afforded by nerves having only very few fibres (2–4 sometimes in the frog), which have, nevertheless, a liberal supply of cells, visible without preparation. Valentin counted twenty-four cells in a nerve which had but two fibres.* Now although it is possible to explain the presence of numerous fibres with rare cells either as due to subdivisions of fibres, or to the fibres having cells elsewhere for their origin, it is not thus that we can explain the presence of numerous cells which have no fibres developed from their processes.

145. With regard to this observation of the cell process

lar to the fibrillar state is the same in the cell substance and the neuroglia. The nerve-fibre, as distinguished from a naked axis cylinder, does not appear till the fourth month. It is at first a bipolar prolongation of the nucleus. As it elongates, the nucleus seems to sit *on* it, and so loosely that it is easily shifted away by pressure on the covering glass. Finally the fibre separates entirely from the nucleus, and *then* begins to clothe itself with the medullary sheath. Very curious is the observation that so long as the axis cylinder is naked it is never varicose, but with the development of the medulla the primitive axis becomes fluid.

* MAYER : *Op. cit.*, 393. I cannot, however, agree with MAYER when he says that the continuity of a nerve-fibre with a cell has *never* been distinctly shown (p. 395) ; in the Invertebrata and in the Electric fishes such a continuity is undeniable ; and it has occasionally been seen in Vertebrata.

running alongside of the fibre, the recent researches of Ranvier may throw some light on it. He describes the cells in the spinal ganglia as all unipolar; each single process pursues a more or less winding course as a fibril, often blending with others, till it reaches one of the fibres from the sensory root. It blends with this fibre at the annular constriction of the fibre, becoming here incorporated with it, so that a T-shaped fibre is the result.* If this should be confirmed, it would reconcile many observations; but it would greatly disturb all current interpretations. Ranvier remarks that it is no longer tenable to suppose that the ganglionic cell is a centre, sensory or motor, receiving the excitation or sending forth a motor impulse; for if the fibril issuing from a cell becomes laterally soldered to a nerve-fibre, there is no possibility of saying in which direction this cell receives the excitation, nor in which it transmits the impulse.

146. We have seen good reason to conclude that the essential element of the nerve—the axis cylinder—is the same substance as the neuroplasm which forms the essential element of the cell. At any rate, we are quite certain that the cell process is neuroplasm. On this ground there is no difficulty in understanding that a cell process may sometimes be drawn out into an axis cylinder (as indeed we see to be the case in the invertebrata and electric fishes); while again in numerous other cases the nerve-fibre has an independent origin, being, in short, a differentiation from the neuroplasm which has become a fibre instead of a cell. It is clear from the observations of Rouget on Development, and of Sigmund Mayer on Regeneration, that fibres, nuclei, and cells become

* RANVIER, in the *Comptes Rendus*, 1875, vol. lxxxi. p. 1276. This observation throws light on the fact that cell processes are sometimes seen entering nerve-roots (§ 124).

The very remarkable observations of Mr. F. BALFOUR, *On the Development of the Spinal Nerves in Elasmobranch Fishes* (*Philos. Trans.*, vol. clxvi. p. 1), show that the spinal root, ganglion, and nerve-trunk arise from histological changes in a mass of cells at first all alike ; *not* that ganglion-cells are formed and from their processes elongate into fibres. The nerve, he says, forms a continuation of its root rather than of its ganglion (p. 181) ; which accords with RANVIER's view.

differentiated from the same neuroplasm, those portions which are not converted into fibres remaining first as lumps of neuroplasm, then acquiring a nucleus, and some of these passing into cells. I mean that between fibres, nuclei, and cells there are only morphological differences in an identical neuroplasm.* If this is in any degree true, it will not only explain how fresh fibres may be developed in the course of fibres, branching from them as from trunks, and branchlets from branchlets, twigs from branchlets, the same conditions of growth being present throughout; it will also completely modify the notion of any physiological distinction between cell and fibre greater than can be assigned to the morphological differences. We shall then no longer suppose that the cell is the fountain whence the fibre draws its nutrition and its "force;" and this will be equally the case even if we admit that a cell is, so to speak, the germ from which a whole plexus of fibres was evolved, for no one will pretend that the "force" of an organism is directly derived from the ovum, or that the ovum nourishes the organism.

147. At this stage of the discussion it is needful to consider a point which will spontaneously occur to every instructed reader, I mean the interesting fact discovered by Dr. Waller, that when a sensory root was divided, the portion which was still in connection with the ganglion remained unaltered, whereas the portion which was only in connection with the spinal cord degenerated; and *vice versâ*, when a motor root was divided, the portion connected with the cord remained unaltered, the portion severed from the cord degenerated. The observation has been frequently confirmed, and the conclusion drawn has been that the cells in the ganglion of the posterior root are the nutritive centres of posterior nerves, the cells in the anterior horn of the cord being the nutritive centres of the anterior nerves. Another interpretation is however needed, the more so because the fact is not constant.† True of some nerves, it is not true of

* In the *Handbuch der menschlichen Anatomie* of W. KRAUSE, which has just appeared, I am pleased to find a similar view, p. 376.

† On this point consult AXEL KEY and RETZIUS, in the *Archiv für*

others. Vulpian found that when he cut out a portion of the lingual nerve, and transplanted it by grafting under the skin of the groin, where of course it was entirely removed from all ganglionic influence, it degenerated, but it also regenerated. Pathological observations convinced Meissner that the ganglia are wholly destitute of an influence on the nutrition of the vagus; and Schiff proved experimentally that other ganglia were equally inoperative, since motor nerves could be separated from the spinal cord without degeneration.* Not however to insist on this, nor on the other facts of regeneration, in the absence of ganglionic influence, let us remark that Dr. Waller's examples would not be conclusive unless the teaching of Embryology could be disproved. That nerves degenerate when separated from ganglia is a fact; but it is also a fact that muscles degenerate when separated from a nerve-centre; yet we do not suppose the nerve-centre to nourish the muscles. And against the fact that the sensory nerve remains unaltered only in that portion which is connected with the ganglion, we must oppose the observations of Kölliker and Schwalbe,† who affirm that none of the fibres which enter the posterior columns of the spinal cord have any direct connection with the cells of the ganglion on the posterior root. The cells of this ganglion they declare to be unipolar (in the higher vertebrates), and the fibres in connection with these cells are not those which pass to the cord, but all of them pass to the periphery. According to Ranvier,

mikros. Anat., 1873, p. 308, where the nutritive disturbance is assigned to the fact that the lymph can no longer take its normal course. WALLER's observations on the degeneration of the optic nerves, with preservation of the integrity of the retina, after division of the nerves (*Proceedings of Royal Society*, 1856, p. 10), cannot be urged in support of his view, because BERLIN and LEBERT's observations are directly contradictory of his. SAEMISCH *und* GRAEFE: *Handbuch der Augenheilkunde*, ii. 346. It is said by KRENCHEL that if the nerves be divided, so as to prevent disturbances in the circulation, no peripheral degeneration takes place (cited by ENGELMANN in *Pflüger's Archiv*, 1875, p. 477).

* SCHIFF: *Lehrbuch der Physiologie*, pp. 120, 121.

† KÖLLIKER: *Gewebelehre*, 317. SCHWALBE: *Archiv für mikros. Anat.*, 1868, p. 51.

the fibres from the cells join the fibres of the posterior root. Schwalbe found that if the spinal nerve be firmly grasped and *steadily* drawn, it will often be pulled from its sheath, and the ganglion laid bare;* in this ganglion all the cells are found undisturbed, which could not be the case had fibres from *those* cells entered the cord, since the traction would necessarily have disturbed them.

RECAPITULATION.

148. At the opening of this chapter mention was made of the besetting sin of the analytical tendency, namely, to disregard the elements which provisionally had been set aside, and not restore them in the reconstruction of a synthetical explanation. Familiar experiences tell us that a stimulus applied to the skin is followed by a muscular movement, or a glandular secretion; sometimes this takes place without any conscious sensation; sometimes we are distinctly conscious of the stimulus; and sometimes we consciously will the movement. These facts the physiologist tries to unravel, and to trace the complicated processes involved. The neurologist of course confines himself exclusively to the neural processes; all the other processes are provisionally left out of account. But not only so: the analytical tendency is carried further, and even in the neural process the *organs* are neglected for the sake of the nervous *tissue*, and the nervous tissue for the sake of the *nerve-cell*. The consequence has been that we have an explanation offered us which runs thus:—

149. The nerve-cell is the supreme element, the origin of the nerve-fibre, and the fountain of nerve-force. The cells are connected one with another by means of fibres, and with muscles, glands, and centres also by means of fibres, which are merely channels for the nerve-force. A stimulus at the

* I was first shown this in 1858 by the late Prof. HARLESS in Munich, who at the same time showed me that the nerve thus bared of its sheath, if left some hours in gastric juice, split up into regular discs, like the sarcous elements of muscles.

surface is carried by a sensory fibre to a cell in the centre; from that point it is carried by another fibre to another cell; and from that by a third fibre to a muscle: a reflex contraction results. This is the elementary "nervous arc." But this arc has also higher arcs with which it is in connection: the sensory cell besides sending a fibre directly to a motor cell, also sends one upwards to the cerebral centres; and here again there is a nervous arc, so that the cerebral centre sends down an impulse on the motor cells, and the contraction which results is due to a volitional impulse. The transmission of the stimulation which in the first case was purely physical, becomes in the latter case psychical. The sensory impression is in one cell transformed into a *sensation*, in another cell into an *idea*, in a third cell into a *volition*.

150. This course is described with a precision and a confidence which induces the inexperienced reader to suppose that it is the transcript of actual observation. I venture to say that it is imaginary from beginning to end. I do not affirm that no such course is pursued, I only say no such course was ever demonstrated, but that at every stage the requisite facts of observation are either incomplete or contradictory. First, be it noted that the actions to be explained are never the actions of organs so simple as the description sets forth. It is not by single fibres and cells that the stimulus is effected, but by complex nerves and complex centres. Only by a diagrammatic artifice can the fibre represent the nerve, and the cell the centre. In reality the cells of the centre (supposing them to be the *only* agents) act in groups, and Anatomy should therefore show them to be mutually united in groups—which is what no Anatomy has succeeded in showing, unless the Neuroglia be called upon. Secondly, be it noted that the current scheme of the relations between cells and fibres is one founded on physiological postulates, not on observation. Thirdly, much of what is actually observed is very doubtful, because we do not know whether the appearances are normal, or due to modes of preparation and post-mortem changes. We cannot at present say, for instance, whether the fibrillated appearance of cell contents

and axis cylinder represents the living structure or not. We may either suppose that the neuroplasmic pulp splits longitudinally into fibrils, or that neuroplasmic threads resolve themselves into a homogeneous pulp—the axis cylinder may be a condensation of many fibrils, or the fibrils may be a resolution of the substance.

151. Let us contrast step by step the Imaginary Anatomy found in the text-books with the Objective Anatomy as at present disclosed by the researches of all the chief workers. Imaginary Anatomy assumes that the sensory fibre passes from a surface into the cells of the posterior horn of the spinal cord. Objective Anatomy sees the fibre pass into the grey substance, but declares that no direct entrance of a fibre into a cell is there visible.

Imaginary Anatomy assumes that from the sensory cells of the grey substance pass fibres in connection with the motor cells of the anterior horn, thus forming a direct channel through which the excitation of a sensory cell is transmitted to a motor cell. Objective Anatomy fails to discover any such direct channel—no such fibres are demonstrable.

Imaginary Anatomy assumes that from the motor cells issue fibres which descend to the muscles and glands, and carry there the motor impulses and the "mandates of the will." Objective Anatomy fails to find at the utmost more than a probability that these cells are continued as fibres, a probability which is founded on the rare facts of cell processes having been seen extending into the roots of the nerves, and of a cell process having occasionally been seen elsewhere continuous with a dark-bordered fibre. Granting, however, that this probability represents the fact, we have thus only one part of the "nervous arc" which can be said to have been verified.

Imaginary Anatomy further assumes that this nervous arc is connected with cerebral centres by means of fibres going upwards from the posterior cells, and fibres descending downwards to the anterior cells. Objective Anatomy sees nothing of the kind. It sees fibres entering the grey substance, and there lost to view in a mass of granular substance, fibrils, neuroblasts, and cells. There *may be* uninterrupted fibres passing upwards and downwards; but it is impossible to see them. And if we are told that physiological interpretations demand such a structure, we may fairly ask if this, and this only, is the structure which is adequate to the propagation of excitation? Now it seems to me that another kind of structure, and one more closely agreeing with what is observed, better answers the demands of Physiology. This will be more evident after the Laws of Nervous Action have been expounded in the succeeding chapter. Meanwhile we may remark that the arrangement of cells and fibres which is imagined as the mechanism of propagation and reflexion is absolutely irreconcilable with the teaching of Experiment: for the spinal cord may be cut through anywhere, without destruction of the transmission of sensory and motor excitations, provided only a small portion of grey substance be left to establish the continuity of the axis. Divide all the substance of the posterior half in one place, and all the substance of the anterior half in another, yet so long as there is a portion of grey substance left as a bridge between the lower and upper segments, the transmission of sensory and motor excitations will take place.

152. In other essential respects we have to note that the anatomical evidence for the current interpretations is absolutely deficient or contradictory. There is no adequate warrant for the assumption that all nerves have their origin in ganglia, all fibres in cells. Such evidence as at present exists is against that supposition, and in favour of the supposition that both cell and fibre are differentiations of a common neuroplasm, sometimes directly, sometimes indirectly continuous. Fibres, and plexuses of fibres, interspersed with cells irregularly distributed—now singly, now in small groups, now in larger and larger groups—constitute the *figured* elements of nerve-tissue; and even if we set aside the *amorphous* substance as indifferent or subordinate, we have still no ground for assigning the supremacy, much less the sole significance, to the cells. The grounds of this denial have been amply furnished in our exposition. For, let it be granted that nerve-cells are the origins of the fibres and the sources of their nutrition—a point which is eminently disputable—this would in no sense help the physiological hypothesis of the cell as the fountain of Neurility. If the fibre is simply the cell-contents drawn out longitudinally, if its essential element is identical with the essential element of the cell, then we can no more ascribe to the cell the exclusive property of Neurility than we can draw a lump of lead out into a wire, and then ascribe different properties to the thin end and the thick end. But on this point it is needless to speculate, since we have experimental evidence proving that the nerve-fibre has its Neurility even when separated from the cell, or even from the ganglion.

153. It is possible—I do not see sufficient evidence for a stronger assertion—that the cells are the nutritive sources of the fibres. They may represent the alimental rather than the instrumental activities of nervous life. (Compare PROBLEM I. § 42.) My contention is that in any case they are not the supreme elements of the active tissue, and in no sense can they be considered as *organs*. Only confusion of ideas could for a moment permit such language, or could assign central functions to cells which are elements of tissue. If the cell be credited with such powers anywhere, it must be credited with them everywhere. Now I ask what conceivable central function can be ascribed to a cell which terminates the fibre in a peripheral ganglion, or which is merely an enlargement in the course of a fibre in a nerve-bundle? Besides the facts already adduced, let attention be called to this: If a nerve-bundle from the *submucosa* of the intestine be examined, there appear among the fibres many nuclei (neuroblasts), and occasionally cells, unipolar and bipolar. These cells—if we may trust the observations of Rouget on the earliest development of nerves, and of Sigmund Mayer on regenerated nerves—are simply more advanced stages of evolution of the neuroblasts; but whatever their genesis may be, there can be nothing in the nature of a central function assigned to them.

154. It may be asked, What part can we assign to cells in neural actions if they are apolar, unipolar, and even when multipolar, isolated from each other, and from fibres? I confess that I have no answer ready, not even an hypothesis. Until some rational interpretation of the cell be given we must be content to hold an answer in suspense. What I would urge is that we are precipitate in assuming that the anatomical connection between one element and another must necessarily be that of a fibre. In a semi-fluid substance, such as neurine, continuity may be perfect without solid fibres: the amorphous substance and the plasmode may as well transmit waves of molecular motion from one part of the tissue to another, and therefore from cell to cell, or from cell to fibre, as a figured substance may. When the posterior root enters the grey substance of the cord, there is no more necessity for its fibres passing directly into the cells of that grey substance, in order to excite their activity, than there is for a wire to pass from the bell to the ear of the servant, who hears the vibrations of the bell through the pulsations of the intervening air upon her tympanum. Look at the structure of the retina, or the cerebellum, and you will find that the ganglionic cells which have processes passing in a direction contrary to that whence the stimulus arrives, have none where continuity of fibre and cell would be indispensable on the current hypothesis. Light stimulates the rods and cones, but there are no nerve-fibres, hitherto discovered, passing from these to the ganglionic cells; instead of that there is a ground-substance thickly interspersed with granules and nuclei. *From* the cells we see processes issue; *to* the cells none are seen arriving. So with the cerebellum. The large cells send their processes upwards to the surface; but downwards towards the white substance the processes are lost in the granular layer, which most histologists regard as connective tissue.

155. A mere glance at nervous tissue in any part will show that cells are far from forming the principal constituents. In the epidermis or a gland the cell is obviously the chief element, forming the bulk of the tissue, and being the characteristic agent. In nerve-tissue, as in connective tissue, the reverse is the case. We must therefore cease to regard

the cell as having the importance now attached to it, and must rather throw the emphasis on the fibres and neuroglia.

156. Before quitting this subject let a word be said on the amazing classification which has attained wide acceptance (although rejected by the most eminent authorities), founded on the size of the cells—the large multipolar cells being specified as motor, the smaller cells as sensory, while those of an intermediate size are sympathetic. I forbear to dwell on the development of this notion which specifies sensational, ideational, and emotional cells, because this does not pretend to have a basis in observation; whereas there are anatomical facts which give a certain superficial plausibility to the original classification. The conception is profoundly unphysiological; yet, if the anatomical evidence were constant, one might give it another interpretation. The evidence is, however, not constant. Large cells are found in regions assigned to sensory nerves, and small cells in motor regions. In the spinal cord of the tortoise Stieda declares that the so-called motor cells are limited to the cervical and lumbar enlargements; all the rest of the motor region being absolutely destitute of them.* Again look at the cells of the retina—no one will assign motor functions to them—yet they are the same as those of the cerebellum and the anterior horns of the spinal cord. (It is worth a passing mention that the structure of the nervous parts of the retina more closely resembles that of the cerebellum than of the cerebrum.)

157. While our knowledge of the cell is thus far indeed from having the precision which the text-books display, and in no sense warrants the current physiological interpretations, our knowledge of fibres and neuroglia is also too incomplete for theoretic purposes. We know that the axis cylinder is the essential element; but we are still at a loss what part is to be assigned to the medullary sheath. There is indeed a popular hypothesis which pronounces it to be the means of *insulating* the fibre, and thus preserving the isolated conduc-

* STIEDA: *Bau des centralen Nervensystem der Amphibien und Reptilien*, 1875, p. 41.

tion of nerve-force. Being of a fatty nature, this insulating office was readily suggested in agreement with the assumption that Neurility was Electricity. Now, without discussing whether Neurility is or is not Electricity, even admitting the former to be satisfactorily proved, I must remark that the admission still leaves the medullary sheath incapable of fulfilling the supposed office, since not only is there no such sheath in most of the invertebrates and in the sympathetic nerves of vertebrates, but even in those nerves which have the sheath it is precisely in places where the insulation would be most needed—namely, just before the terminations of the fibres in muscles and in centres—that the sheath is *absent*. This is as if we tried to conduct water through a pipe which fell short at both ends—before it left the cistern, and before it reached the spot to be watered. If there is a tendency in Neurility to spread wherever it is not insulated by a medullary sheath, then before reaching the centres and the muscles, it must, on the insulating hypothesis, dribble away!

158. The facts expressed in the "law of isolated conduction" are important, and are difficult of explanation; but it is obvious that they cannot be referred to the presence of the medullary sheath. Nor indeed will any insight into the propagation of stimulation through the central axis be intelligible until we have reformed our anatomical theories, and taken the Neuroglia into account. The theory which connects every fibre directly with a cell, and every cell with another by anastomosis—even were it demonstrated—would not explain the law of isolated conduction. Butzke cogently remarks * that such a disposition of the elements should render all neural paths invariable; whereas the fact is that they are very variable. We learn to perform actions, and then we unlearn them; the paths are traversed now in one direction, now in another. Fluctuation is the characteristic of central combinations. And for this fluctuating combination of elements a corresponding diversity is required in the possible channels. This seems to be furnished by the

* Butzke, in *Archiv für mikroskopische Anatomie*, Bd. iii. Heft 3, p. 596.

network of the Neuroglia. See the representation copied from Butzke's plate, and note how the cell-process blends

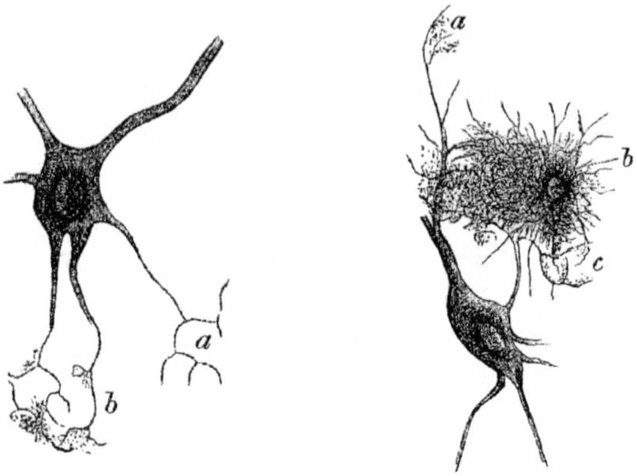

Fig. 26.—*Nerve-cells with processes terminating in neuroglia.*

with the meshes of the Neuroglia. Is it fanciful to regard this network of fibrils as having somewhat the relation of capillaries to blood-vessels? Did we not experimentally know that the capillaries are terminal blood-vessels, we should not suspect it from mere examination of the structure.

159. Having insisted that our knowledge is insufficient for any explanation of the "law of isolated conduction," I can only suggest a path of research which may lead to some result. What we know is that some stimulations are propagated from one end of the cerebro-spinal axis to the other in definitely *restricted* paths, while others are *irradiated* along many paths. In the succeeding chapter this will be more fully considered; what we have here to note is that the manifold irradiations of a stimulation have an anatomical substratum in the manifold subdivisions of the network of fibrils and the amorphous substance in which they penetrate.

160. In conclusion, I would say, let no one place a too great confidence in the reigning doctrines respecting the elementary structure of the nervous system, but accept every statement as a "working hypothesis" which has its value in so far as it links together verified facts, or suggests new research, but is wholly without value in so far as it is made a basis of deductions not otherwise verified. Hypotheses are indispensable to research, but they must be accompanied by vigilant scepticism. Imagination is only an enemy to Science when Scepticism is asleep.

CHAPTER VIII.

THE LAWS OF NERVOUS ACTIVITY.

161. THE foregoing remarks have had the object of showing how little substantial aid Psychology can at present derive from what is known of the elementary structure of the nervous system, indispensable as an accurate knowledge of that structure must be to a complete analysis of its functions. This caution has been specially addressed to those medical and psychological students whose researches leave them insufficient leisure to pursue microscopical investigations for themselves, and who are therefore forced to rely on second-hand knowledge, which is usually defective in the many qualifying considerations which keep scepticism vigilant. Relying on positive statements, and delusive diagrams which only display what the observer *imagines*, not what he actually *sees*, they construct on such data theories of disease, or of mental processes; or else they translate observed facts into the terms of this imaginary anatomy, and offer the translation as a new contribution to Science.

162. But little aid as can at present be derived from the teaching of the microscope, some aid Psychology may even now derive from it. The teaching will often serve, for instance, to correct the precipitate conclusions of subjective analysis, which present artificial distinctions as real distinctions, separating what Nature has united. It will show certain organic connections not previously suspected; and since whatever is organically connected cannot functionally be separated, such sharply-marked analytical distinctions as those of periphery and centre, or of sensation and motion, must be only regarded as artificial aids. The demonstration of the indissoluble union of the tissues is a demonstration of

their functional co-operation. So also the anatomical demonstration of the similarity and continuity of all parts of the central system sets aside the analytical separation of one centre from another, except as a convenient artifice; proving that cerebral substance is one with spinal substance, having the same properties, the same laws of action.

For the present, Psychology must seek objective aid from Physiology and Pathology rather than from elementary Anatomy. In the paragraphs which are to follow I shall endeavour to select the chief laws of nervous activity which the researches of physiologists and pathologists disclose. By these laws we may direct and control psychological research.

THE ENERGY OF NEURILITY.

163. Vitality is characterised by incessant molecular movement, both of composition and decomposition, in the building up of structure and the liberation of energy. The life of every organism is a complex of changes, each of which directly or indirectly affects the statical and dynamical relations, each being the resultant of many co-operant forces. In the nourishment of every organite there is an accumulation of molecular *tension*, that is to say, stored-up energy in a latent state, ready to be expended in the activity of that organite; and this expenditure may take place in a steady flow, or in a sudden gush. The molecular movements under one aspect may be called convergent, or *formative:* they build the structure, and tend to the state of equilibrium which we call the statical condition of the organite, *i.e.*, the condition in which it is not active, but ready to act. Perfect equilibrium is of course never attained, owing to the incessant molecular change: indeed Life is inconsistent with complete repose. Under another aspect the molecular movements may be called *discharging:* they constitute the dynamic condition of the organite, in which its functional activity appears. The energy is now diverted, liberated, and the surplus, over and above that which is absorbed in formation, instead of slowly dribbling off, gushes forth in a directed stream. The slow formation of a secretion in a gland-cell, and the discharge of that secretion, will illustrate this; or (if muscular *tone* be admitted) the incipient contraction of the chronic state, and the complete contraction of the dynamic state, may also be cited.

164. The discharge which follows excitation may thus be viewed as a *directed quantity* of molecular movement. Because it is always strictly relative to the energy of tension, and is inevitable when that tension attains a certain surplus over what is required in construction, there is a limit, 1°, to the growth and evolution of every organite, and every organism (comp. Problem I. § 118), and, 2°, to its dynamical effect. When there is no surplus, the organite is incapable of discharge: it is then exhausted, *i.e.*, will not respond to stimulus.

165. The speciality of nerve-tissue is its pre-eminence in directive energy. Like all other tissues, it grows, develops, and dies; but above all others it has what we call *excitability*, or readiness in discharging its energy in a directed stream. By its topographical distribution it plays the functional part of exciting the activity of other tissues: it transmits molecular disturbance from periphery to centre, from centre to centre, and from centre to muscles, vessels, and glands. When a muscle is excited it moves, and when a gland is excited it secretes; but these actions end, so to speak, with themselves; the muscle does not directly move any other muscle;* the gland does not directly excite any other gland.

* Except in the rare cases where there is anastomosis of the muscle-fibres; as, for example, in the heart. [According to ENGELMANN'S remarkable researches, the muscles of the heart form a continuum, so that irritation is propagated from one to the other: *Pflüger's Archiv*, 1875, p. 465. This is indubitably the case in the embryonic heart, as ECKHARD pointed out.] This I hold to be the main cause of its rhythmic pulsation after removal from the body. Whatever influence the ganglia may have in exciting this pulsation, such influence would be powerless were not the muscles so connected; as may be seen in the other organs which are richly supplied with ganglia, yet do not move spontaneously; and in organs (such as the ureter or the embryonic heart, and the hearts of invertebrata) which move spontaneously, yet have no ganglia.

The nerve, on the contrary, has always a widespreading effect: it excites a centre which is continuous with other centres; and in exciting one muscle, usually excites a group. Hence the nervous system is that *which binds the different organs into a dynamic unity.* And Comparative Anatomy teaches that there is a parallelism between the development of this system and the efficient complexity of the organism. As the tissues become more and more specialised, and the organs more and more individualised, they would become more and more unsuited to the general service of the organism, were it not that a corresponding development of the nervous system brought a unifying mechanism.

The great instability of neurine, in other words, its high degree of tension, renders it especially apt to disturb the tension of other tissues. It is very variable; and this variability will have to be taken into account in explaining the restriction of discharges to particular centres. A good example of exaggerated tension is furnished by strychnine poisoning. The centres are then so readily excitable that a touch, or a puff of cold air on the skin, will determine convulsions. And it is worthy of remark that for some hours after this convulsive discharge the centres return to something like their normal state; and the animal may then be stroked, pinched, or blown upon without abnormal reactions. But during this interval the centres are slowly accumulating excess of tension from the poisoned blood; and at the close, convulsions will again follow the slightest stimulus. This alternation of exhaustion and recrudescence is noticed by Schröder van der Kolk in the periodicity of the phenomena exhibited in spinal disease.*

THE PROPAGATION OF EXCITATION.

166. Understanding, then, that the propagation of an excitation depends on the state of tension of the tissue, and always follows the line of least resistance, whichever that

* SCHRÖDER VAN DER KOLK: *Bau und Funktionen der Med. Spinalis* p. 67.

may be at the moment, we have to inquire whether the transmission takes place only in one direction, from periphery to centre in sensory nerves, and from centre to periphery in motor nerves? By most physiologists this is answered affirmatively. Indeed a special property has been assigned to each nerve, in virtue of this imaginary limitation of centripetal and centrifugal conduction. The "nerve-current" (accepted as a physical fact, and not simply a metaphor) is supposed to "flow" from the central cells along the motor nerve to the muscles; but by a strange oversight the current is also made to "flow" *towards* the central cells which are said to produce it! Now although the fact may be, and probably is, that normally the sensory nerve, being stimulated at its peripheral end, propagates the stimulation towards the centre, and the motor nerve propagates its central stimulation towards the periphery, the question whether each nerve is not capable of transmission in both directions is not thus answered. *A priori* it is irrational to assert that nerves fundamentally alike in composition and structure are unlike in properties; and we might as well suppose that a train of gunpowder could only be fired at one end, as to suppose that a nerve could only be excited at one end. And how does the evidence support this *a priori* conclusion? Dubois Reymond proved that each nerve conducted electricity in both directions; but as Neurility has not been satisfactorily shown to be identical with the electric current, this may not be considered decisive. Such a doubt does not hang over the following facts. M. Paul Bert, pursuing John Hunter's curious experiments on animal *grafting*, has grafted the tail of a rat under the skin of the rat's back, the tip of the tail being inserted under the skin, its base rising into the air, so that there is here an inversion of the normal position. In the course of time Sensibility gradually reappears in this grafted tail; and at the end of about twelvemonths the rat not only feels when the tail is pinched, but knows *where* the irritation lies, and turns round to bite the pincers.* Here

* It is very instructive to learn that for some six months or so the rat is quite incapable of correctly *localising* the pain.

we have a case of a sensory nerve reversed, yet transmitting stimulation from the base to the tip of the tail, instead of from the tip to the base, as in a normal organ. Vulpian and Philippeaux having divided two nerves, united the central end of the sensory nerve with the peripheral end of the motor nerve; when the organic union was complete, and each nerve was formed out of the halves of two different nerves, the effect of pinching one of these was to produce simultaneously pain and movement, showing that the excitation was transmitted upwards to the centre, and downwards to the muscles.* It may be compared with a train of gunpowder having a loaded cannon at one end and a bundle of straw at the other, when if a spark be dropped anywhere on this train, the flame runs along in both directions, explodes the cannon, and sets alight the straw.

167. Indeed we have only to remember the semi-liquid nature of the axis cylinder to see at once that it must conduct a wave of motion as readily in one direction as in another. A liquid transmits waves in any direction according to the initial impulse. There is consequently no reason for asserting that because the usual direction is centripetal in a sensory nerve, and centrifugal in a motor nerve, each nerve is *incapable* of transmitting excitations in both directions. And I think many phenomena are more intelligible on the assumption that neural transmission is in both directions. If the eye is fixed steadfastly on a particular colour during some minutes, the retina becomes exhausted, and no longer responds to the stimulus of that colour: here the stimulation is of course centripetal. But if instead of looking intently on the colour, the mind (in complete absence of light) pictures it intently, *this cerebral image is equally capable of exhausting the retina;* and unless we believe that colour is a

* VULPIAN: *Leçons sur le Système Nerveux*, p. 288. The experiment has been confirmed by ROSENTHAL, and by BIDDER (*Archiv für Anatomie*, 1865, p. 246), who first (in 1842) attempted this union of different nerves, but arrived at negative results; as did SCHIFF (*Lehrbuch der Physiol.*, 1859, p. 134) and GLUGE *et* THIERNESSE (*Annales des Sciences Naturelles*, 1859, p. 181).

cerebral, not a retinal phenomenon (which is my private opinion), we must accept this as proof of a centrifugal excitation of a sensory tract. Another illustration may be drawn from the muscular sense. There may be a few sensory fibres distributed to muscles; but even if the observations of Sachs * should be confirmed, I do not think that all muscle sensations can be assigned to these fibres, but that the so-called motor fibres must also co-operate. When a nerve acts upon a muscle, the muscle reacts on the nerve; and when a nerve acts on a centre, the centre reacts on the nerve. The agitation of the central tissue cannot leave the nerve which blends with it unaffected; the agitation of the muscular tissue must also by a reversal of the "current" affect its nerve. Laplace points out how the movement of the hand which holds a suspended chain is propagated along the chain to its terminus, and if when the chain is at rest we once more set that terminus in motion, the vibration will remount to the hand.† The contraction of a muscle will not only stimulate the sensory fibres distributed through it, but also, I conceive, stimulate the very motor fibres which caused the contraction, since these fibres blend with the muscle.‡

168. To understand this, it is necessary to remember that the stimulation of a nerve does not arise § in the *changed state* of that nerve, but in the *process of change*, *i.e.*, the disturb-

* SACHS, in the *Archiv für Anat.*, 1874, pp. 195, *sq.*

† LAPLACE: *Essai Philos. sur les Probabilités*, p. 239.

‡ The mode of termination of nerves in muscles is still a point on which histologists disagree; probably because there is no abrupt termination, but a blending of the one tissue with the other. In the Tardigrades, for example, there is actually no appreciable distinction between nerve and muscle at the point of insertion of the nerve; and if in the higher animals there is an appreciable difference between nerve and muscle, there is an inseparable blending of undifferentiated substance at their point of junction. [According to ENGELMANN's recent researches, there seems good reason to suppose that muscles are composed of contractile substance and a substance which is a modification of axis-cylinder substance: the first being doubly refracting, the second isotropic: *Pflüger's Archiv*, 1875, p. 432.]

§ SCHIFF: *Lehrbuch*, p. 73.

ance of the tension. The duration of the stimulation is that of the changing process, and the intensity increases with the differential of the velocity of change. So that when a nerve which has been excited by a change of state returns to its former state, this return—being another change—is a new excitation. That it is not the changed state, but the change, which is operative, explains the fact noted by Brown Séquard: a frog poisoned by strychnine, when decapitated and all respiration destroyed, will remain motionless for days together, if carefully protected from all external excitation; but its nervous system is in such a state of tension all this time that the first touch produces general convulsions. Freusberg also notes that if a brainless frog be suspended by the lower jaw, and one foot be pinched, the other leg is moved at first, then quickly droops again, and remains at rest until the pincers are removed from the pinched foot, when suddenly all four legs are violently moved by the *stimulation which the simple removal produces.* Let us also add the well-known and significant fact that if a nerve be divided rapidly by a sharp razor, neither sensation nor motion is produced, because the intensity of a stimulus being, to speak mathematically, *the function of the changing process,* the duration of the process is in this case too brief. On the same ground the application of a stimulus will excite no movement, if the force be very slowly increased from zero to an intensity which will destroy the nerve; but at any stage a *sudden* increase will excite a movement.

169. We may group all the foregoing considerations in this formula:

LAW I. Every neural process is due to a sudden disturbance of the molecular tension. The liberated energy is discharged along the lines of least resistance.

The conditions which determine the lines of least resistance are manifold and variable. The nervous system is a continuous whole, each part of which is connected with diverse organs; but in spite of this anatomical diversity, the deeper uniformity causes the activity of each part to depend on and involve the activity of every other, more or less. By "more or less" is meant, that although the excitation of one part necessarily affects the state of all the others, because of their structural community, so that *each sensation and each motion really represents a change in the whole organism,* yet the responsive discharge determined in each organ by this change, depends on the tension of the organ and its centre at that moment. A bad harvest really affects the whole nation; but its effect is conspicuous on the welfare of the poor rather than of the rich, although the price of bread is the same to rich and poor. Nervous centres, and muscular or glandular organs, differ in their excitability; one condition of this greater excitability being the greater frequency with which they are called into activity. The medulla oblongata is normally more excitable than the medulla spinalis; the heart more than the limbs. Hence a stimulus which will increase the respiration and the pulse may have no *appreciable* effect on the limbs; but some effect it must have.

170. Imagine all the nerve-centres to be a connected group of bells varying in size. Every agitation of the connecting wire will more or less agitate all the bells; but since some are heavier than others, and some of the cranks less movable, there will be many vibrations of the wire which will cause some bells to sound, others simply to oscillate without sounding, and others not sensibly to oscillate. Even some of the lighter bells will not ring if any external pressure arrests them; or if they are already ringing, the added impulses, not being rhythmically timed, will *arrest* the ringing. So the stimulus of a sensory nerve agitates its centre, and through it the whole system; usually the stimulation is mainly reflected on the group of muscles innervated from that centre, because this is the readiest path of discharge; but it sometimes does not mainly discharge along this path, the line of least resistance lying in another direction; and the discharge never takes this path without also irradiating upwards and downwards through the central tissue. Thus irradiated, it falls into the general stream of neural processes; and according to the state in which the various centres are at the moment it modifies their activity. A nervous shock—

physical or mental—sensibly affects all the organs. A severe wound paralyses, for a time, parts far removed from the wounded spot. A blow on the stomach will arrest the heart; a fright will do the same. Terror relaxes the limbs, or sets them trembling; so does a concussion: if a frog be thrown violently on the ground, all its muscles are convulsed; but if the nerves of one limb be divided before the shock, the muscles of that limb will not be convulsed.

171. We are apt to regard the discharge on the moving organs as if that were the sole response of a stimulation; but although the most conspicuous, it is by no means the most important effect. Besides exciting the muscles, more or less, every neural process has its influence on the organic processes of secretion, and effects thermal and electrical changes. Schiff has demonstrated that every sensation raises the temperature of the brain; Nothnagel, that irritation of a sensory nerve causes constriction of the cerebral arteries, and hence cerebral anæmia. Brown Séquard and Lombard find the temperature of a limb raised when its skin is pinched, and lowered when the skin *elsewhere* is pinched. Georges Pouchet has shown that fishes change colour according to the brightness or darkness of the ground over which they remain; and these changes are dependent on nervous stimulation, mainly through the eye, division of the optic nerves preventing the change. These are so many *a posteriori* confirmations of what *a priori* may be foreseen. They are cited here merely to enforce the consideration, seldom adequately kept before the mind, that every neural process is a change which causes other changes in the whole organism.

STIMULI.

172. Stimuli are classed as external and internal, or physical and physiological. The one class comprises all the agencies in the External Medium which *appreciably* affect the organism; the other class all the changes *in* the organism which appreciably disturb the equilibrium of any organ. Although the pressure of the atmosphere, for example, unquestionably affects the organism, and determines organic processes, it is not reckoned as a stimulus unless the effect become appreciable under sudden variations of the pressure. In like manner the blood is not reckoned among the internal stimuli, except when sudden variations in its composition, or its circulation, determine appreciable changes. Because the external stimuli, and the so-called Senses which respond to them, are more conspicuous than the internal stimuli and the Systemic Senses, they have unfortunately usurped too much attention. The massive influence of the Systemic Sensations in determining the desires, volitions, and conceptions of mankind has not been adequately recognised. Yet every one knows the effect of impure air, or a congested liver, in swaying the mental mood; and how a heavy meal interferes with muscular and mental exertion.* What is conspicuous in such marked effects, is less conspicuously, but not less necessarily, present in slighter stimuli.

173. A constant pressure on the tympanum excites no sound; only a rhythmic alternation of pressures will excite the sensation. A constant temperature is not felt; only changes in temperature. If Light and Sound were as uniform as the circulation of the blood, or the pressure of the atmosphere, we should be seldom conscious of the existence of these stimuli. But because the changes are varied and marked, our attention is necessarily arrested by them. The changes going on within the tissues are too graduated to fix the attention; it is only by considering their cumulative effects that we become impressed with their importance. For example, the development of the sexual glands determines conspicuous physical and moral results—we note consequent effects on voice, hair, horns, structure of the skull and size of the muscles, no less than the rise of new feelings, desires, instincts, ideas. Any organic interference with the

* FREUSBERG observed that the reflex movements in the legs of a dog whose spine had been divided were considerably lessened after food or drink. They fell from 95 to 46 pendulum-beats in a minute after a *litre* of water had been drunk. See his instructive memoir, *Reflex-Lähmungen beim Hunde*, in *Pflüger's Archiv*, 1874, p. 369.

activity of the ovaries will alter the moral disposition of the animal: suppression of this organic process means non-development of the feelings of maternity; the moral superstructure is absent because its physical basis is wanting.

174. Blood supplies the tissues with their plasmodes; a constant supply of oxygenated blood is therefore necessary to the vitality of the tissues. But it is an error to suppose that oxygen is the special stimulus of nerve-centres, or that their activity depends on their oxidation; on the contrary, the deficiency of oxygen or surplus of carbonic acid is that which stimulates. When saturated with oxygen, the blood paralyses respiration; when some of the oxygen is withdrawn, respiration revives. Here—as in all other cases—we have to remember that differences in degree readily pass into differences in kind, so that an excess of a stimulus produces a reversal of the effect; thus although surplus of carbonic acid excites respiratory movements, excess of carbonic acid causes Asphyxia. Abundance of blood is requisite for the continuous activity of nerve-centres; but while a temporary deficiency of blood renders them more excitable, too great a deficiency paralyses them. Anæmia, which causes great excitability, and convulsions (so that nerves when dying are most irritable), may easily become the cause of the death of the tissue. There are substances which can only be dissolved by a given quantity of liquid; if this quantity be in excess, they are precipitated from the solution. There are vibrations of a given order which cause each string to respond; change the special order, and the string returns to its repose.

In the stillness and darkness of the night we are excluded from most of the external stimuli, yet a massive stream of systemic sensations keeps the sensitive mechanism active, and in sleep directs the dreams. The cramps and epileptiform attacks which occur during sleep are most probably due to the over-excitability produced by surplus carbonic acid. To temporary anæmia may be assigned the strange exaggeration of our sensations during the moments which precede awakening; and the greater vividness of dream-images.

It is only needful to mention in passing the varied stimuli by which cerebral changes act upon the organism. The mention of a name will cause a blush, a brightening of the eye, a quickening of the pulse. The thought of her absent infant will cause a flow of milk in the mother's breast.

175. We may formulate the foregoing considerations in another law:

LAW II. The neural excitation, which is itself a change, directly causes a change in the organ innervated, and indirectly in the whole organism.

The significance of this law is, that although for the convenience of research and exposition we isolate one organ from the rest of the organism, and one process from all the co-operant processes, we have to remember that this is an artifice, and that in reality there is no such separation.

STIMULATION.

176. Passing now from these general considerations to their special application, we may formulate the law of stimulation:

LAW III. A faint or moderate stimulation increases the activity of the organ; but beyond a certain limit, increase of stimulation diminishes, and finally arrests, the activity. Duration of stimulation is equivalent to increase.

A muscle stimulated contracts; if the stimulation be repeated, the muscle becomes tetanised, and in this state has reached its limit; a fresh stimulation then *relaxes* the muscle. A very faint stimulation of the vagus quickens the pulsation of the heart, but a slight increase, or duration of the stimulation, slackens and arrests the heart.* Every one

* M. HERZEN thus describes the effects of stimulating the vagus with varying intensities: "Si l'on se sert de l'appareil de Dubois Reymond, on commence par appliquer une irritation tellement faible qu'elle ne produit aucun effet; on rapproche alors peu à peu les deux bobines de l'appareil avec le plus grand soin, par fractions de centimètres, par *millimètres* s'il le faut, et l'on trouve ainsi le degré d'irritation qui accelère les battements du cœur et qui produit le maximum de pulsa-

knows how a moderate feeling of surprise, pleasure, or pain quickens the heart and the respiration; and how a shock of surprise, joy, grief, or great physical pain depresses, and even arrests them. Excess of light is blinding; excess of sound deafening.

177. The nervous system is incessantly stimulated, and variably. Hence a great variation in the excitability of different parts. While the regular and moderate activity of one part is accompanied by a regular flow of blood to it, so that there is a tolerably constant rhythm of nutrition and discharge, any irregular or excessive activity exhausts it, until there has been a nutritive restoration. We can thus understand how one centre may be temporarily exhausted while a neighbouring centre is vigorous. Cayrade decapitated a frog, and suspended light weights to each of its hind legs; when either leg was stimulated, the weight attached to it was raised. After each repetition the weight was raised less and less, until finally the weight ceased to be raised: the centre had been exhausted. But now when the other leg, which had been in repose, was stimulated, it energetically contracted, and raised its attached weight; showing that its centre was not exhausted by the action of the other.*

178. This seems in contradiction with the principle that the excitation of one centre is an excitation of all. It also seems in contradiction with the principle urged by Herzen, that irritation of one sciatic nerve *diminishes* the excitability

tions dans l'unité de temps admise pour l'expérience. Quand on est là il suffit *d'un millimètre* de plus pour faire disparaître l'augmentation, un autre millimètre peut produire une diminution, et un *troisième* peut arrêter le cœur complètement. En reculant alors, en éloignant peu à peu les deux bobines, *on rêtourne à la force qui produit l'augmentation des battements.*" HERZEN: *Expériences sur les Centres Modérateurs de l'Action Réflexe,* 1864, p. 68. There have been serious doubts thrown on these experiments; but several experimenters have confirmed their exactness. Quite recently they have been confirmed by BULGHERI: *Il Morgagni,* viii.; and by ARLOING and TRIPIER: *Archives de Physiologie,* 1872, iv. p. 418. It must be confessed, however, that the whole subject of the heart's innervation is at present very imperfectly understood.

* CAYRADE: *Recherches sur les Mouvements Réflexes,* 1864, p. 58.

of the opposite leg; and this again seems contradicted by the principle urged by Setschenow, that although moderate excitation of one sciatic nerve will diminish the excitability of the other, a powerful excitation will increase it.

179. All three principles are, I believe, exact expressions of experimental evidence; and their seeming contradictions may be reconciled on a wider survey of the laws of neural activity, interpreted according to the special conditions of each case. These laws may be conveniently classified as Laws of Discharge, and Laws of Arrest; the second being only a particular aspect of the first.

THE LAW OF DISCHARGE.

180. The physiological independence of organs, together with their intimate dependence in the organism, and the fact that this organism is incessantly stimulated from many sides at once, assure us *a priori* that the "waves" of molecular movement due to each stimulus must sometimes interfere and sometimes blend with others, thus diverting or neutralising the final discharge in the one case, and in the other case swelling the current and increasing the energy of the discharge. We are accustomed to speak of one part "playing on another," sympathising with another, and so on; but what is the process expressed in these metaphors? When an idea, or a painful sensation, quickens the pulse, or increases the flow of a secretion, we are not to imagine that from a spot in the cerebrum, or the surface, there is a nerve-fibre going directly to the heart, or the gland, transmitting an impulse; in each case the central tissue has been agitated by a sudden change at the stimulated point, and the discharge on heart and gland is the resultant of this agitation along the lines of least resistance. The nerves of the great toe, for example, pass into the spinal cord at a considerable distance from the spot where the nerves of the arm enter it; when, therefore, the great toe is pinched, the arm does not move by direct stimulation of its nerves, but by the indirect stimulation which has traversed the whole central substance.

181. This is intelligible when we know that the whole central substance is continuous throughout; but the difficulty arises when we have to explain why, if this central substance is stimulated throughout, *only* arms and legs respond; in other words, why the toe-centre "plays upon" the arm-centre, and not on the others? When a frog is decapitated, if we gently touch one leg with the point of the scalpel, the leg will move, but only this leg. Prick more forcibly, and both legs will move. Keep on pricking, and all four legs are drawn up, and the frog hops away. Each excitation was propagated along the cord; but the discharge was restricted in the first case to one limb, in the second to two, in the third it involved all the muscles of the trunk. At the sight of a friend a dog wags his tail gently: as there is no *direct* connection between the optic nerves and the tail, this playing of one centre on another must be by the agency of intermediate centres; and we know that if the dog's spinal cord be divided, this excitation from the optic centre is no longer possible, yet the tail will wag if the abdomen be tickled, or the leg pinched. Now compare the effect on the dog produced by the sight of his master, or of a friend accustomed to take him out. There is no longer a gentle wagging of the tail, but an agitation of the whole body: he barks, leaps, and runs about; the central stimulation is discharged through many outlets; and could we test the effect, we should find an appreciable alteration in the thermal and electrical condition of the whole organism, with corresponding changes in circulation, secretion, &c. So different are the consequences of two slightly different retinal impressions mingling their stimulations with the same mass of central substance!

182. The discharge is determined by two conditions: the state of tension, and the energy of the stimulation. *The state of tension is increased by every stimulation which falls short of a discharge;* that is to say, faint and frequent stimulation augments the excitability, whereas powerful stimulation exhausts it. When, therefore, one wave succeeds another in the same direction, it reaches a centre more disposed to discharge; or, as Cayrade expresses it, "a certain agitation of the cells is necessary for the manifestation of their property of reaction, in the same way that the concentric circles produced on the surface of water by a falling stone are more rapid and more numerous if a stone has already agitated the surface."

183. So much for the tension. What has been called the energy of the stimulation is more complicated. It is not measurable as a simple physical process; we cannot say that a given quantity of any external force will determine a given discharge. It is mostly complicated by psychical processes, and these so modify the result that instead of the predicted discharge there is arrest, or discharge from another centre. Press a dog's skin with increasing violence, and the effect increases from pleasurable to painful irritation; but whether the dog will cry out and bite, or cry out and struggle to escape, depends upon whether the pincher is a stranger or a friend. If you hurt a dog while removing a thorn from its foot it will cry out, but although the pain causes it to initiate a biting movement, by the time your hand is reached that movement will have been changed, and the dog will lick the hand which he knows is hurting him in the endeavour to relieve him of the thorn. The co-operation of the mind is here evident enough. A purely psychical process has interfered with the purely physiological process. And I shall hereafter endeavour to show that psychical processes analogous in kind though simpler in degree are really co-operant in actions of the spinal cord. The dog would be said to discriminate between the pain inflicted by a friend, and the same pain inflicted by a stranger. In other words, the sensitive mechanism would be differently determined in the direction of discharge, although the initial stimulation was the same in each case. If we admit that the resulting action is in each case the consequence of the particular group of elements co-operating, there will be no ground for denying that analogous *discrimination* is manifested by the brainless animal, who also responds differently to different external stimuli, and differently to the same stimulus under different central conditions. The brainless frog croaks if its back be

gently stroked with the handle of a scalpel; but if the point be used, or if the handle be roughly pressed, instead of croaking, the frog raises his leg in defence. Here the difference in the peripheral irritation has excited a different reaction in the centre; and this might be interpreted as purely physical; if now the leg be fastened, and the movement of defence be thus prevented, the frog will employ the other leg; or adopt some other means of relieving itself from the irritation. It was a mass of registered experiences which determined the dog not to bite his master. An analogous registration of experiences determines the changed reactions of the brainless frog. But this is a point which can only be touched on in passing here, and it is touched on merely to facilitate our exposition of the complicated conditions of neural discharge. These may be formulated in

184. Law IV. The simultaneous influence of several stimuli, each of which separately excites the same centre, is cumulative: stimuli then assist each other, and their resultant is their *arithmetical* sum.

Simultaneous stimuli, each of which excites a different centre, *interfere* with each other's energy, and their resultant is their *algebraical* sum.

In this law there is a condensed expression of that composition of forces which may either result in Discharge or Arrest. By simultaneity is not to be understood merely the coincidence of impressions, but also the reverberations of impressions not yet neutralised by others. Thus when Sensibility is tested by the now common method,* it is found that if one leg is withdrawn after a lapse of, say, ten pendulum beats, the other leg, which has not been irritated, will nevertheless, on irritation, be withdrawn in less than ten beats, provided the central agitation caused by the first stimulation has *not yet subsided*. But, on the contrary, the withdrawal will be considerably deferred, or even prevented altogether, if at the same time that the leg is acted on by the

* A frog's brain is removed, and the body then suspended by the lower jaw, the legs are allowed to dip into a slightly acidulated liquid, the chemical action of which stimulates the skin.

acid, a more powerful excitation takes place in some other part of the body. In the one experiment we see simultaneous excitation in the same centre and the same direction. In the other simultaneous excitation in different centres. The more powerful excitation suppresses the discharge from the less powerful; but although it prevails, it loses just as much force as it arrests.*

185. There is another very interesting experiment by Freusberg, which must be cited here.† When the sciatic nerve is divided, the frog's leg is of course not withdrawn from the acidulated water, because in that case no sensory excitation is propagated from the skin to the centre; but although there is no stimulation from the skin, there is one from the muscles, as appears in the fact that if a small weight be suspended on this leg, the other leg is more rapidly withdrawn from the acidulated water—the action of the muscles having affected the centre and increased its excitability.

186. When the motor group of one leg is moderately stimulated, the discharge is confined to the muscles of that one leg; and according to Herzen the excitability of the motor group of the other leg is thereby somewhat diminished. But if the stimulation be increased, there is an irradiation to the other group, which irradiation, although not sufficient to excite a discharge, renders it much more *ready* to discharge, so that a feeble stimulus suffices. This accords with Setschenow's observations, and is confirmed by Freusberg's experiment, in which, when one leg was stimulated by acid, if the acid were not wiped off but allowed to keep up the irritation, the other leg moved without being irritated; and this other

* I saw a patient in the Berlin *Charité* whose face and left hand were in a constant state of convulsive twitching, but no sooner was a scar on the left hand (where the nerve had been divided) firmly pressed than the twitchings ceased, and *pain* was felt; on removal of the pressure, pain ceased and the twitchings returned.

† *Pflüger's Archiv*, 1875. No one interested in the Reflex Theory should omit a careful study of the papers by FREUSBERG and GOLTZ. I have drawn freely from them.

leg having come to rest, when in its turn dipped in the acid, was more rapidly withdrawn than the first leg had been on first being stimulated; showing that the central groups had become more excitable by the stimulation of either leg.

187. While it is intelligible that an excitation of one group should increase the activity of neighbouring groups, by an increase of the vascular activity of the region, it is not so readily intelligible why the feebler excitation of one group should diminish the excitability of its neighbour; yet the facts seem to warrant both statements.

188. The conditions which determine Discharge are obscure. We may, however, say that anatomical and physiological data force the conclusion that whenever the central tissue is powerfully stimulated in any one part, there is either a discharge, or a greater tension (tendency to discharge) in every other part; in consequence of which, every fresh stimulus in the *same* direction finds the parts more prepared to react; while every fresh stimulus in a *contrary* direction meets with a proportional resistance. Stated thus generally, the principle is clear enough; but the immense complication of stimulations, and the statical variableness of the organs, renders its application to particular cases extremely obscure. Why does the ticking of a clock arrest the attention, even with unpleasant obtrusiveness, at one time, and presently afterwards cease to be heard at all? Why does the cut of a knife cause intense pain, and a far greater cut received during the heat and agitation of a quarrel pass unfelt? Why will the same external force excite convulsions in all the muscles, and at another time scarcely be distinguishable? These are consequences of the temporary condition of the centres; but there are permanent conditions which in some organisms determine equally variable results. Thus the shock of terror which will simply agitate one person, will develop an epileptic attack in another, and insanity in a third; just as exposure to cold will in one person congest the liver, in another the lungs. A loud and sudden sound causes winking in most persons, and in many a sort of convulsive shock. The harsh noise of a file causes a shiver in some persons, and

in others "sets the teeth on edge," while in others it causes an increased flow of saliva.

189. Nerves and centres have different degrees of excitability. The nerve-terminals in the skin are more sensitive to impressions than those in the mucous membrane; those in the alimentary canal are more sensitive than those in the peritoneum; and all nerve-terminals are more sensitive than nerve-trunks. A touch on the surface of the larynx will produce a cough, but the nerve-trunk itself may be pinched or galvanised without producing any such reflex. Moreover, there is the difference of grouping. If the skin of the abdomen be tickled, there is a reflex on the adductor and extensor muscles of the leg; but these movements are reversed if the skin of the back be tickled. Nor indeed are these movements invariable in either case; the one series will sometimes quite suddenly change to the other, if the irritation is kept up. That one and the same stimulus applied to the same spot should now excite this group and now the other, shows that *both* motor groups are affected, and that the discharge takes place from the one which at the time being is in the highest tension. The alternation of tension explains rhythmical discharge.

THE LAW OF ARREST.

190. The Law of Arrest is only another aspect of the Law of Discharge, and may be regarded as the conflict of excitations. If a stranger enters the room where a woman lies in labour, there will often be caused a sudden cessation of the uterine contractions.* Again, every one knows how the breathing and the beating of the heart are arrested by the idea of danger. The arrest is in each of the three cases only temporary, because when the shock of the new stimulus has caused its discharge (arrest), the peripheral irritation which

* Sir JAMES PAGET has an interesting collection of facts which illustrate this Law of Arrest, in his paper on "Stammering with other Organs than those of Speech," *British Medical Journal*, 1868, vol. ii. p. 437, reprinted in his *Clinical Lectures and Essays*, 1875, p. 77.

caused the former discharges resumes its influence, and uterus, heart, and diaphragm begin to move again, even more energetically. Note, moreover, that not only will the cerebral excitation arrest the spinal discharge—an idea check the contractions of the uterus or the heart—but the reverse also takes place. The brain of the woman may be intently occupied with some scheme for the education or welfare of her expected child, but no sooner do the labour pains set in, than all these cerebral combinations are arrested.

191. One sensation arrests another; one idea displaces another. If the foreleg of a headless frog be irritated, the hind-leg will also be moved by the stimulation; or *vice versa.* Here there has been a propagation of the excitation in either direction. But if while the legs are thus irritated, and the centres are ready to discharge, another and more powerful irritation reach the centre—say by pinching the skin of the back—there will be no discharge on the legs. If the vagus be irritated, the heart is arrested; but this does not take place if at the same time, or immediately before, the foot has been sharply pinched. A few gentle taps on the abdomen suffice to stop the heart; but if a drop of acid be previously placed on the skin, we tap in vain, the heart continues to beat. Brown Séquard cites several cases in which convulsions were arrested by irritation of sensitive surfaces;* and Dr. Crichton Browne records a case of a patient in whom there was abolition of spinal reflex, due to cerebral irritation: tickling the soles of the feet, or pricking the toes, which normally excites reflex movements, in this case excited none whatever. "This seems to prove that nerve currents, set in motion by irritation of the brain, or some of its convolutions, transmitted down the cord, may inhibit reflex action."† Examples might indefinitely be multiplied. Pinch the skin of a rabbit between the eyes, and you will observe that pulse and respiration are slackened; but if the tail, which is very sensitive, be pinched, this slackening is only momentary, and is succeeded by a quickening—unless the pain be great. Even

* *Archives de Physiol.*, 1868, p. 157.

† *West Riding Lunatic Asylum Reports*, 1874, p. 200.

the effect of intense pain may be neutralised by stimulating the vagus—just as the effect of stimulating the vagus may be neutralised by pain. Claude Bernard found that having dropped ammonia on the eyelid of a dog, the pain caused a convulsive closure of the lid; but on galvanising the vagus, the lid opened again, to be closed when the galvanism ceased.* When the heart is beating faintly (as in syncope), any irritating vapour applied to the nostrils will cause a more energetic pulsation; yet a very irritating vapour lowers the action of the heart beating normally, and will even arrest that of a rabbit. Over-stimulation has almost always the opposite effect of moderate stimulation.

192. While there seems every reason to believe that an excitation necessarily affects the whole cerebro-spinal axis, there is no doubt that there is a certain restriction of this irradiation to definite paths, *i.e.*, the responsive discharge is confined to definite groups. Some of these restrictions are connate pathways: we bring them with us at birth; but most of them are pathways acquired after birth. The boy who sheds tears at parting from his mother when he goes to school, will shed no tears when he parts from her to go to college, nay, perhaps will shed none when he parts from her for ever: not that his love has lessened, but that the idea of such expression of it as "unmanly" has become an organised tendency and arrests the tears. A youth of southern race, who has not learned to be ashamed of tears, weeps freely under such circumstances.

193. The pathways organised at birth are not many. Examples are the inspiration which follows expiration; the movements of coughing when the larynx is tickled; the movements of swallowing, sneezing, &c. Even these may be arrested for a brief time by what is called "the will;" but when once the discharge begins in any part of the mechanism, the whole group is necessarily involved and the action is then inevitable. Many of the reflex actions which are universal are nevertheless acquired. Winking, for instance, when an object approaches the eye, is universal among us,

* CLAUDE BERNARD: *Système Nerveux*, i. 383.

but is never seen in infants, nor in animals. It is even doubtful whether the drawing up of the leg when the toes are pinched is not an acquired reflex. Doubtful, I mean, in this sense, that although the fact of non-withdrawal is observable in infants, who cannot localise their sensations, this may be due to the imperfect development of their nervous system. Mr. Spalding has proved that although the callow bird cannot fly, the mechanism of flight is no sooner developed than the action follows at once, without any previous tentative experiences.

194. By experience we learn to restrict the paths of irradiation, so as to wink with one eye while the other is unmoved, to bend one finger while the rest are extended, to move one limb, or one group of muscles, while the others are at rest; in short, to execute any one particular action, and not at the same time agitate superfluously many other organs. The boy when first learning to write is unable to prevent the simultaneous motions of tongue and legs, which are ludicrously irrelevant to the purpose of writing; but he learns to keep all his organs in subjection, and only the eyes and hands active.* An analogous restriction takes place in thinking. A train of thought is kept up by the exclusion of all suggestions which are not pertinent; and the power of the thinker is precisely this power of concentration.

THE HYPOTHESIS OF INHIBITORY CENTRES.

195. The facts and their formulated laws which have just been adduced furnish a sufficient explanation of all the phenomena of arrest which of late years have been detached and assigned to a special mechanism of inhibitory nerves and centres. In spite of the eminent authorities countenancing the hypothesis of a particular set of inhibitory nerves, and particular centres of inhibition, I must confess that the hypothesis appears to me inadmissible; and that I side with those

* See the excellent remarks of Dr. LAUDER BRUNTON on this point in his paper on Inhibition in the *West Riding Lunatic Asylum Reports*, 1874, p. 180.

physiologists who hold that each nerve and each centre has its inhibitory action. Indeed, if the action of arrest be, as I maintain, only another aspect of the action of discharge, the result of the conflict of forces, to say that all centres have the property of excitation, is to say that all have the properties of discharge and arrest: the discharge is only the resultant of the conflict along the line of least resistance; the arrest is the effect of the conflict along the line of greatest resistance. The observed phenomena of arrest are so varied and numerous that the upholders of the inhibitory hypothesis have been forced to invent not only arresting centres, but centres which arrest these arresting centres! Dr. Lauder Brunton candidly remarks: "At present our notions of nervous action seem to be getting as involved as the Ptolemaic system of astronomy, and just as epicycles became heaped upon cycles, so nerve-centres are being added to nerve-centres. And yet, clumsy though the system may be, it serves at present a useful purpose, and may give real aid until a better is discovered." I do not think a Copernicus is needed to discover a better. The Law of Arrest as a general neural law suffices, when the right conception of a *centre* as a physiological rather than an anatomical designation is admitted. (See p. 153.)

196. It would be out of place here to consider the conflicting evidence which at present renders the question of the movements of the heart one of the most unsatisfactory in the whole range of experimental physiology. After devoting much time to it, and after writing a long chapter on it, I suppress what I had written, and content myself with the statement that no advantage whatever is derived from the hypothesis of a special mechanism of arrest, unless perhaps in giving a temporary precision to the direction of research. I mean that the search for special centres may lead to the discovery of the particular paths to which an impulse is restricted in any one action: as, for instance, the vagus in retarding the pulsation of the heart. If the cerebrum can determine a movement, and combine various movements, it is a centre of arrest; if the cerebellum can determine and regulate movements, it is a centre of arrest; if the medulla oblongata can determine and regulate movements, it is a centre of arrest; if the medulla spinalis can determine and combine movements, it is a centre of arrest; if a nerve can dilate a constricted blood-vessel, or constrict a dilated one, it is a nerve of arrest. In other words, every centre exerts its action either in discharging, or in arresting the discharge of some other centre.

The physiological process of Arrest may be physically interpreted as Interference;* not that the process in nerve-tissue is to be understood as the *same* as that observed in fluids, or that the metaphor of neural waves is to be taken for more than an intelligible picturing of the process; the difference in the two agents forbids our admitting the resemblance to be more than analogical. Thus interpreted, however, we see that not only will one centre arrest the action of another, but one nerve may be made to arrest itself! I mean that, under similar conditions of interference, the stimulation which normally follows on external stimulus may be inhibited by a previous, or a counter stimulation. Thus the nerve which will be stimulated by a chemical or mechanical stimulus, wholly fails to react if a constant current is passing through it, although this constant current does not itself cause a constant contraction. Remove the electrodes, and then the chemical or mechanical stimulus takes effect. Or the experiment may be reversed: let the nerve be placed in a saline solution, and the muscles will be at once thrown into violent contraction; if the electrodes are now applied to the nerve, the contractions suddenly cease, to begin again directly the electrodes are removed.

ANATOMICAL INTERPRETATION OF THE LAWS.

197. The problem for the anatomist is twofold: First,

* The interesting question of interference has been experimentally treated by WUNDT in his recently-published *Mechanik der Nerven*, 1876, and theoretically as wave-movement by MEDEM: *Grundzüge einer exakten Psychologie*, 1876.

given the organ, he has to determine its function, or *vice versa*, given the part of an organ, to determine its functional relation; secondly, given the function, he has to determine its organ. The structural and functional relations of nerves and centres have been ascertained in a general way; we are quite sure that the posterior nerves carry excitations from sensitive surfaces, that the anterior nerves carry excitations to muscles and glands; and that the central grey substance not only reflects a sensory excitation as a motor excitation, but propagates an excitation along the whole cerebro-spinal axis. But when we come to a more minute analysis of the functional activities, and endeavour to assign their respective values to each part of the organic mechanism, the excessive complexity and delicacy of the mechanism baffles research. We are forced to grope our way; and the light of the hypothetic lamps which we hold aloft as often misdirects as helps us. The imaginary anatomy which at present gains acceptance, no doubt seems to simplify explanations; but this seeming turns out to be illusory when closely examined. The imagined arrangement of fibres and cells we have seen to be not in agreement with observation; and were it demonstrable, it would not account for the laws of propagation. Suppose sensory fibres to terminate in cells, and fibres from these to pass *upwards* to other sensory cells and *transversely* to motor cells, how in such a connected system could irradiations take place, if the law of isolated conduction were true? And how could isolated conduction take place, if the excitation of a part were necessarily the excitation of the whole? Why, for example, is pain not always irradiated? Why is it even localised in particular spots, determining movements in particular muscles; and when irradiation takes place, why is it circumscribed, or—and this is very noteworthy—manifested in two widely different places, the intercostal and trigeminal nerves? Why does the irritation of intestinal worms manifest itself now by troubles of vision, now by noises in the ear, and now by convulsions?

198. Answers to such questions must be sought elsewhere. Our first search should be directed to the anatomical data, which have hitherto been so imprudently disregarded. Under the guidance of the laws formulated in this chapter, let us accept the anatomical fact of a vast network forming the ground-substance in which cells and fibres are embedded, and with which they are continuous; let us accept the physiological principle of similarity of property with similarity of composition and structure; let us accept the hypothesis that the discharge of neural energy is dependent on the degree of stimulus and the degree of tension at the time being—and we shall have at least a general theory of the process, though there will still remain great obscurities in particular applications. We shall have before us a vast network of pathways, all equally capable of conducting an excitation, but not all equally and at all moments open. It will always be difficult to determine what are the conditions which at any moment favour or obstruct particular openings. Paths that have been frequently traversed will of course be more readily traversed again; but this very facility will *sometimes* be an obstacle, since it will have caused that path to be preoccupied, or have fatigued the organ to which it leads.

199. Since the escape of an excitation must always be along the lines of least resistance, an obvious explanation of the restriction to certain paths has been to assume that some fibres and cells have naturally greater resistance than others. But this explanation is simply a restatement of the fact in other words. What is this greater resistance? Why is it present in one fibre rather than in another? We should first have to settle whether the resistance was in the nervous pathway itself, or in the centre, or in the organ innervated; an excitation might pass along the nervous tract, yet fail to change the state of the centre, or the organ, sufficiently to produce an appreciable response; and only those parts where an appreciable response was produced would then be considered as having had the pathways of propagation open.

200. When we reflect on the innumerable stimulations to which the organism is subjected from so many various points, and remember further that *each stimulation leaves behind it a tremor which does not immediately subside,* we shall conceive something of the excessive complexity of the mechanism, and marvel how any order is established in the chaos. What we must firmly establish in our minds is that the mechanism is essentially a *fluctuating* one, its elements being combined, recombined, and resolved under infinite variations of stimulation. If it were a mechanism of fixed relations, such as we find in machines, or in the "mechanism of the heavens," we might accept the notion of certain organites having greater resistance as a consequence of their structure, just as one muscle resists being moved by the impulse which will move another. Nor is it doubtful that such differences exist in nervous organites; but the laws of central excitation are not interpretable by any such hypothesis, since we know that the paths which were closed against an impulse of considerable energy may be all open to an impulse of feebler energy, and that a slight variation in the stimulus will be followed by a wide irradiation. For example, a grain or two of snuff will excite the violent and complex act of sneezing, but the nerves of the nasal cavity may be pinched, cut, or rubbed, without producing any such result. One group of nervous organites will fail to involve the activity of neighbouring groups; and the simple movement of a single organ is then all that appreciably follows the stimulation; yet by a slight change in the stimulation, the organites are somewhat differently grouped, and the result is a complex movement of many organs. It is this fluctuation of combination in the organites which renders education and progress possible. Those combinations which have very frequently been repeated acquire at last an automatic certainty.

We are now in a position to examine with more precision the extremely important laws of nervous action which are involved in the phenomena designated by the terms Reflex Action, Automatic Action, and Voluntary Action.

PROBLEM III.

ANIMAL AUTOMATISM.

"L'organisme le plus complexe est un vaste mécanisme qui résulte de l'assemblage de mécanismes secondaires."

CLAUDE BERNARD.

"Les corps vivants sont machines à l'infini."

LEIBNITZ.

"Noi lamentiamo con Majendie che nel linguaggio fisiologico siensi intruse le preopinioni psicologiche col trascico inevitabile dei vocaboli, ai quali codeste preopinioni si trovano legate. Probabilmente questa fu una delle principali cagioni degli errori e degli equivoci anatomofisiologici, da cui non poterono svincolarsi, a loro insaputa, i cultori sperimentali della scienza, perchè nell' interpretare i fenomeni osservati erano obbligati ad usare il linguaggio di una falsa moneta in corso."

LUSSANA e LEMOIGNE: *Fisiologia dei Centri Nervosi*, 1871, i. 16.

ANIMAL AUTOMATISM.

CHAPTER I.

THE COURSE OF MODERN THOUGHT.

1. MODERN Philosophy has moved along two increasingly divergent lines. One, traversed by Galileo, Descartes, Newton, and Laplace, had for its goal the absolute disengagement of the physical from the mental, *i.e.*, the objective from the subjective aspect of phenomena, so that the physical universe, thus freed from all the complexities of Feeling, might be interpreted in mechanical terms. As a preliminary simplification of the problem this was indispensable; only by it could the First Notion of primitive speculation be replaced by the Theoretic Conception of scientific speculation.* The early thinker inevitably invested all external objects with properties and qualities similar to those he assigned to human beings, and their actions he assigned to human motives. Sun, moon, and stars seemed living beings; flames, streams, and winds were supposed to be moved by feelings such as those known to move animals and men. Nor was any other conception then possible: men could only interpret the unknown by the known, and their standard of all action was necessarily drawn from their own actions. Not having analysed Volition and Emotion, above all not having localised these in a neuro-muscular system, men could not suspect that the movements of planets and plants, and of streams and stones,

* On the distinction between first notions and theoretic conceptions, see *Problems of Life and Mind*, vol. ii. p. 251.

had motors of a different kind from the movements of animals. The scientific conception of inert insensible Matter was only attained through a long education in abstraction; and is assuredly never attained by animals, or by savages. But no sooner were vital conditions recognised, than the difference between vital and mechanical movements emerged. When men learned that many of their own actions were unaccompanied either by Love or Hate, by Pleasure or Pain, and that many were unprompted by conscious intention, while others were unaccompanied by conscious sensation, they easily concluded that wherever the special conditions of Feeling were absent, the actions must have some other motors. Intelligence, Emotion, Volition, and Sensation being one by one stripped away from all but a particular class of bodies, nothing remained for the other bodies but insensible Matter and Motion. This was the Theoretic Conception which science substituted for the First Notion. It was aided by the observation of the misleading tendency of interpreting physical phenomena by the human standard, substituting our fancies in the place of facts, manipulating the order of the universe according to our imagination of what it might be, or ought to be. Hence the vigilance of the new school in suppressing everything pertaining to the subjective aspect of phenomena, and the insistance on a purely objective classification, so that by this means we might attain to a knowledge of things as they are. By thus withdrawing Life and Mind from Nature, and regarding the universe solely in the light of Motion and the laws of Motion, two great scientific ends were furthered, namely, a classification of conceptions, and a precision of terms. Objective phenomena made a class apart, and the great aim of research was to find a mathematical expression for all varieties under this class. Masses were conceived as aggregates of Atoms, and these were reduced to mathematical points. Forces were only different modes of Motion. All the numberless differences which perception recognised as *qualities* in things, were reduced to mere variations in *quantity*. Thus all that was particular and concrete became resolved by analysis into what was general and abstract. The Cosmos then only presented a problem of Mechanics.

2. During this evolution, the old Dualism (which conceived a material universe sharply demarcated from the mental universe) kept its ground, and attained even greater precision. The logical distinction between Matter and Mind was accepted as an essential distinction, *i.e.*, representing distinct reals. There was on the one side a group of phenomena, Matter and Force ; on the other side an unallied group, Feeling and Thought: between them an impassable gulf. How the two were brought into relation, each acting and reacting on the other, was dismissed as an "insoluble mystery" —or relegated to Metaphysics for such minds as chose to puzzle over questions not amenable to experiment. Physics, confident in the possession of mathematical and experimental methods which yielded definite answers to properly restricted questions, peremptorily refused to listen to any suggestion of the kind. And the career of Physics was so triumphant that success seemed to justify its indifference.

3. In our own day this analytical school has begun to extend its methods even to the mental group. Having reduced all the objective group to mathematical treatment, it now tries to bring the subjective group also within its range. Not only has there been more than one attempt at a mathematical Psychology; but also attempts to reduce Sensibility, in its subjective no less than in its objective aspect, to molecular movement. Here also the facts of Quality are translated into facts of Quantity; and all diversities of Feeling are interpreted as simply quantitative differences.

4. Thus far the one school. But while this Theoretic Conception stripped Nature of consciousness, motive, and passion, rendering it a mere aggregate of mathematical relations, a critical process was going on, which, analysing the nature of Perception, was rapidly moving towards another goal. Locke, Berkeley, Hume, and Kant, directing their analysis exclusively to the subjective aspect of phenomena, soon broke down the barriers between the physical and mental, and gradually merged the former in the latter. Matter and its

qualities, hitherto accepted as independent realities, existing where no Mind perceived them, were now viewed as the creations of Mind—their existence was limited to a state of the percipient. The old Dualism was replaced by Idealism. The Cosmos, instead of presenting a problem of Mechanics, now presented a problem of Psychology. Beginning with what are called the secondary qualities of Matter, the psychological analysis resolved these into modes of Feeling. "The heat which the vulgar imagine to be in the fire and the colour they imagine in the rose are not there at all, but are in us—mere states of our organism." Having gained this standing-place, there was no difficulty in extending the view from the secondary to the primary qualities. These also were perceptions, and only existed in the percipient. Nothing then remained of Matter save the hypothetical unknown x—the postulate of speculation. Kant seemed for ever to have closed the door against the real Cosmos when he transformed it into a group of mental forms —Time, Space, Causality, Quantity, &c. He propounded what may be called a theory of mental Dioptrics whereby a pictured universe became possible, as Experience by its own *a priori* laws moulded *itself* into a consistent group of appearances, which produced the illusion of being a group of realities. He admitted, indeed, that by the operation of Causality we are compelled to believe in a Real underlying the appearances; but the very fact that this Causality is a *subjective law*, is proof, he said, of its not being an *objective truth*. Thus the aim of the mechanical conception was to free research from the misleading complexities of subjective adulterations, and view *things as they are* apart from their *appearances;* but this aim seemed illusory when Psychology showed that Time, Space, Matter, and Motion were themselves not objective reals except in so far as they represented subjective necessities; and that, in short, things *are* just what they *appear*, since it is only in the relation of external reals to internal feelings that objects exist for us.

5. Idealism has been the outcome of the psychological method. It has been of immense service in rectifying the

dualistic conception, and in correcting the mechanical conception. It has restored the subjective factor, which the mechanical conception had eliminated. It has brought into incomparable clearness the fundamental fact that all our knowledge *springs from*, and is *limited by*, Feeling. It has shown that the universe represented in that knowledge, can only be a picture of the system of things as these exist in relation to our Sensibility. But equally with the mechanical conception it has erred by incomplete analysis. For a complete theory of the universe, or of any one phenomenon, those elementary conditions which analysis has provisionally set aside must finally be restored. When Quality is replaced by Quantity, this is an artifice of method, which does not really correspond with fact. The quality is the fact given in feeling, which we analytically refer to quantitative differences, but which can never be wholly resolved into them, since it must be presupposed throughout. One colour, for example, may be distinguished from another as having more or fewer undulations; and so we may by abstraction, letting drop all qualitative characters, make a scale of undulations to represent the scale of colours. But this is an ideal figment. It is the representation of one series of feelings by another series of different feelings. No variation of undulations will really correspond with variation in colour, unless we reintroduce the suppressed *quality* which runs through all colour. Attempt to make one born blind feel, or even understand, Colour by describing to him the kind of wave-movement which it is said to be, and the vanity of the effort will be manifest. Movement he knows, and varieties of movement as given in *tactile and muscular sensations;* but no combination and manipulation of such experiences can give him the specific sensation of Colour. That is a purely subjective state, which he is incapable of experiencing, simply because one of the essential factors is absent. One set of objective conditions is present, but the other set (his sense-organ) is defective. Without the "greeting of the spirit" undulations cannot become colours (nor even undulations, for these also are forms of feeling). Besides the sense-organ there is needed the feeling of Difference, which is itself the product of past and present feelings. The reproduction of other colours, or other shades of colour, is necessary to this perception of difference; and this involves the element of Likeness and Unlikeness between what is produced and reproduced. So that a certain mental co-operation is requisite even for the simplest perception of quality. In fact, psychological analysis shows that even Motion and Quantity, the two objective terms to which subjective Quality is reduced, are themselves Fundamental Signatures of Feeling;* so that here, as elsewhere, it is only by analytical artifice that the objective can be divorced from the subjective. Matter *is* for us the Felt; its Qualities are differences of Feeling.

6. Not that this result is to be interpreted as freeing our Theoretic Conception from its objective side, and landing us in Idealism, which suppresses the real universe. The denial of all reality apart from our minds, is a twofold mistake: it confounds the conception of general relations with particular relations, declaring that because the External in its relation to the sentient organism can only be what it is felt to be, therefore it can have no *other* relations to other individual reals. This is the first mistake. The second is the disregard of the constant presence of the objective real in every fact of Feeling: the Not-Self is emphatically present in every consciousness of Self.

The legitimate conclusion is neither that of Dualism nor of Idealism, but what I have named Reasoned Realism (*Problems*, vol. i. p. 176), which reconciles Common Sense with Speculative Logic, by showing that although the *truth* of things (their *Wahrheit*) is just what we perceive in them (our *Wahrnehmung*), yet their *reality* is this, and much more than this. *Things* are what they are felt to be; and what they are thought to be, when thoughts are symbols of the perceptions. Idealism declares that they are *nothing but* this. It is against this *nothing but* that Common Sense protests; and the protest is justified by Reasoned Realism,

* Not transcendental and *a priori*, as Kant teaches; but immanent in Feeling.

which, taking a comprehensive survey of the facts, thus answers the idealist: "Your synthesis is imperfect, since it does not include *all* the data—notably it excludes the fact of an objective or Not-Self element in every feeling. You may, conceivably, regard the whole universe as nothing but a series of changes in your consciousness; but you cannot hope to convince me that I myself am simply a change in yourself, or that my body is only a fleeting image in your mind. Hence although I conclude that the Not-Self is to you, as to me, undivorceable from Self, inalienable from Feeling, in so far as it is felt, yet there must nevertheless be for both of us an existence not wholly coextensive with our own. *My* world may be my picture of it; *your* world may be your picture of it; but there is something common to both which is more than either—an existent which has different relations to each. *You* are not *me*, nor is the pictured Cosmos *me*, although I picture it. Looking at you and it, I see a vast whole of which you are a small part; and such a part I conclude myself to be. It is at once a picture and the pictured; at once subjective and objective. To me all your modes of existence are objective aspects, which, drawing from my own experience, I believe to have corresponding subjective aspects; so that your emotions, which to me are purely physical facts, are to you purely mental facts. And psychological analysis assures me that all *physical facts are mental facts expressed in objective terms*, and *mental facts are physical facts expressed in subjective terms*."

7. But while Philosophy thus replaces the conceptions of Dualism and Idealism by the conception of the Twofold Aspect, the special sciences in their analytical career have disregarded the problem altogether. The mechanical theory of the universe not only simplified research by confining itself solely to the objective aspect of phenomena, but by a further simplification set aside all vital and chemical relations, to deal exclusively with mechanical relations. In ascertaining the mathematical relations of the planetary system, no elucidation could possibly be gained from biological or chemical conceptions; the planets therefore were provisionally stripped of everything not mechanical. In systematising the laws of motion, it was necessary to disengage the abstract relations from everything in any way resembling spontaneity, or extra-mechanical agency: Matter was therefore, by a bold fiction, declared to be inert, and its Motion regarded as something superadded from without.

7*a*. And this was indispensable for the construction of those ideal laws which are the objects of scientific research. Science, as we often say, is the systematisation of Experience under the forms of ideal constructions. Experience implies Feeling, and certain fundamental Signatures, all reducible to the primary discernment of Likeness and Unlikeness. Hence Science is first a *classification* of qualities or discerned likenesses and differences; next a *measurement* of quantities of discerned likenesses and differences. Although measurement is itself a species of classification, it is distinguished by the adoption of a standard unit of comparison, which, being precise and unvarying, enables us to express the comparisons in precise and unvarying symbols. Whether the unit of length adopted be an inch, a foot, a yard, a mile, the distance of the earth from the sun, or the distances of the fixed stars, the quantities thus measured are symbols admitting of one invariable interpretation. The exactness of the mathematical sciences is just this precision and invariability of their symbols, and is not, as commonly supposed, the source of any superior certainty as to the facts. The classificatory sciences, which deal with qualities rather than with quantities, may be equally *certain,* and represent fuller *knowledge,* because involving more varied feelings, but they cannot pretend to exactness. Even on the quantitative side, certainty is not identical with exactness. I may be quite certain that one block of marble is larger than another—meaning that it affects me more voluminously—but I cannot know how much larger it is, without interpreting my feelings by the standard of quantity—the how-muchness as represented by that standard. The immense advantages of exact measurement need not be insisted on. The Biological Sciences, which are predominantly classificatory, can never rival the Cosmological

Sciences in exactness; but they may reach a fuller knowledge; and their certainty will assume more and more the character of exactness as methods of measurement are applied to their classifications of qualities. The qualitative and quantitative aspects of phenomena are handled by the two great instruments, Logic and Mathematics, the second being only a special form of the first. These determine the general conceptions which are derived from our perceptions, and the whole constitute Experience.

8. What is the conclusion to which these considerations lead? It is that the separation of the quantitative from the qualitative aspect of phenomena—the objective mechanical from the subjective psychological—is a logical artifice indispensable to research; but it is only an artifice.* In pursuance of this artifice, each special science must be regarded as the search after special analytical results; and meanwhile this method should be respected, and no confusion of the boundaries between one science and another should be suffered. Mechanical problems must not be confused by the introduction of biological relations. Biological problems must not be restricted to mechanical relations. I do not mean that the mechanical relations present in biological phenomena are not to be sought, and, when found, to be expressed in mechanical terms; I mean that such an inquiry must be strictly limited to mechanical relations. Subjective relations are not to be denied, because they are provisionally set aside, in an inquiry into objective relations; but we must carefully distinguish which of the two orders we are treating of, and express each in its appropriate terms. This is constantly neglected. For example, nothing is more common than to meet such a phrase as this: "A *sensory impression* is transmitted as a *wave* of *motion* to the brain, and there being transformed into a state of *consciousness*, is again reflected as a *motor* impulse."

The several sciences having attained certain analytical

* The reader will understand that although mechanical relations are modes of Feeling, as all other relations are, yet their aspect is exclusively objective, referring to objects ideally detached from subjects.

results, it remains for Philosophy to co-ordinate these into a doctrine which will furnish general conceptions of the World, Man, and Society. On the analytical side a mechanical theory of the universe might be perfected, but it would still only be a theory of mechanical relations, leaving all other relations to be expressed in other terms. We cannot accept the statement of Descartes that Nature is a vast mechanism, and Science the universal application of mathematics. The equation of a sphere, however valuable from a geometrical point of view, is useless as an explanation of the nature and properties of the spherical body in other relations. And so a complete theory of the mechanical relations of the organism, however valuable in itself, would be worthless in the solution of a biological problem, unless supplemented by all that mechanical terms are incompetent to express.

9. The course of biological speculation has been similar to the cosmological. It also began with a First Notion, which compendiously expressed the facts of Experience. Nor can any Theoretic Conception be finally adopted which does away with these facts, known with positive certainty, and popularly expressed in the phrase: "I have a body, and a soul." We may alter the phrase either into, "I *am* a body, and I *am* a soul;" or into, "My body is only the manifestation of my soul;" or, "My soul is only a function of my body;" but the fundamental experiences which are thus expressed are of absolute authority, no matter how they may be interpreted. That I have a body, or am a body, is not to be speculatively argued away. That I move my arm to strike the man who has offended me, or stretch out my hand to seize the fruit which I see, is unquestionable; that these movements are determined by these feelings, and are never thus effected unless thus determined, is also unquestionable. Here are two sets of phenomena, having well-marked differences of aspect; and they are grouped respectively under two general heads, Life and Mind. Life is assigned to the physical organism, or Body—all its phenomena are objective. Mind is assigned to the psychical organism, or Soul—all its phenomena are subjective. Although what is called my Body is shown to be a group of qualities which are feelings—its

colour, form, solidity, position, motion—all its physical attributes being what is felt by us in consequence of the laws of our organisation; yet inasmuch as these feelings have the characteristic marks of objectivity, and are thereby referred to some objective existence, we draw a broad line of demarcation between them and other feelings having the characteristic marks of subjectivity, and referring to ourselves as subjects. Psychological analysis shows us that this line of demarcation is artificial, only representing a diversity of aspect; but as such it is indispensable to science. We cannot really separate in a sensation what is objective from what is subjective, and say how much belongs to the Cosmos apart from Sensibility, and how much to the subject pure and simple; we can only view the sensation alternately in its objective and subjective aspects. What belongs to extramental existence in the phenomenon of Colour, and what to the "greeting of the spirit," is utterly beyond human knowledge: for the ethereal undulations which physicists presuppose as the cosmic condition are themselves subjected to this same greeting of the spirit: they too are ideal forms of sensible experiences.

10. This conclusion, however, was very slowly reached. The distinction of aspects was made the ground of a corresponding distinction in agencies. Each group was personified and isolated. The one group was personified in Spirit—an existent in every respect opposed to Matter, which was the existent represented in the other group. One was said to be simple, indestructible; the other compound, destructible. One was invisible, impalpable, beyond the grasp of Sense; the other was visible, tangible, sensible. One was of heaven, the other of earth. Thus a biological Dualism, analogous to the cosmological, replaced the First Notion. It was undermined by advances in two directions. Psychology began to disclose that our conception of Matter was, to say the least, *saturated* with Mind, its Atoms confessedly being ideal figments; and that all the terms by which we expressed *material qualities* were terms which expressed *modes of Feeling;* so that whatever remained over and above this was the unknown *x*, which speculation required as a postulate.

Idealism, rejecting this postulate, declared that Matter was simply the projection of Mind, and that our Body was the objectivation of our Soul. Physiology began to disclose that all the mental processes were (mathematically speaking) *functions* of physical processes, *i.e.*, varying with the variations of bodily states; and this was declared enough to banish for ever the conception of a Soul, except as a term simply expressing certain functions.

11. Idealism and Materialism are equally destructive of Dualism. The defects of particular idealist and materialist theories we will not here touch upon; they mainly result from defects of Method. Not sufficiently recognising the primary fact testified by Consciousness, namely, that Experience expresses both physical and mental aspects, and that a Not-Self is everywhere indissolubly interwoven with Self, an objective factor with a subjective factor, the idealist reduces Existence to a mere panorama of mental states, and the Body to a group in this panorama. He is thus incapable of giving a satisfactory explanation of all the objective phenomena which do not follow in the same order as his feelings, which manifest a succession unlike his expectation, and which he cannot class under the order of his mental states hitherto experienced. He conceives that it is the Mind which *prescribes* the order in Things; whereas experience assures us that the order is *described*, not prescribed by us: described in terms of Feeling, but determined by the laws of Things, *i.e.*, the genesis of subjective phenomena is determined by the action of the Cosmos on our Sensibility, and the reaction of our Sensibility. He overlooks the evidence that the mental forms or laws of thought which determine the character of particular experiences, were themselves evolved through a continual action and reaction of the Cosmos and the Soul, precisely as the laws of organic action which determine the character of particular functions were evolved through a continual adaptation of the organism to the medium. These immanent laws are declared to be transcendental, antecedent to all such action and reaction.

A similar exclusiveness vitiates the materialist doctrine.

Overlooking the primary fact that Feeling is indissolubly interwoven with processes regarded as purely physical because they are considered solely in their objective aspect, the materialist fails to recognise the operation of psychological laws in the determination of physiological results; he hopes to reduce Biology to a problem of Mechanics. But Vitality and Sensibility are coefficients which must render the mechanical problem insoluble, if only on the ground that mechanical principles have reference to quantitative relations, whereas vital relations are qualitative. His error is the obverse of the vitalist's error. The vitalist imagines that the speciality of organic phenomena proves the existence of a cause which has no community with the forces operating elsewhere; so, turning his back on all the evidence, he attempts to explain organic phenomena without any aid from Physics and Chemistry. The materialist, turning his back on all the evidence of quite special conditions only found at work in living organisms, tries to explain the problem solely by the aid of Physics and Chemistry. It is quite certain that physiological and psychological problems are not to be solved if we disregard the laws of Evolution through Epigenesis. The mental structure is evolved, as the physical structure is evolved. It is quite certain that no such evolution is visible in anorganisms, nor will any one suppose it to be possible in machines. From the biological point of view we must therefore reject both Idealism and Materialism. We applaud the one when it says, "Don't confuse mental facts by the introduction of physical hypotheses;" and the other when it says, "Don't darken physical facts with metaphysical mists." We say to both: "By all means make clear to yourselves which aspect of the phenomena you are dealing with, and express each in its own terms. But in endeavouring to understand a phenomenon you must take into account all its ascertainable conditions. Now these conditions are some times only approachable from the objective side; at other times only from the subjective side."

12. While it is necessary to keep the investigation of a process on its objective side, limited to objective conditions,

and to express the result in objective terms, we must remember that this is an artifice; above all, we must remember that even within the objective limits our analyses are only provisional, and must be finally rectified by a restoration of all the elements we have provisionally set aside. Thus rectified, the objective interpretation of vital and mental phenomena has the incomparable advantage of simplifying research, keeping it fixed on physical processes, instead of being perturbed by suggestions of metaphysical processes. And as all physical investigation naturally tends to reduce itself to a mechanical investigation, because Mechanics is the science of motion, and all physical processes are motions, we may be asked, Why should not the mechanical point of view be the rational standing-point of the biologist? Our answer is, Because Mechanics concerns itself with abstract relations, and treats of products without reference to modes of production, *i.e.*, with motions without reference to all the conditions on which they depend. Every physical change, if expressed in physical terms, is a change of position, and is determined by some preceding change of position. It is a movement having a certain velocity and direction, which velocity and direction are determined by the velocity and direction of a force (a pressure or a tension) compounded with the forces of resistance, *i.e.*, counter-pressures. Clearly, the nature of the forces in operation must be taken into account; and it is this which the mechanical view disregards, the biological regards. The mechanical view is fixed on the ascertained adjustment of the parts, so that the working of the organism may be explained as if it were a machine, a movement here liberating a movement there. The biological view includes this adjustment of parts, but takes in also the conditions of molecular change in the parts on which the adjustment dynamically depends. Mechanical actions may be expressed as the enlargement or diminution of the angle of two levers; but chemical actions are not thus expressible; still less vital and mental actions.

13. The organism is on the physical side a mechanism, and so long as the mechanical interpretation of organic phenomena is confined to expressing the mechanical principles

involved in the mechanical relations, it is eminently to be applauded. But the organism is something more than a mechanism, even on the physical side; or, since this statement may be misunderstood, let me say, what no one will dispute, that the organism is a mechanism of a very special kind, in many cardinal points unlike all machines. This difference of kind brings with it a difference of causal conditions. In so far as the actions of this mechanism are those of a dependent sequence of material positions, they are actions expressible in mechanical terms; but in so far as these actions are dependent on vital processes, they are not expressible in mechanical terms. Vital facts, especially facts of sensibility, have factors neither discernible in machines nor expressible in mechanical terms. We cannot ignore them, although for analytical purposes we may provisionally set them aside.

In the course of the development of the mechanical theory, the history of which has just been briefly sketched, biological problems have more and more come under its influence. There has always been a fierce resistance to the attempt to explain vital and sentient phenomena on mechanical, or even physical principles, but still the question has incessantly recurred, How far is the organism mechanically interpretable? And while the progress of Biology has shown more and more the machine-like adjustment of the several parts of which the organism is composed, it has also shown more and more the intervention of conditions not mechanically interpretable. We shall have to consider the question therefore under two forms. First, whether animals are machines, and if not, by what characters do we distinguish them from machines? Secondly, in what sense can we correctly speak of Feeling as an agent in organic processes?

CHAPTER II.

THE VITAL MECHANISM.

14. No answer can be successfully attempted in reply to the first of the questions which closed the last chapter until we have given precision to certain terms of incessant recurrence. I have often to remark on the peculiar misfortune of Psychology, that all its principal terms are employed by different writers, and are understood by different readers, in widely different senses: they denote and connote meanings of various significance. All physicists mean the same thing when they speak of weight, mass, momentum, electricity, heat, &c. All chemists mean the same thing when they speak of affinity, decomposition, oxygen, carbonic acid, &c. All physiologists mean the same thing when they speak of muscle, nerve, nutrition, secretion, &c. But scarcely any two psychologists mean precisely the same thing when they speak of sensation, feeling, thought, volition, consciousness, &c.; and the differences of denotation and connotation in their uses of such terms lead to endless misunderstanding. As Rousseau says, "Les définitions pourraient être bonnes si l'on n'employait pas les mots pour les faire." But since we must employ words as our signs, our utmost care should be given to clearly marking what it is the signs signify.

15. The question we have now before us, whether animal actions are interpretable on purely mechanical principles? can only be answered after a preliminary settlement of the terms. The first of these terms to be settled is that of mechanism, when applied to the vital organism. If the organism is a mechanism, its actions must of course be interpretable on mechanical principles. But this general truth requires a special interpretation, if on inquiry we find that

the organism is a particular kind of mechanism, one which is *not* to be classed under the same head as inorganic machines. And this we do find. In Problem I. § 22, will be found a statement of the radical difference between organic and inorganic mechanisms, due to the differences in their structures. But the differences there noted do not affect the operation of abstract mechanical principles, which are of course manifested *wherever* there is a dependent sequence of material changes; and which are the same abstract principles in the mechanism of the heavens, the mechanism of a paper-mill, or the mechanism of an animal body. In other words, the principles are abstract, and are abstracted from all concrete cases by letting drop what is special to each case, retaining only what is common to all. This procedure is indispensable to the ideal constructions of Science. But we cannot rightly interpret any concrete case by abstract principles alone; we must restore the special characters which the abstraction has eliminated. The most lucid explanation of the mechanism of the heavens will leave us quite in the dark respecting the action of a paper-mill, until we have studied the mill at work, ascertained its structure and mode of operation, and therein detected what is common both to its mechanism and to the mechanism of the heavens. Thus equipped, we approach the study of the animal mechanism, but find ourselves wholly in the dark until we have also ascertained its structure and mode of operation; then we may recognise in it the principles of dependent sequence which had been abstracted from the paper-mill and the heavens. To neglect this concrete study, and to argue from Machinery to Life in disregard of special conditions, is not more rational than to assume that the movement of a piston is prompted by volition.

16. The recognition of special differences is no denial of fundamental identities. We do not deny the presence of phenomena in organisms which belong to physical and chemical agencies, but we assert that organisms have other phenomena besides these, dependent on conditions not present in physical and chemical phenomena. The same material elements and forces may be recognised in a moving inorganic body, and a moving organic body; but in the latter there is a speciality of combination with a speciality of result. Just as the same words and laws of grammatical construction may be recognised in prose and poetry; yet poetry is not prose, but has special rules of its own, and special effects. In an organism, as in a machine, the adjustment of the parts is a condition of the mechanical action; the one enables us to explain the other. But the parts adjusted, and the consequences of the adjustment, are unlike in the two cases. This unlikeness is pervading and profound. One cardinal difference is that the combination of the parts is in the machine a fixed, in the organism a fluctuating adjustment; and this fluctuation is due to certain vital processes subjectively known as *sensitive guidance.* Hence machines have fixed and calculated mechanisms; whereas organisms are variable and to a great extent incalculable mechanisms.

17. I conceive, therefore, that a theory which reduces vital activities to purely physical processes is self-condemned. Not that we are to admit the agency of any extra-organic principle, such as the hypothesis of Vitalism assumes (Prob. I. § 14); but only the agency of an intra-organic principle, or the abstract symbol of *all* the co-operant conditions—the special combination of forces which result in organisation. This assures us that an organism is a peculiar kind of mechanism, the processes in which are peculiar to it; and among those processes there is one which results in what we call Sensibility. This Sensibility is a factor which raises the phenomena into another order. To overlook its presence is fatal to any explanation of the organic mechanism. Yet it is overlooked by those who tell us that when an impression on a nerve is conveyed to the brain, and is thence reflected on the limbs—as when the retina of a wolf is stimulated by the image of a sheep, and the spring of the wolf upon the sheep follows as a "purely mechanical consequence—the whole process has from first to last been physical." Unless the term *physical* is here used to designate the *objective sequence,* as contemplated by an onlooker, who likens the process to the sequence observable in a machine, I should say that from first to last the process has been *not* physical, but *vital*, involving among its essential conditions the peculiarly vital factor named Sensibility. The process taking place in the wolf's organism is one which involves conditions never found in purely physical processes. We may indeed analytically disregard these. We may view the process in its purely physical relations, or in its purely chemical relations, or in its purely mathematical (mechanical) relations. But this is the artifice of the analytical method. In reality the process is no one of these, for it is all of these; it is a process in a living organism, and depends on conditions only found in living organisms—nay, in this particular case the process depends on conditions only found in organisms like that of the wolf; for the image of the sheep will stimulate the brain of a goat, horse, or elephant without producing any such movement in the organism.

18. The importance of this point must excuse my reiteration of it. We must make clear to ourselves that the organism is in its objective aspect a physiological mechanism, in its subjective aspect a psychological mechanism: in both aspects it is to be radically demarcated from all inorganic mechanisms. In it the combination and co-ordination of movements involve conditions never present in machines; among these conditions, there are combinations and co-ordinations of Sensibility, which, although material processes on the objective side, are processes believed to be only present in organisms. We have the strongest reasons for concluding that every feeling, every change in Sensibility, has its correlative material process in the organism—is, in short, only the subjective aspect of the objective organic change. What in Physiology is called Co-ordination and has reference to movements, in Psychology may be called Logic, having reference to feelings. But be this latter point accepted or rejected, the one point which admits of no dispute is that an organism is radically distinguishable from every inorganic mechanism in that *it acquires through the very exercise of its primary constitution, a new constitution with new powers.* Its

adjustment is a changing and developing mechanism. That is to say, a machine, however complex its structure, is constructed once for all, and this primary constitution is final, the adjustment of parts remaining unaltered; and although by exercise the machine may come to work more easily, with less friction, it never comes to work differently, to *readjust* its parts, and develop new capabilities. It has no *historical* factor manifest in its functions. It has no experience. It reacts at last as at first. How different the organism! This has not only variable adjustments due to internal fluctuations, it has experience which develops new parts, and new adjustments of old parts. Every organism has its *primary* constitution in the adjustment of parts peculiar to the species; it has also its *secondary* or modified constitution, in the adjustment which has been more or less altered by individual experiences; it has, thirdly, its *temporary* constitution in the variable adjustment due to the varying state of tension which results from varying stimulation.

19. A word on each. There is a structural disposition of the parts which is common to large groups of organisms, so that a corresponding similarity is observable in the reactions of these organisms. Thus all quadrupeds use their limbs for locomotion in very similar ways; birds use their wings for flight in similar ways. All vertebrates swallow their food, defend themselves, shrink when hurt, &c., in ways that are very similar. In so far as their organisations are alike, their actions and reactions are alike. In so far as their organisations differ, their actions and reactions differ. The goose and the vulture are alike in the main lines of structure; still more alike are duck and hen; yet, owing to certain unlike characters of structure, they manifest some marked differences in action and reaction: the goose will starve in the presence of food which the vulture gluttonously devours, and the vulture will refuse the vegetable food which the goose devours; the duck plunges into the water, the hen not only refuses to enter it, but is greatly agitated when she sees the ducklings she has hatched plunging into it. That peculiar instincts, habits, and feelings are rigorously determined by peculiarities in the organism, no one doubts, when animals are in question. If this is less obvious in the case of men, the reason is that there the influence of other factors somewhat masks the operation of the primary constitution—these factors are the modified and the temporary constitutions. Yet even in man it is true to say that his feelings and actions are the result of his organisation, native and acquired.

20. No two men are organised in all respects alike. There are individual variations in structure, both native and acquired. These may be too slight to be appreciable by any other test than the difference of reaction under similar external stimuli; but the variations in the sensibility to music, colour, temperature, sexual influence, moral influence, &c., betray corresponding differences in the organisms. Any one variation in structure, seemingly trivial, may be the origin of well-marked diversity in physical and moral characters. Compare the bull with the ox, or the predatory aggressive eagle with the cowardly vulture. Nor are the temporary modifications to be overlooked. Antoine Cros mentions the case of a patient, a young girl, suffering from congested liver and spleen, which of course altered the state of her blood, and thus for a time modified her constitution. Her moral character was greatly altered by it. She ceased to feel any affection for father or mother; would play with her doll, but could not be brought to show any delight in it; could not be drawn out of her apathetic sadness. Things which previously had made her shriek with laughter, now left her uninterested. Her temper changed, became capricious and violent.* Congestion of the lungs, if unaccompanied by congestion of the liver, never produces such effects, because not thus altering the blood. The effects of liver congestion are familiar. Cros cites the case of a magistrate whose liver was enlarged, and whose skin showed a markedly bilious aspect, and in whom all affection seemed to be dead: he did not exhibit any perversion or violence, only want of emotive reaction. If he went to the theatre he could not feel the slightest pleasure in it.

* ANTOINE CROS: *Les Fonctions supérieures du Système nerveux*, 1875, p. 85.

The thoughts of his home, his absent wife and children, were, he declared, as unaffecting to him as a problem in Euclid.

21. Owing to the recognised dependence of peculiar instincts and modes of reaction on peculiarities of structure, comparative anatomists are quite confident, when they find a portion of a skull with two occipital condyles, that the animal to which this skull belonged had red blood-corpuscles without nuclei, and (if a female) suckled its young. If in that fragment of skull there remain a single tooth, it will prove that the animal was carnivorous or herbivorous, and had, or had not, retractile claws. From such data a general conclusion may be formed as to the instincts and habits of the animal. The data disclose much of the primary constitution, that is to say, the mechanism which the animal brought with it into the world, ready prepared to react in definite ways on being stimulated. The connate mechanism has correlative tendencies of reaction. Some of these tendencies are inevitably called into play by external conditions, and they continue unaltered amid great varieties of circumstances, provided none of these variations directly deprive them of their appropriate stimulation. Such tendencies of the connate mechanism are styled *automatic* (an unfortunate metaphor, which has led to the theory of Automatism), and include, besides the visceral reactions, the more complex reactions of winking, breathing, swallowing, coughing, flying, walking, &c. It is true that we learn to walk, and learn to wink, whereas the other actions require no tentative efforts directed by experience; but the mechanism of all these actions is already laid down in the primary constitution, and is inevitably called into play.

22. The instincts also belong to the connate mechanism, and in the course of the normal experience of the animal inevitably come into play; but, unlike the automatic tendencies of breathing, swallowing, and coughing, they are capable of modification, or even suppression, by alterations in the course of individual experience. The connate mechanism of the cat determines its dread of water, and its enmity to the dog and mouse; yet a cat will by the modifications of certain experiences become as ready as an otter to take to the water, and become so fond of a dog that she will allow him to tend upon her kittens; and so indifferent to the mouse that she will let it run over her body. All this implies a new adjustment in the nervous centres, with new modes of reaction on sensory impressions: the inherited mechanism has been modified. I need not dwell on the profound modifications which the human inherited mechanism undergoes in the course of experience—how social influences and moral and religious teachings redirect, or even suppress, many primary tendencies; so that "moral habits" become organised, and replace the original tendencies of the organism. These, when organised, become the inevitable modes of reaction, and are sometimes called secondarily-automatic. It is important to recognise this organisation of experiences, this acquisition of a secondary or modified constitution, if we would explain psychological processes by physiological processes. Thus the processes of Logic are automatic, they belong to the connate primary mechanism, and their action is inevitable, invariable. The elements of a judgment, like the elements of a perception, may vary, and we therefore say that one judgment is false, and one perception incomplete; but the judging process is always the same, and the perceiving process is always the same. We may breathe pure air or impure air, but the breathing process is in each case the same; and judgment is as automatic as breathing, not to be altered, not to be suppressed. Again, the moral terror at wickedness of any recognised kind is as automatic as the instinctive terror at danger. The one has its roots in the primary disposition called love of approbation and its correlative dread of disapprobation: the social instinct. The other has its root in the primary disposition called "instinct of self-preservation," which is really the reflex shrinking from pain: the physiological instinct.

23. Besides the connate and acquired mechanism, we have now to consider the temporary and fluctuating adjustments which represent the statical condition of the organism at each moment. The automatism of the primary constitution is such that previous experience and conscious effort are not needed; nor will any experience or any effort alter the mode of reaction. If a strong light falls on the eye, the iris contracts; if the eyeball is dry, the eyelid drops; if sound-waves beat upon the tympanum, the stapedius muscle contracts; if the lining of the throat be tickled, the muscles involved in coughing or in vomiting contract. No experience is necessary for these actions, some of which are so complicated that if we had to learn them, as we learn far simpler actions, the organism would perish before the power was attained. Yet all of these presuppose a certain normal state of the mechanism, any considerable variation in which will modify or suppress them.

24. Secondarily-automatic actions are those which have been acquired through experiences that have modified the organism, and produced a new adjustment of parts. We learn to shield the eyes against a strong glare of light by raising the hand; by winking we learn to shield the eye against an approaching body; we also learn to turn the head in the direction of a sound, and to thrust away with our hands the object that is irritating our skin. Experience has been necessary for all these actions, and has finally organised the tendencies to perform them, so that the reaction is invariable, inevitable, unless controlled by the will. If you tickle my throat, I may, or may not, push aside your hand; but if the inside of my throat be tickled, I must cough. Here we see the difference between the automatic and secondarily-automatic actions. The second being due to individual experience, are more or less controllable; and whether they are or are not controlled depends on the condition of the nerve-centres at the moment. You may tickle my throat, or irritate my skin, without causing any movement of my hands to thwart you, either because my nerve-centres are preoccupied by other stimulations, and I am not conscious of the irritation, or because I do not choose to thwart you.

25. It should be added that some secondarily-automatic actions have become so firmly organised that we can only with great difficulty interfere with them. Others never enter into consciousness, and are therefore often supposed to be purely mechanical. The movement of the eye towards the brightest light, and the convergence of the axes of both eyes, are reflexes which, although involuntary and unconscious, are the products of education. They do not belong to the connate constitution, although they are so inevitably acquired by experience that they belong to every normal child. At first the infant stares with a blank gaze, and its eyes, though moving under the stimulus of light, move incoherently; the axes never converge except by accident. Very early, however, the infant's eyes are observed to follow the movements of a bright light; and at last they acquire so certain and rapid a power of adjustment that the eyes shift from spot to spot, always "fixing" the object by bringing the most sensitive part of the retina to bear on it. The incoherent movements have become precisely-regulated movements. It is the same with speech. The vocal organs are exercised in an incoherent babble. By degrees these movements become regulated so as to respond definitely to definite stimuli, and words are formed, then sentences, till finally fluent speech becomes in a great degree automatic. The vocal muscles respond to an auditory stimulus, and the child repeats the word it has heard, just as the eye-muscles respond to a retinal stimulus. That we acquire the power of converging the axes, and accommodating the lens to near objects, is not only proved by observation of infants, but also by cases of disease. After the reflex mechanism has been long established, so that it acts with inevitable precision, a slight paralysis of one of the muscles has the effect of making all objects appear in a different position; the patient trying to touch an object, then always moves his hand on one side of it. Von Graefe relates the case of a stonebreaker who always struck his hand with the hammer when he tried to strike the stone. Yet this very man *learned* to accommodate his movements to the new impressions; so that if his paralysis had been cured, his modified mechanism would have been ill adapted to the new conditions, and he would once more have struck his hand instead of the stone.

26. This digression on the native and acquired dispositions of the organism, while it has brought into strong light all

that can be cited in favour of regarding animal bodies as mechanisms, and their actions as the direct consequences of mechanical adjustments, has also made conspicuous the radical difference between an organism and a machine. We cannot too emphatically insist on this radical difference. Between the group of conditions involved in the structure and action of a machine, and the group of conditions involved in the structure and action of an organism, there are contrasts as broad as any that can be named. To overlook these in taking account solely of the conditions common to both groups is a serious error. On such grounds we might insist that a tiger is a violet, because both are organisms.

The biologist will admit that an organism is a mechanism, and (in so far as its bodily structure is concerned) a material mechanism. All the actions of this structure are therefore mechanical, in the two senses of the term: first, as being the actions of material adjustments; secondly, as being movements, and thereby included under the general laws of motion represented in Mechanics; the abstract laws of movement for an organic body are not different from the abstract laws of movement for an inorganic body. So far we have been considering the abstract relations only. No sooner do we consider the phenomena as concrete wholes, than we find great diversity in the modes of production of the movements in organisms and machines. Now it is precisely the modes of production which have interest for us. We never understand a phenomenon so as to gain any practical control over it, or any theoretical illumination from it, unless we have mastered some of its conditions; our knowledge of these conditions is the measure of our power.

CHAPTER III.

THE RELATION OF BODY AND MIND.

27. THE second question proposed was, In what sense can Feeling be correctly spoken of as an Agent in organic processes? This brings us face to face with a much-debated topic, the relation of Body and Mind; and demands a theoretic interpretation of that First Notion which expresses universal experience, namely, that what I know as Myself is a Body, in one aspect, and a Soul, in the other. What I call my Body is a persistent aggregate of objective phenomena; and my Soul is a persistent aggregate of subjective phenomena: the one is an individualised group of experiences expressible in terms of Matter and Motion, and therefore designated *physical;* the other an individualised group of experiences expressible in terms of Feeling, and therefore designated *psychical.* But, however contrasted, they are both simply embodiments of Experience, that is to say, are Modes of Feeling. All Existence—as known to us—is the Felt. The laws of our organism compel us, indeed, to postulate an Existent which is *extra mentem*—a Real not Ourselves—but the same laws debar us from any knowledge whatever of what this *is*, or is *like*. We know Things absolutely *in so far* as they exist in relation to us; and that is the only knowledge which can have any possible significance for us.

28. It is impossible for me to doubt that I am a Body, though I may doubt whether what is thus called is anything more than a group of feelings. It is impossible for me to doubt that I am a Soul; though I may doubt whether what is thus called is more than a group of bodily functions. In separating what is unquestionable from what is questionable, we separate the fundamental facts of consciousness from the theoretic interpretations of those facts: no theoretic interpretation can efface or alter the facts. Whatever Philosophy may discover, it cannot displace the fact that I know I am a Soul, *in every sense in which that phrase represents Experience:* I know the Soul in knowing its concretes (feelings), and in knowing it as an abstraction which condenses those concretes in a symbol. The secondary question is, Whether this abstraction represents one Existent, and the abstraction Body another and wholly different Existent, or the two abstractions represent only two different Aspects? this may be debated, and must be answered according to theoretic probabilities.

29. What are the probabilities? We are all agreed that Consciousness is the final arbiter. Its primary deliverance is simply that of *a* radical distinction. It is silent on the nature of the distinction—says nothing as to whether the distinction is one of agents or of aspects. It says, "I am a Soul." With equal clearness it says, "I am a Body." It does *not* say, "I am two things." Nor does the fact of a radical distinction imply more than a contrast of aspects, such as that of convex and concave. The curve has at every point this contrast of convex and concave, and yet is the identical line throughout. A mental process is at every point contrasted with the physical process assumed to be its correlate; and this contrast demands equivalent expression in the terms of each. The identity underlying the two aspects of the curve is evident to Sense. The identity underlying the mental and physical process is not evident to Sense, but may be made eminently *probable* to Speculation, especially when we have explained the grounds of the difference, namely, that they are apprehended through different modes. But although I admit that the conclusion is only one of probability, it is one which greatly transcends the probability of any counter-hypothesis. Let us see how this can be made out.*

* The solution offered in the present chapter was first offered in *Problems of Life and Mind*, 1875, ii. 457, *sq.* I mention this because since the publication of that volume other writers have expressed the same ideas, sometimes using my language and illustrations; *e.g.*, M. TAINE in the *Revue Philosophique*, January 1877, art.: *Les Vibrations cérébrales et la Pensée.*

30. We start from the position that a broad line of demarcation must be drawn between the mental and the physical aspect of a process, supposing them to be identical in reality. Nothing can be more *unlike* a logical proposition than the physical process which is its correlate; so that Philosophy has hitherto been forced to forego every attempt at an explanation of how the two can be causally connected: referring the connection to a mystery, or invoking two different agents, spiritual and material, moving on parallel lines, like two clocks regulated to work simultaneously. But having recognised this difference, can we not also discern fundamental resemblances? First and foremost, we note that there is common to both the basis in Feeling: they are both modes of Consciousness. The Mind thinking the logical proposition is not, indeed, in the same *state* as the Mind picturing the physical process which is the correlate of that logical proposition—no more than I, who see you move on being struck, have the same feelings as you who are struck. But the Mind which pictures the logical proposition as a process, and pictures the physical process as a bodily change, is contemplating one and the same event under its subjective and objective aspects; just as when I picture to myself the feelings you experience on being struck I separate the subjective aspect of the blow from its objective aspect. Secondly, between the logical proposition and the physical process there is a community of causal dependence, *i.e.*, the mode of grouping of the constituent elements, whereby this proposition, and not another, is the result of this grouping, and not another. In fact, what in subjective terms is called Logic, in objective terms is Grouping.

31. Let us approach the question on a more accessible side. Sensation avowedly lies at the basis of mental manifestations. Now, rightly or wrongly, Sensation is viewed alternately as a purely subjective fact—a psychological process—and as a purely objective fact—the physiological reaction of a sense-organ. It is so conspicuously a physiological process that many writers exclude it from the domain of Mind, assign it to the material organism, and believe that it is explicable on

purely mechanical principles. This seems to me eminently disputable; but the point is noticed in proof of the well-marked objective character which the phenomenon assumes. In this aspect a sensation is simply the reaction of a bodily organ. The physiologist describes how a stimulus excites the organ, and declares its reaction to be the sensation. Thus viewed, and expressed in terms of Matter and Motion, there is absolutely nothing of that subjective quality which characterises sensation. Yet without this quality the objective process cannot be a sensation. Exclude Feeling, and the excitation of the auditory organ will no more yield the sensation of Sound by its reaction, than the strings and sounding-board of a piano when the keys are struck will yield music to a deaf spectator. Hence the natural inference has been that inside the organism there is a *listener:* the Soul is said to listen, transforming excitation into sensation. This inference only needs a more systematic interpretation and it will represent the biological theory, which demands something *more* than the reaction of the sensory organ—namely, the reaction of the whole organism *through* the sensory organ. I mean, that no organ isolated from the organism is capable of a *physiological* reaction—only of a physico-chemical reaction; and sensation depends on (*is*) the physiological reaction. When a sense-organ is stimulated, this stimulation is a vital process, and is raised out of the class of physico-chemical processes by virtue of its being the indissoluble part a of complex whole. Interfere with any one of the co-operant conditions—withdraw the circulation, check respiration, disturb secretion—and the sense-organ sinks from the physiological to the physical state; it may then be brought into contact with its normal stimuli, but no stimulation (in the vital sense) will take place, there will be no vital reaction.

Condensing all vital processes in the symbol Vitality, we may say Vitality is requisite for every physiological process. A parallelism may be noted on the subjective side: all the sentient processes may be condensed in the one symbol Sensibility (Feeling), and we must then say, No psychological process is possible as an isolated fact, but demands the co-operation of others—it is a *resultant* of all the contemporaneous conditions of Sensibility in the organism. In ordinary language this is what is meant by saying that no impression can become a sensation without the intervention of Consciousness—an ambiguous phrase, because of the ambiguity of the term Consciousness, but the phrase expresses the fact that in Sensation a process in the organism is necessary to the reaction of the organ.

32. Having recognised the distinction between the two processes objective and subjective, physical and mental, we have recognised the vanity of attempting to assign their limits, and to say where Motion ends and Feeling begins, or how Feeling again changes into Motion. The one does *not* begin where the other ends. According to the two-clock theory of Dualism, the two *agents* move on parallel lines. On the theory of Monism the two *aspects* are throughout opposed. Both theories explain the facts; which explanation is the most congruous with experience? Against the first we may object that the hypothesis of two Agents utterly unallied in nature wants the cardinal character of a fertile hypothesis in its unverifiableness: it may be true, we can never know that it is true. By the very terms of its definition, the Spirit—if that mean *more* than an abstract expression of sentient states—is beyond all sensible experience. This is indeed admitted by the dualists, for they postulate a Spirit merely because they cannot otherwise explain the phenomena of Consciousness. Herein they fail to see that even their postulate brings no explanation, it merely restates the old problem in other terms.

33. Up to the present time these same objections might have been urged with equal force against Monism. Indeed, although many philosophers have rejected the two-clock theory of Leibnitz, they have gained a very hesitating acceptance for their own hypothesis of identity. To most minds the difficulty of imagining how a physical process could *also* be a psychical process, a movement also be a feeling, seemed not less than that of imagining how two such distinct Agents as Matter and Mind could co-operate, and react on each other, or move simultaneously on parallel lines. Although for many years I have accepted the hypothesis of Monism, I have always recognised its want of an adequate reply to such objections. Unless I greatly deceive myself, I have now found a solution of the main difficulty; and found it in psychological conditions which are perfectly intelligible. But knowing how easily one may deceive oneself in such matters, I will only ask the reader to meditate with open-mindedness the considerations now to be laid before him, and see if he can feel the same confidence in their validity.

34. One of the early stages in the development of Experience is the separation of Self from the Not-Self. I look out on "the vast extern of things," and see a great variety of objects, included in a visible hemisphere. All these objects in various positions, having various forms and colours, I believe to be wholly detached from, and in every way unallied to, Myself. And what is that Self? It is my Body as a visible and tangible object, separated from all other visible and tangible objects by the constant presence of feelings connected with it and its movements, and not connected with the other objects. This constant presence of feelings is referred to a Soul, which I then separate from my Body, as an Inner Self; and from this time onwards I speak of the Body as *mine*, and learn to regard it in much the same light as other outer objects. In my naïve judgment the external objects are supposed to exist *as* I see and touch them, whether I or any one else see and touch them or not: they in no sense belong to the series of feelings which constitute the Me. And since my Body resembles these objects in visible and tangible qualities, and also in being external to my feelings, it also takes its place in the objective world. Thus arises the hypothesis of Dualism which postulates a *Physis*, or object-world, and an *Æsthesis*, or subject-world: two independent existents, one contemplated, the other contemplating.

35. Philosophy, as we know, leads to a complete reversal of this primitive conclusion, and shows that the *contemplated* is a *synthesis of contemplations*, the Physis being *also* the

Æsthesis. Psychological investigation shows that the objects supposed to *have* forms, colours, and positions within an external hemisphere, have these only in virtue of the very feelings from which they are supposed to be separated. The *visible* universe exists only *as seen:* the objects are Reals conditioned by the laws of Sensibility. The space in which we see them, their geometrical relations, the light and shadows which reveal them, the forms they affect, the lines of their changing directions, the qualities which distinguish them,—all these are but the externally-projected signs of feelings. They are signs which we interpret according to organised laws of experience; each sign being itself a feeling connected with other feelings. We project them outside according to the "law of eccentric projection"—which is only the expression of the fact that one feeling is a sign of some other, and is thereby *ideally detached* from it. According to this law I say, "my Body;" just as I say, "my House;" or, "my Property." Misled by this, Dualism holds that in the very fact of detaching my Body from my Self, calling it *mine,* is the revelation of a distinct entity within the body. But that this is illusory, appears in the application of this same law of eccentric projection to sensations and thoughts, which are called *mine,* as my legs and arms are mine. If it is undeniable that I say *my* Body—and thus ideally detach the Body from the Soul—it is equally undeniable that I say *my* Soul; and from what is the Soul detached? In presence of this difficulty, the metaphysician may argue that neither Body nor Soul can be coextensive with its manifestations, but demands a noumenal Real for each —a *substratum* for the bodily manifestations, and a *substratum* for the mental manifestations. This, however, is an evasion, not a solution of the difficulty. If we postulate an unknown and unknowable noumenon, we gain no insight: first, because Philosophy deals only with the known functions of unknown quantities, and therefore leaves the x out of the calculation; secondly, because, granting the existence of these noumena, we can have no rational grounds for asserting that they are not of one and the same nature; for we have no grounds for *any* assertion whatever about them. And if it be urged against this, that Consciousness testifies to a distinction, I answer that on a closer scrutiny it will be found to testify to nothing more than a diversity of manifestation. All therefore that comes within the range of knowledge is, How does this diversity arise?

36. There are two ways, and there are only two, in which differences arise. These are, 1°, the *modes of production* of a product, and, 2°, our *modes of apprehension* of the product. Things may be very different, and yet to our apprehension indistinguishable, so that we regard them as identical; and they may be identical, yet appear utterly unlike. A mechanical bird may seem so like a living bird, and their actions so indistinguishable to the spectator, that he will not suspect a difference, or suspecting it, will not be able to specify it. Of both objects, so long as his modes of apprehending them are circumscribed, he can only say what these imply: he sees familiar forms, colours, and movements, which he interprets according to the previous experiences of which these are the signs. But by varying the modes of apprehension, and gaining thus a fuller knowledge, he finds that the two products have very different modes of production; hence he concludes the products to be different: the mechanism of the one is not the organism of the other; the actions of the mechanical bird are not the actions of the living bird. The fuller knowledge has been gained by viewing the objects under different relations, and contemplating them *in* their modes of production, not as merely visible products. He sees the mechanism performing by steel springs, wheels, and wires, the work which the organism performs by bones, muscles, and nerves; and the farther his analysis of the modes of production is carried, the greater are the differences which he apprehends.

37. Now consider the other side. One and the same object will necessarily present very different aspects under different subjective conditions, since it is *these* which determine the aspect. The object cannot be to Sight what it is to Hearing, to Touch what it is to Smell. The vibrations of a tuning-fork are seen as movements, heard as sounds. In

current language the vibrations are said to cause the sounds. Misled by this, philosophers puzzle themselves as to how a material process (vibration) can be transformed into a mental process (sensation), how such a cause can have so utterly different an effect. But I have formerly * argued at some length that there is no transformation or causation of the kind supposed. The tuning-fork—or that Real which in relation to Sense is the particular object thus named—will, by one of its modes of acting on my Sensibility through my optical apparatus, determine the response known as *vibrations;* but it is not this response of the optical organ which is transformed into, or causes the response of the auditory organ, known as *sound.* The auditory organ knows nothing of vibrations, the optical nothing of sounds. The responses are both modes of Feeling determined by organic conditions, and represent the two different relations in which the Real is apprehended. The Real *is* alternately the one and the other. And if the one mode of Feeling has a physical significance, while the other has a mental significance, so that we regard the vibrations as objective facts, belonging to the external world, and the sounds as subjective facts, exclusively belonging to the internal world, this is due to certain psychological influences presently to be expounded. Meanwhile let us fix clearly in our minds that both vibrations and sounds are modes of Feeling. My consciousness plainly assures me that it is I who see the one, and hear the other; not that there are two distinct subjects for the two distinct feelings. Add to which, manifold uncontradicted experiences assure me that the occasional cause — the objective factor—of the one feeling, is also the cause of the other, and not that the two feelings have two different occasional causes. From both of these undeniable facts we must conclude that the difference felt is simply a difference of aspect, determined by some difference in the modes of apprehension.

38. Assuming then that a mental process is only another aspect of a physical process—and this we shall find the more probable hypothesis—we have to explain by what influences

* *Problems of Life and Mind*, vol. ii. pp. 417 and 466.

these diametrically opposite aspects are determined. From all that has just been said we must seek these in the modes of apprehension. There can be no doubt that we express the fact in very different terms; the question is, What do these terms *signify?* Why do we express one aspect in terms of Matter and Motion, assigning the process to the objective world; and the other aspect in terms of Feeling, assigning the process to the subjective world?

Let the example chosen be a logical process as the mental aspect, and a neural process as its physical correlate. The particular proposition may be viewed logically, as a grouping of experiences, or physiologically, as a grouping of neural tremors. Here we have the twofold aspect of one and the same reality; and these different aspects are expressed in different terms. We cannot be too rigorous in our separation of the terms; for every attentive student must have noted how frequently discussions are made turbid by the unconscious *shifting of terms* in the course of the argumentation. This is not only the mistake of opponents who are unaware of the shifting which has occurred in each other's minds, so that practically the adversaries do not meet on common ground, but cross and recross each other; it is also the mistake of the solitary thinker losing himself in the maze of interlacing conceptions instead of keeping steadily to one path. Only by such shifting of terms can the notion of the physical process causing, or being transformed into, the mental process for a moment gain credit; and this also greatly sustains the hypothesis of Dualism, with its formidable objections: How can Matter think? How can Mind act on Matter causing Motion?

39. Those who recognised that the terms Matter and Mind were abstractions mutually exclusive, saw at once that these questions, instead of being formidable, were in truth irrational. To ask if Matter could think, or Mind move Matter, was a confusion of symbols equivalent to speaking of a yard of Hope, and a ton of Terror. Although Measure and Weight are symbols of Feeling, and in *this* respect are on a par with Hope and Terror, yet because they are objec-

tive symbols they cannot be applied to subjective states, without violation of the very significance they were invented to express. No one ever asks whether a sensation of Sound can be a sensation of Colour; nor whether Colour can move a machine, although Heat can, yet the one is no less a sensation than the other. On similar grounds no one should ask whether Matter can think, or Mind move Matter. The only rational question is one preserving the integrity of the terms, namely, whether the living, thinking organism presents itself to apprehension under the twofold aspect—now under the modes of Feeling classified as objective or physical; now under the modes classified as subjective or mental.

40. We are told that it is "impossible to imagine Matter thinking," which is very true; only by a gross *confusion* of terms can Thought be called a property of cerebral tissue, or of Matter at all. We may, indeed, penetrate beneath the terms which relate to aspects, and recognise in the underlying reality not two existences, but one. Our conceptions of this reality, however, are expressed in symbols representing different classes of feelings, objective and subjective; and to employ the terms of one class to designate the conceptions of the other is to frustrate the very purposes of language. Matter and Mind, Object and Subject, are abstractions from sentient experiences. We know them as abstractions, and know the concrete experiences from which they are abstracted. Philosophers, indeed, repeatedly assure us that we neither know what Matter is nor what Mind is, we only know the *phenomenal products* of the action and reaction of these two unknown noumena. Were this so, all discussion would be idle; we could not say whether Matter was or was not capable of thinking, whether Mind was or was not the same as Matter, we could only abstain from saying anything whatever on the topic. What should we reply to one who asked us to name the product of two unknown quantities? So long as x and y are without values their product must be without value. If the value of x be known, and that of y unknown, then the product still remains unknown: $x + y = x + 0 = x$. Therefore, unless

the Objective aspect were the *equivalent* of the Subjective aspect, it could never be subjectively present. Feeling is but another aspect of the Felt.

41. It is because we do know what Matter is, that we know it is *not* Mind: they are symbols of two different modes of Feeling. If we separate the conception of citizenship from the conception of fatherhood, although the same man is both citizen and father, how much more decisively must we separate the conception of Matter, which represents one group of feelings, from the conception of Mind, which represents another? One element in the former is common to the whole group, namely, the reference to a Not-Self, induced by the sensation of Resistance, which always ideally or sensibly accompanies the material class. The axiom, I feel, *ergo* I exist, has its correlative:—I act, *ergo* there are other existents on which I act; and these are not wholly Me, for they resist, oppose, exclude me; yet they are also one with Me, since they are felt by me. In my Feeling, that which is not Me is Matter, the objective aspect of the Felt, as Mind is the subjective aspect.

But since Hunger and Thirst, Joy and Grief, Pain and Terror, are also *felt,* yet are never classed under the head of Matter, the grounds of the classification of feelings have to be expressed. Professor Bain makes the distinction between Matter and Mind to rest solely on the presence or absence of Extension: this is the decisive mark: Matter he defines as the Extended. The definition is inadequate. When I see a dog and its image reflected in a pool, or see a dog and think of another, in the three cases dog, image, and idea have Extension; but I recognise the dog as a material fact, the idea as a mental fact; and although the image of the dog has material conditions by which I am optically affected, just as the idea has material cerebral conditions, I recognise a marked difference between them and the dog, due to the different modes of apprehension. The dog is known as a persistent reality, which, when Sight is supplemented by Touch, will yield sensations of Resistance, and thus disclose its materiality. The image vanishes if I attempt to touch it;

I see its outlines waver and become confused with every disturbance of the surface of the pool; the idea vanishes when another idea arises; whence I conclude that neither has material reality, because neither has the Resistance which characterises the Not-Self. The image and the idea may be referred to material conditions, but so may pains, terrors, volitions, yet these are all without Extension, simply because they are not visual feelings.

42. Matter does not represent all feelings, but only the objective sensibles; and these are not all characterised by Extension, but only those which directly or indirectly involve optico-tactical experiences accompanied by muscular experiences. Matter is primarily the Visible and Resistent; and secondarily, whatever can be imagined as such; so that ether, molecules, and atoms, although neither visible nor tangible, are ranged under the head of Matter. Colour is a feeling as Sound and Scent are feelings, and although material conditions are equally presupposed in all three, yet Colour alone has Extension, and because it can be imaged it has a more objective character than the others, which having no lines and surfaces, want the optical conditions for the formation of images, and are less definitely connected with tactical and muscular experiences. Nevertheless, since Sound and Scent are obviously associated with objects seen and touched, they have a degree of materiality never assigned to such feelings as Hunger and Thirst, Pleasure, Terror, and Hope.

43. When we refer feelings to material conditions, we follow the natural tendency to translate the little known in terms of the better known, and employ the symbols Matter and Motion, because these furnish the intellect with images, *i.e.*, definite and exact elements to operate with. In hearing a sound, there is nothing at all like "vibrations," nothing like "aerial waves" and "neural processes," given in that feeling; but on attempting to *explain* it, we remove it from the sphere of Sensation to carry it into the sphere of Intellect, and we must change our symbols in changing our problem; here our only resource is to translate the subjective state into an *imaginable* objective process, which can only be expressed

in terms of Matter and Motion. What we *heard* as Sound is then *seen* as Vibration. When we are optically or mentally contemplating vibrations and neural processes, we are supplanting one source of feeling by another, translating an event in another set of symbols. But we can no more hear the sound in seeing the vibrations, than a blind man can see the fly in the amber which he feels with his fingers, or than we can feel the amber he holds, while we are only looking at it. The phrase "material conditions of Feeling" sometimes designates the objective aspect of the subjective process, and sometimes the agencies in the external medium which cooperate with the organism in the production of the feelings. In each case there is an attempt to explain a feeling by intelligible symbols.

44. The Animal probably never attempts such explanation; satisfied with the facts, it is careless of their factors. Man is never satisfied: is restless in the search after factors; and having found them, seeks factors of these factors; so that Lichtenberg felicitously calls him "*das rastlose Ursachenthier*"—"the animal untiring in the search for causes." And thus sciences arise: we translate experiences into geometrical, physical, chemical, physiological, and psychological terms—different symbols of the different modes of apprehending phenomena.

45. "I see an elephant." In other words, I am affected in a certain way, and interpret my affection by previous similar experiences, expressing these in verbal symbols. But I want an explanation, and this the philosopher vouchsafes to me by translating my affection into his terms. He takes me into another sphere—tells me of an undulating Ether, the waves of which beat upon my retina—of lines of Light refracted by media and converged by lenses according to geometric laws—of the formation thereby of a tiny image of the gigantic elephant on my retina as on the plate of a camera-obscura—this, and much more, is what *he* sees in *my* visual feeling, and he bids me see it also. Grateful for the novel instruction, I am compelled to say that it does not alter my vision of the elephant, does not make the fact a

whit clearer, does not indeed correspond with what I feel. It is outside knowledge, valuable, as all knowledge is, but supplementary. It is translation into another language. And when I come to examine the translation, I find it very imperfect. I ask my instructor: Is it the tiny image on my retina which I see, and not the big elephant on the grass? And how do I see this retinal image, which you explain to be upside down?—how is it carried from my retina to my mind? I have no consciousness of tiny reversed image, none of my retina, only of a fact of feeling, which I call "seeing an elephant." The camera-obscura has no such feeling—it reflects the image, it does not see the object. Here my instructor, having reached the limit of his science,* hands me over to the physiologist, who will translate the fact for me in terms not of Geometry, but of Anatomy and Physiology. The laws of Dioptrics cease at this point: the image they help to form on the retina is ruthlessly dispersed, and all its beautiful geometric construction is lost in a neural excitation, which is transmitted through semifluid channels of an optic tract to a semifluid ganglion, whence a thrill is shot through the whole brain, and is there *transformed* into a visual sensation. Again I fancy I have gained novel instruction of a valuable kind; but it does not affect my original experience that I am enabled to translate it into different terms; the less so because I cannot help the conviction that the translation is imperfect, leaving out the essential points. If a phrase be translated for me into French or German, I gain thereby an addition to my linguistic knowledge, but the experience thus variously expressed remains unaffected. When the fact is expressed in geometrical or physiological terms, the *psychical process* finds no adequate expression. Neither in the details, nor in the totals, do I recognise any of

* "The retinal image is the last effect known of the action of objects on us; what happens beyond the retina we know not; our knowledge of the objective process has at present here its limit."—EWALD HERING: *Beiträge zur Physiologie*, 1862, p. 166. That is to say, we have a definite translation of the process in geometric terms as far as the retina, and thence onwards Geometry fails us, and Neurology and Psychology are invoked.

the qualities of my state of feeling in seeing the elephant. I do not see the geometrical process, I do not see the anatomical mechanism, I see the elephant, and am conscious only of that feeling. You may consider my organism geometrically or anatomically, and bring it thus within the circle of objective knowledge; but my subjective experience, my spiritual existence, that of which I am most deeply assured, demands another expression. Nay more, on closely scrutinising your objective explanations, it is evident that a psychical process is *implied* throughout—such terms as undulations, refractions, media, lenses, retina, neural excitation, overtly refer, indeed, to the material objective aspect of the facts, but they are themselves the modes of Feeling by which the facts are apprehended, and would not exist *as such* without the 'greeting of the spirit."

46. What, then, is our conclusion? It is, that to make an adequate explanation of psychical processes by material conditions we must first establish an equivalence between the subjective and objective aspects; and, having taken this step, we must complete it by showing wherein the difference exists; having established this identity and diversity, we have solved the problem.

Let us attempt this solution. When I speak to you, the spoken words are the same to you and to me. You hear what I hear, you apprehend what I apprehend. But there were muscular movements of articulation felt by me and not felt by you; to feel these you also must articulate the words; but so long as you merely hear the words, there is a difference in our states of feeling. Some of my movements you can see, others you can imagine; but this is not my feeling of them, it is your optical equivalent of my muscular feeling. On a similar assumption of equivalence, a neural process is made to stand for a logical process. In thinking a proposition, we are logically grouping verbal symbols representative of sensible experiences; and this is a quite peculiar state of Consciousness, wholly unlike what would arise in the mental or visual contemplation of the neural grouping, which is its physiological equivalent. But this diversity does not discredit the idea of their identity; and although some of my readers will protest against such an idea, and will affirm that the logical process is not a process taking place in the organism at all, but in a spirit which uses the organism as its instrument, I must be allowed in this exposition to consider the identity established, my purpose being to explain the diversity necessarily accompanying it. Therefore, I say, that although a logical process is identical with a neural process, it must appear differently when the modes of apprehending it are different. While you are thinking a logical proposition, grouping your verbal symbols, I, who mentally *see* the process, am grouping a totally different set of symbols: to you the proposition is a subjective state, *i.e.*, a *state* of feeling, not an *object* of feeling: to become an object, it must be apprehended by objective modes: and this it can become to you as to me, when we see it as a process, or imagine it as a process. But obviously your state in seeing or imagining the process must be different from your state when the process itself is passing, since the modes of apprehension are so different. There may be every ground for concluding that a logical process has its correlative physical process, and that the two processes are merely two aspects of one event; but because we cannot apprehend the one aspect as we apprehend the other, cannot *see* the logical sequence as we *see* the physical sequence, this difference in our modes of apprehension compels us to separate the two, assigning one to the subjective, the other to the objective class. Between the sensible perception of an object and the reproduced image of the object there is chiefly a quantitative difference in the physiological and psychological processes: the image is a faint sensation. Yet this quantitative difference brings with it the qualitative distinction which is indicated in our calling the one a sensation, the other a thought. The consequence has been that while all philosophers have admitted the sensation to be—at least partly—a process in the bodily organism, the majority have maintained that the thought is no such process in the organism, but has its seat in a spirit independent of the organism.

47. The states of Feeling which are associated with other states characterised as objective because overtly referring to a Not-Self, we group under the head of Matter: we assign material conditions as their antecedents. Whereas states of Feeling which are not thus associated we group under the head of Mind, and assign internal conditions as their antecedents. Colour and Taste are very different states of Feeling, yet both are spontaneously referred to external causes, because they are associated with visual and tactical states; whereas Hunger, Nausea, Hope, &c., have no such associations, and their material conditions are only theoretically assigned.

Our intelligible universe is constructed out of the elements of Feeling according to certain classifications, the broadest of which is that into external and internal, object and subject. The abstractions Matter and Mind once formed and fixed in representative symbols, are easily accredited as two different Reals. But the separation is ideal, and is really a distinction of Aspects. We know ourselves as Body-Mind; we do not know ourselves as Body *and* Mind, if by that be meant two coexistent independent Existents; and the illusion by which the two Aspects appear as two Reals may be made intelligible by the analysis of any ordinary proposition. For example, when we say "this fruit is sweet," we express facts of Feeling—actual or anticipated—in abstract terms. The concrete facts are these: a coloured feeling, a solid feeling, a sweet feeling, &c., have been associated together, and the coloured, solid, sweet group is symbolised in the abstract term "fruit." But the colour, solidity, and sweetness are also abstract terms, representing feelings associated in other groups, so that we find "fruit" which has no "sweetness;" and "sweetness" in other things besides "fruits." Having thus separated ideally the "sweetness" from the "fruit"—which in the concrete sweet-fruit is not permissible—we easily come to imagine a real distinction. This is the case with the concrete living organism when we cease to consider it in its concrete reality, and fix our attention on its abstract terms—Body and Mind. We then think of Body apart from Mind, and believe in them as two Reals, though neither exists apart.

There is no state of consciousness in which object and subject are not indissolubly combined. There is no physical process which is not indissolubly bound up with the psychical modes of apprehending it. Every idea is either an image or a symbol—it has therefore objective reference, a material aspect. Every object is a synthesis of feelings—it has therefore subjective reference, a material aspect. Thus while all the evidence points to the identity of Object and Subject, there is ample evidence for the logical necessity of their ideal separation as Aspects. This I have explained as a case of the general principle which determines all distinctions—namely, the diversity in the modes of production of the products, which—subjectively—is diversity in the modes of apprehending them. The optico-tactical experiences are markedly different from the other experiences, as being more directly referred to the Not-Self which resists; and because these lend themselves to ideal constructions by means of images and symbols, it is these experiences into which we translate all the others when we come to explain them and assign their conditions. For—and this is the central position of our argument—all interpretation consists in translating one set of feelings in the terms of another set. We condense sets of feelings in abstract symbols; to *understand* these we must reduce them to their concrete significates. They are signs; we must show what they are signs of.

Now the symbols Object and Subject are the most abstract we can employ. Because they are universal, they represent what cannot in reality be divorced. We can, indeed, ideally separate ourselves from the Cosmos; in the same way we can ideally separate our inner Self or Soul from our outer Self or Body; and again our Soul from its sentient states, our Body from its physical changes. But not so in reality. The separation is a logical artifice, and a logical necessity for Science.

The necessity will be obvious to any one who reflects how

the ideal constructions of Science demand precision and integrity of terms. The problem of Automatism brings this very clearly into view. The question is, Can we translate all psychological phenomena in mechanical terms? If we *can*, we ought; because these terms have the immense advantage of being *exact*, dealing as they do with quantitative relations. But my belief is that we cannot—nay, that we cannot even translate them all into physiological terms. The distinction between quantitative and qualitative knowledge (p. 314) is a barrier against the mechanical interpretation. Physiology is a classificatory science, not a science of measurement. Nor can the laws of Mind be deduced from physiological processes, unless supplemented by and interpreted by psychical conditions individual and social.

CHAPTER IV.

CONSCIOUSNESS AND UNCONSCIOUSNESS.*

48. SCIENCE demands precision of terms; and in this sense Condillac was justified in defining it, *"une langue bien faite."* The sciences of Measurement are exact because of the precision of their terms, and are powerful because of their exactness. The sciences of Classification cannot aspire to this precision, and therefore, although capable of attaining to a fuller knowledge of phenomena than can be reached by their rivals, this advantage of a wider range is accompanied by the disadvantage of a less perfect exposition of results. While physicists and chemists have only to settle the significance of the facts observed, biologists and social theorists have over and above this to settle the significance of the terms they employ in expressing the facts observed. Hence more than half their disputes are at bottom verbal.

This is markedly the case in the question of Automatism. One man declares that animals are automata; another that they are conscious automata; and while it is quite possible to hold these views and not practically be in disagreement with the views of ordinary men, or indeed with the views of spiritualist and materialist philosophers, we can never be sure that the advocates of Automatism do not mean what they are generally understood to mean. If a man says that by an automaton he does not here mean a machine, such as a steam-engine or a watch, but a vital mechanism which has its parts so adjusted that its actions resemble those of a machine; and if he adds that this automaton is also conscious of some of its actions, though unconscious of others, we can only object to his using terms which have misleading

* Compare *Problem II. chap.* 4.

connotations. If he mean by "conscious automata," that animals are mechanisms moved on "purely mechanical principles," their consciousness having nothing whatever to do with the production of their actions, then indeed our objection is not only to his use of terms, but to his interpretation of the facts.

49. The questions of fact are two: Are animal mechanisms rightfully classed beside machines? and, Is consciousness a coefficient in the actions of animal mechanism? The first has already been answered; the second demands a preliminary settlement of the terms "conscious," "unconscious," "voluntary," and "involuntary." The aim of Physiology is to ascertain the particular combinations of the elementary parts involved in each particular function—in a word, the mechanism of organic phenomena; and the modern Reflex Theory is an attempt to explain this mechanism on purely mechanical principles, without the co-operation of other principles, especially those of Sensation and Volition. It is greatly aided by the ambiguity of current terms. We are accustomed to speak of certain actions as being performed unconsciously or involuntarily. We are also accustomed to say that Consciousness is necessary to transform an impression into a sensation, and that Volition is the equivalent of conscious effort. When, therefore, unconscious and involuntary actions are recorded, they seem to be actions of an insentient mechanism. The Reflex Theory once admitted, a rigorous logic could not fail to extend it to all animal actions.

50. I reject the Reflex Theory, on grounds hereafter to be urged, but at present call attention to the great ambiguity in the terms "conscious" and "unconscious." In one sense no definition of Consciousness can be satisfactory, since it designates an ultimate fact, which cannot therefore be made more intelligible than it is already. In another sense no definition is needed, since every one knows what is meant by saying, "I am conscious of such a change, or such a movement." It is here the equivalent of Feeling. To be conscious of a change, is to feel a change. If we desire to express it in physiological terms, we must define Consciousness—

"a function of the organism;" and this definition we shall find eminently useful, because the organism being a vital mechanism, and the integrity of that mechanism being necessary for the integrity of the function, while every variation of the mechanism will bring a corresponding variation of the function, we shall have an objective guide and standard in our inquiries. Organisms greatly differ in complexity, yet because they also agree in the cardinal conditions of Vitality, among which Sensibility is one, we conclude that they all have Feeling; but the Feeling of the one will differ from that of another, according to the complexity of the sentient mechanism in each. The perfection of this mechanism lies in the co-ordination of its parts, and the consensus of its sentient activities; any disturbance of that consensus must cause a modification in the total consciousness; and when the disturbance is profound the modification is marked by such terms as "insanity," "loss of consciousness," "insensibility." These terms do not imply that the sentient organs have lost their Sensibility, but only that the disturbed mechanism has no longer its normal consensus, no longer its normal state of Consciousness. Each organ is active in its own way so long as its own mechanism is preserved; but the united action of the organs having been disturbed, their *resultant* function has been altered. Hence in a fit of Epilepsy there is a complete absence of some normal reactions, with exaggeration of others. In a state of Coma there is no spontaneity—none of the manifold adaptations of the organism to fluctuating excitations, external and internal, observable in the normal state. The organism still manifests Sensibility—but this is so unlike the manifestations when its mechanism is undisturbed (and necessarily so since the Sensibility varies with the mechanism) that it is no longer called by the same name. In the normal organism Sensibility means Feeling, or Consciousness; but in the abnormal organism there is said to be a "loss of Consciousness." What the physiologist or the physician means by the phrase "loss of Consciousness" is intelligible, and for his purposes unobjectionable. He observes many organic processes going on undisturbed—the unconscious patient breathes, secretes, moves his limbs, &c. These processes are referred to the parts of the mechanism which are not disturbed; they are obviously independent of that adjustment of the mechanism which by its *consensus* has the special resultant named Consciousness; he therefore concludes that these, and many other organic processes, which are neither accompanied nor followed by *discriminated* feelings, are the direct consequences of the stimulated mechanism. He never hesitates to adopt the popular language, and say, "We sometimes act unconsciously, perceive unconsciously, and even think unconsciously, all by the simple reflex of the mechanism."

Now observe the opening for error in this language. The actions are said to go on unconsciously, and, because unconsciously, as pure reflexes, which are then assigned to an insentient mechanism, and likened to the actions of machines. But, as I hope hereafter to make evident, the reflex mechanism necessarily involves Sensibility; and therefore reflex actions may be unaccompanied by Consciousness—in one meaning of that term—without ceasing to be sentient: the feelings are operative, although not discriminated. On the other hand, there is another and very general meaning of the term Consciousness, which is the equivalent of Sentience.

51. In discussing Automatism, or the Reflex Theory, it is absolutely necessary that we should first settle the meaning we assign to the term Consciousness. The laxity with which the term is used may be seen in the enumeration occupying six pages of Professor Bain's account of the various meanings. Psychology is often said to be "the science of the facts of Consciousness;" and the Brain is often assigned as "the organ of Consciousness." Yet there are many mental processes, and many cerebral processes, which are declared to be unconscious. Obviously if Consciousness is the function of the Brain, there can be no cerebral activity which is unconscious; just as there can be no activity of the lungs which is not respiratory. Usage therefore points to a general and a special sense of the term. The general usage identifies it with Sensibility, in its subjective aspect as Sentience, including

all psychical states, both those classed under Sensation, and those under Thought. These states are the "facts of consciousness" with which Psychology is occupied. In the special usage it is distinguished from all other psychical states by a peculiar reflected feeling of Attention, whereby we not only *have* a sensation, but also *feel* that we have it; we not only think, but are conscious that we are thinking; not only act, but are conscious of what we do. It is this which Kant indicates when he defines it "the subjective form accompanying all our conceptions (*Begriffe*);" and Jessen when he defines it "the internal knowing of our knowing, an in itself reflected knowing." *

52. We shall often have to recur to this general and this special meaning, both of which are too firmly rooted for any successful attempt to displace them. The fact that some organic processes and some mental processes take place now consciously and now unconsciously, *i.e.*, now with the feeling of reflected attention, and now with no such feeling, assuredly demands a corresponding expression; nor, in spite of inevitable ambiguities, is there ground for regretting that the expression chosen should be only an extension of the expression already adopted for all other states of Sentience. A sentient or conscious state can only be a state of the sentient organism, itself the unity of many organs, each having its Sensibility. There is more or less consensus, but there is no introduction of a new agent within the organism, converting what was physical impression into mental reaction. From first to last there has been nothing but neural processes, and combinations of such processes—which, viewed subjectively, are sentient processes. Thus the gradations of sensitive reaction are Sentience, Consentience, and Consciousness, which are represented in the Logic of Feeling and the Logic of Signs. The familiar term Conscience will then represent the

* "Das Bewusstwerden ist nichts Anderes als ein weiter fortgeschrittenes Erinnern oder Neuwerden des von aussen aufgenommenen Wissens, ein innerliches Wissen dieses Wissens oder ein in sich reflectirtes Wissen."—JESSEN: *Versuch einer Wissenschaftlichen Begründung der Psychologie*, 1855, p. 477.

Logic of Conduct. Thus understood, we may say that a man sometimes acts unconsciously, or thinks unconsciously, although his action and thought are ruled by Consentience, as he sometimes acts and thinks unconscientiously, although he is not without obedience to Conscience on other occasions. The feeling which determines an action is *operative*, although it may not be *discriminated* from simultaneous feelings. When this is the case, we say the feeling is unconscious; but this no more means that it is a purely physical process taking place outside the sphere of Sentience, than the immoral conduct of a man would be said to be mechanical, and not the conduct of a moral agent. There is undoubtedly a marked distinction expressed in the terms Consciousness and Unconsciousness, but it is not that of contrasts such as Mental and Physical, it is that of grades such as Light and Darkness. Just as Darkness is a positive optical sensation very different from mere privation—just as it replaces the sensation of Light, blends with it, struggles with it, and in all respects differs from the *absence* of all optical sensibility in the skin; so Unconsciousness struggles with, blends with, and replaces Consciousness in the organism, and is a positive state of the sentient organism, not to be confounded with a mere negation of Sentience; above all, not to be relegated to merely mechanical processes.

52*a*. Remember that, strictly speaking, Consciousness is a psychological not a physiological term, and is only used in Physiology on the assumption that it is the subjective *equivalent* of an objective process. To avoid the equivoque of "unconscious sensation," we may substitute the term "unconscious neural process;" and as all neural processes imply Sensibility, which in the subjective aspect is Sentience, we say that Sentience has various modes and degrees—such as Perception, Ideation, Emotion, Volition, which may be conscious, sub-conscious, or unconscious. When Leibnitz referred to the fact of "obscure ideas," and modern writers expressed this fact as "unconscious cerebration," the first phrase did not imply a process that was other than mental, the second phrase did not imply a process that was other than physiological: both indicated a mode of the process known as Consciousness under other modes. There are different neural elements grouped in Ideation and Emotion; there are different neural elements grouped in Consciousness, Sub-consciousness, and Unconsciousness; but one tissue with one property is active in all.

53. The nervous organism is affected as a whole by every affection of its constituent parts. Every excitation, instead of terminating with itself—as is the case in most physical processes—or with the motor impulse it excites, is propagated throughout the continuous tissue, and thus sends a *thrill* throughout the organism. The wave of excitation in passing onwards beats against variously-grouped elements—temporary and permanent centres—disturbing their balance more or less, and liberating the energy of some, increasing the tension of others, necessarily affecting all. Those groups which have their energy liberated set up processes that are either *discriminated* as sensations, or are blended with the general stream, according to their *relative* energy in the consensus. Thus the impulse on reaching the centres for the heart, lungs, legs, and tail excites the innervation of these organs; but as these are only parts of the organism, and as all the parts enter the consensus, and Consciousness is the varying resultant of this ever-varying consensus, the thrill which any particular stimulus excites will be unconscious, sub-conscious, or conscious, in proportion to the extent of the *irradiated* disturbance, which will depend on the statical conditions of the centres at the moment. A sound sends a thrill which excites emotion, causes the heart to beat faster, the muscles to quiver, the skin-glands to pour forth their secretion; yet this same sound heard by another man, or the same man under other conditions, physical or historical, merely sends a faint thrill, just vivid enough to detach itself as a sensation from the other simultaneous excitations; and the same sound may excite a thrill which is so faint and fugitive as to pass unconsciously. Physiological and psychological inductions assure us that these are only differences of degree. The same kind of physiological effect accompanies the

conscious and unconscious state. Every sensory impression, no matter whether discriminated or not, affects the circulation and develops heat. The blood-vessels of the part impressed expand, vessels elsewhere contract—a change in the blood pressure has been effected, which of course implies that the whole organism has been affected. Delicate instruments show that at the time a sensation is produced the temperature of the brain is raised. The same is true of ideation. Mosso has invented a method of registering the effect of thought on the circulation. He finds ideation accompanied by a contraction of the peripheral vessels proportionate to the degree of intellectual effort. A young man translating Greek showed greater contraction than when he was translating Latin. During sound sleep—when we are said to be unconscious—sudden noises always cause contraction of the peripheral vessels. Psychological observation assures us that the conscious and unconscious states were both consentient, and were both operative in the same degree. The absorbed thinker threads his way through crowded streets, and is sub-conscious and unconscious of the various sights, sounds, touches, and muscular movements which make up so large a portion of his sentient excitation at the time; yet he deftly avoids obstacles, hears the sound of a hurried step behind him, recognises an interesting object directly it presents itself, and can even recall in Memory many of the uninteresting objects which he passed in sub-conscious and unconscious indifference.

54. On all grounds, therefore, we must say that between conscious, sub-conscious, and unconscious states the difference is only of degree of complication in the neural processes, which by relative preponderance in the consensus determine a relative discrimination. We can only discriminate one thrill at a time; but the neural excitations simultaneously pressing towards a discharge are many; and the conditions which determine now this, and now the other excitation to predominate by its differential pressure, are far beyond any mechanical estimate. I mention this because the advocates of the Reflex Theory maintain that the neural processes are

the same whether a sensation be produced or not; and that since the same actions follow the external stimulation whether sensation be produced or not, this proves the actions to be purely mechanical. I reply, the neural processes are *not* the same throughout in the two cases—otherwise the effects would be the same. You might as well say, "Since the explosion of the gun is the same, whether shotted or not, a blank cartridge will kill;" but if you tell me that your gun killed the bird, I declare that the cartridge was *not* a blank one. Whether the explosion of the gun *also* produced terror in one bystander, curiosity in a second, and attracted no notice from a third, will be altogether another matter. In like manner the sensory impression which determines a movement may or may not be accompanied or followed by *other* sentient states; the fact of such movement is evidence of its sentient antecedent; and an external stimulus that will produce *this* neural process, and this consequent movement, must produce a feeling, although not necessarily a discriminated sensation. Now since, for discrimination, *other* neural processes must co-operate, we cannot say that in the two cases *all* the neural processes have been the same throughout; nor because of this difference can we say that the process of the undiscriminated sensation is a mechanical, not a sentient process. In the next problem this point will be argued more fully.

55. The need of recognising Consciousness and Consentience as degrees of energy and complexity in sentient states is apparent when we consider animal phenomena. Has a bee consciousness? Has a snail volition? or are they both insentient mechanisms? All inductions warrant the assertion that a bee has thrills propagated throughout its organism by the agency of its nerves; and that some of these thrills are of the kind called sensations—even discriminated sensations. Nevertheless we may reasonably doubt whether the bee has sentient states resembling otherwise than remotely the sensations, emotions, and thoughts which constitute human Consciousness, either in the general or the special sense of that term. The bee feels and reacts on feelings; but its feelings

cannot closely resemble our own, because the conditions in the two cases are different. The bee may even be said to think (in so far as Thought means logical combination of feelings), for it appears to form Judgments in the sphere of the Logic of Feeling—τὸ νοητικὸν; although incapable of the Logic of Signs—τὸ διανοητικὸν. We should therefore say the bee has Consentience, but not Consciousness—unless we accept Consciousness in its *general* signification as the equivalent of Sentience. The organism of the bee differs from that of a man, as a mud hut from a marble palace. But since underlying these differences there are fundamental resemblances, the functions of the two will be fundamentally alike. Both have the function of Sentience; as mud hut and palace have both the office of sheltering.

56. The question of Volition will occupy us in the next chapter. Restricting ourselves here to that of Consciousness, and recalling the distinction of the two meanings of the term, we now approach the question of Unconsciousness. Are we to understand this term as designating a purely physical state in contrast to the purely mental state of Consciousness; or only as designating a difference of degree? This is like asking whether Light and Darkness are both optical feelings, or one an optical feeling and the other a physical process? On the Reflex Theory, no sooner does a vital and mental process pass from the daylight of Consciousness, or twilight of Subconsciousness, into the darkness of Unconsciousness, than the whole order of phenomena is abruptly changed, they cease to be vital, mental, and lapse into physical, mechanical processes. The grounds of this conclusion are, first, the unpsychological assumption that the unconscious state is out of the sphere of Sentience; and secondly, the unphysiological assumption that the Brain is the only portion of the nervous system which has the property of Sensibility. Restate the conclusion in different terms and its fallacy emerges: "organic processes suddenly cease to be organic, and become purely physical by a slight change in their *relative* position in the consensus; the organic process which was a conscious sensation a moment ago, when its energy was not balanced by

some other process, suddenly falls from its place in the group of organic phenomena—sentient phenomena—to sink into the group of inorganic phenomena now that its energy is balanced." Consider the parallel case of Motion and Rest in the objective sphere. They are two functions of the co-operant forces, one dynamic, the other static; although markedly distinguishable as functions, we know that they are simply the co-operant forces now unbalanced and now balanced; what we call Rest is also a product of moving forces, each of which is operant, and will issue in a definite resultant when its counter-force is removed. Motion and Rest are correlatives, and both belong to the sphere of Kinetics. In like manner Consciousness and Unconsciousness are correlatives, both belonging to the sphere of Sentience.* Every one of the unconscious processes is operant, changes the general state of the organism, and is capable of at once issuing in a discriminated sensation when the force which balances it is disturbed. I was unconscious of the scratch of my pen in writing the last sentence, but I am distinctly conscious of every scratch in writing this one. Then, as now, the scratching sound sent a faint thrill through my organism, but its relative intensity was too faint for discrimination; now that I have redistributed the co-operant forces, by what is called an act of Attention, I hear distinctly every sound the pen produces.

57. The inclusion of Sub-consciousness within the sentient sphere is obvious; the inclusion of Unconsciousness within that sphere may be made so, when we consider its modes of production, and compare it with the extra-sensible conception of molecules and atoms. The Matter which is sensible as masses, may be resolved into molecules, which lie beyond the discrimination of sense; and these again into atoms, which are purely ideal conceptions; but because molecules are *proved*, and atoms are *supposed*, to have material properties,

* In common language a stone or a tree is said to be unconscious; but this is an anthropomorphic extension of the term. In strictness we should no more speak of unconsciousness outside the sphere of Sentience than of darkness outside the sphere of Vision.

and to conform to sensible canons of the objective world, we never hesitate to class them under the head of Matter; nor do we imagine that in passing beyond the discrimination of Sense they lose their objective significance. They are still physical, not mental facts. So with Sentience: we may trace it through infinite gradations from Consciousness to Sub-consciousness, till it fades away in Unconsciousness; but from first to last the processes have been those of a sentient organism; and by this are broadly distinguished from all processes in anorganisms. The movement of a limb has quite different modes of production from the movement of a wheel; and among its modes must be included those of Sensibility, a peculiarly vital property. Oxidation may be slow or rapid, manifesting itself as combustion, heat, or flame, but it is always oxidation—always a special chemical phenomenon. And so the neural process of Sentience, whether conscious, sub-conscious, or unconscious, is always a state of the sentient organism. If a material process does not change its character, and become spiritual, on passing beyond the range of sensible appreciation, why should a psychical process become material on passing beyond the range of discrimination? If we admit molecules as physical units, sentient tremors are psychical units. The extra-sensible molecules have indeed their subjective aspect, and only enter perception through the "greeting of the spirit." The sentient tremors have also their objective aspect, and cannot come into existence without the neural tremors, which are their physical conditions.

58. It is only by holding fast to such a conception that we can escape the many difficulties and contradictions presented by unconscious phenomena, and explain many physiological and psychological processes. Descartes—followed by many philosophers—identified Consciousness with Thought. To this day we constantly hear that to have a sensation, and to be conscious of it, is one and the same state; which is only admissible on the understanding that Consciousness means Sentience, and Sentience the activity of the nervous system viewed subjectively. Leibnitz pointed out that we have many psychical states which are unconscious states—to have an

idea and be conscious of it, are, he said, not one but two states. The Consciousness by Descartes erected into an essential condition of Thought, was by Leibnitz reduced to an accompaniment which not only may be absent, but in the vast majority of cases is absent. The teaching of most modern psychologists is that Consciousness forms but a small item in the total of psychical processes. Unconscious sensations, ideas, and judgments are made to play a great part in their explanations. It is very certain that in every conscious volition—every act that is so characterised—the larger part of it is quite unconscious. It is equally certain that in every perception there are unconscious processes of reproduction and inference—there is much that is *implicit*, some of which cannot be made explicit—a "middle distance" of sub-consciousness, and a "background" of unconsciousness. But, throughout, the processes are those of Sentience.

59. Unconsciousness is by some writers called *latent* Consciousness. Experiences which are no longer manifested are said to be stored up in Memory, remaining in the Soul's picture-gallery, visible directly the shutters are opened. We are not conscious of these feelings, yet they exist as latent feelings, and become salient through association. As a metaphorical expression of the familiar facts of Memory this may pass; but it has been converted from a metaphor into an hypothesis, and we are supposed to *have* feelings and ideas, when in fact we have nothing more than a modified *disposition* of the organism—temporary or permanent—which when stimulated will respond in this modified manner. The modification of the organism when permanent becomes hereditary; and its response is then called an instinctive or automatic action. And as actions pass by degrees from conscious and voluntary into sub-conscious and sub-voluntary, and finally into unconscious and involuntary, we call them volitional, secondarily automatic, and automatic. If any one likes to say the last are due to latent consciousness, I shall not object. I only point to the fact that the differences here specified are simply differences of degree—all the actions are those of the sentient organism.

60. Picture to yourself this sentient organism incessantly stimulated from without and from within, and adjusting itself in response to such stimulations. In the blending of stimulations, modifying and arresting each other, there is a fluctuating "composition of forces," with ever-varying resultants. Besides the stream of direct stimulations, there is a wider stream of indirect or reproduced stimulations. Together with the present sensation there is always a more or less complex group of revived sensations, the one group of neural tremors being organically stimulated by the other. An isolated excitation is impossible in a continuous nervous tissue; an isolated feeling is impossible in the consensus or unity of the sentient organism. The term Soul is the personification of this complex of present and revived feelings, and is the substratum of Consciousness (in the general sense), all the particular feelings being its *states*. To repeat an illustration used in my first volume, we may compare Consciousness to a mass of stationary waves. If the surface of a lake be set in motion each wave diffuses itself over the whole surface, and finally reaches the shores, whence it is reflected back towards the centre of the lake. This reflected wave is met by the fresh incoming waves, there is a blending of the waves, and their product is a pattern on the surface. This pattern of stationary waves is a fluctuating pattern, because of the incessant arrival of fresh waves, incoming and reflected. Whenever a fresh stream enters the lake (*i.e.*, a new sensation is excited from without), its waves will at first pass over the pattern, neither disturbing it nor being disturbed by it; but after reaching the shore the waves will be reflected back towards the centre, and there will more or less modify the pattern.

CHAPTER V.

VOLUNTARY AND INVOLUNTARY ACTIONS.

61. Much of what has been said in the preceding chapter respecting the passive side of the organism is equally applicable to the active side. Our actions are classed as voluntary and involuntary mainly in reference to their being consciously or unconsciously performed; but not wholly so, for there are many involuntary actions of which we are distinctly conscious, and many voluntary actions of which we are at times sub-conscious and unconscious. I do not propose here to open the long and arduous discussion as to what constitutes Volition, my present purpose being simply that of fixing the meaning of terms, so that the question of Automatism may not be complicated by their ambiguities. "Voluntary" and "involuntary" are, like "conscious" and "unconscious," correlative terms; but commonly, instead of being understood as indicating differences of degree in phenomena of the same order, they are supposed to indicate differences of kind—a new agent, the Will, being understood in the one case to direct the Mechanism which suffices without direction in the other.

62. This interpretation is unphysiological and unpsychological, since it overlooks the fact that both voluntary and involuntary actions belong to the same *order* of phenomena, *i.e.*, those of the sentient organism. Both involve the same *efficient* cause, *i.e.*, co-operant conditions. We draw a line of demarcation between the two abstractions—as between all abstractions—but the concrete processes they symbolise have no such demarcation. Just as the thought which at one moment passes unconsciously, at another consciously, is in itself the same thought, and the same neural process; so the

action which at one moment is voluntary, and at another involuntary, is itself the same action, performed by the same mechanism. The incitation which precedes, and the feeling which accompanies the action, belong to the accessory mechanisms, and may be replaced by other incitations and other feelings; as the fall of an apple is the same event, involving the same conditions, *i.e.*, efficient cause, whether the *occasional* cause be a gust of wind or the gardener's scissors, and whether the fall be seen and heard or not. I may utter words intentionally and consciously, and I may utter the same words automatically, unconsciously; I may wink voluntarily, and wink involuntarily. There are terms to express these differences; but they do not express a difference in the efficient agencies.

63. Many writers seem to think that the involuntary actions belong to the physical mechanical order, because they are not stimulated by cerebral incitations, and cannot be regulated or controlled by such incitations—or as the psychologists would say, because Consciousness in the form of Will is no agent prompting and regulating such actions. But I think this untenable. The actions cannot belong to the mechanical order so long as they are the actions of a vital mechanism, and so long as we admit the broad distinction between organisms and anorganisms. Whether they have the special character of Consciousness or not, they have the general character of sentient actions, being those of a sentient mechanism. And this becomes the more evident when we consider the gradations of the phenomena. Many, if not all, of those actions which are classed under the involuntary were originally of the voluntary class—either in the individual or his ancestors; but having become permanently-organised dispositions—the pathways of stimulation and reaction having been definitely established—they have lost that volitional element (of hesitation and choice) which implies regulation and control. But even here a slight change in the habitual conditions will introduce a disturbance in the process which may awaken Consciousness, and the sense of effort, sometimes even causing control. An instinctive or an automatic

action may be thus changed, or arrested. Take as an example one of the unequivocally automatic actions, that of Breathing. It is called automatic because, like the actions of an automaton, it is performed by a definitely-constructed mechanism, always working in the same way when stimulated and left to itself. There must of course be a sense of effort in every impulse which has resistance to overcome, organs to be moved; but the mechanism of Breathing is so delicately adjusted, that the sense of effort is reduced to a minimum, and we are unconscious of it, or sub-conscious of it. Nevertheless, without altering the rate or amplitude of the inspirations and expirations, we become distinctly conscious of them, and, moreover, within certain limits we can control them, so that the Breathing passes from the involuntary to the voluntary class.

64. Pass on to other examples. What action can be more involuntary than the rhythmic movements of the heart and the contractions of the iris? Compared with the actions of the tongue or limbs, these seem riveted by an iron necessity, freed from all consciousness and control. Yet the movements of the heart are not only stimulated by sensations and thoughts, they are also capable of being felt; and the movements both of heart and iris are not wholly removed from our control. That we do not habitually control (that is, *interfere* with) the action of the heart, the contraction of the iris, or the activity of a gland, is true; it is on this account that such actions are called involuntary; they obey the immediate stimulus. But it is an error to assert that these actions *cannot* be controlled, that they are altogether beyond the interference of other centres, and cannot by any effort of ours be modified. It is an error to suppose these actions are essentially distinguished from the voluntary movement of the hands. We have acquired a power of definite direction in the movements of the hands, which renders them obedient to our will; but this acquisition has been of slow laborious growth. If we were asked to use our toes as we use our fingers—to grasp, paint, sew, or write with them, we should find it not less impossible to control the movements of the

toes in these directions, than to contract the iris, or cause a burst of perspiration to break forth. Certain movements of the toes are possible to us; but unless the loss of our fingers has made it necessary that we should use our toes in complicated and slowly-acquired movements, we can do no more with them than the young infant can do with his fingers. Yet men and women have written, sewed, and painted with their toes. All that is requisite is that certain links should be established between sensations and movements; by continual practice these links *are* established; and what is impossible to the majority of men, becomes easy to the individual who has acquired this power. This same power can be acquired over what are called the organic actions; nevertheless the habitual needs of life do not *tend* towards such acquisition, and without some strong current setting in that direction, or some peculiarity of organisation rendering it easy, it is never acquired. In ordinary circumstances the number of those who can write with their toes is extremely rare, the urgent necessity which would create such a power being rare; and rare also are the examples of those who have any control over the movement of the iris, or the action of a gland; but both rarities exist.

It would be difficult to choose a more striking example of reflex action than the contraction of the iris of the eye under the stimulus of light;* and to ordinary men, having no link established which would guide them, it is utterly impossible to close the iris by any effort. It would be not less impossible to the hungry child to get on the chair and reach the food on the table, until that child had *learned* how to do so. Yet there are men who have learned how to contract the iris. The celebrated Fontana had this power; which is possessed also by a medical man now living at Kilmarnock—Dr. Paxton—a fact authenticated by no less a person than Dr. Allen Thomson.† Dr. Paxton can contract or expand

* The contraction may be effected in the eye out of the organism. See p. 204. It is then no reflex.

† *Glasgow Medical Journal*, 1857, p. 451. See also further on, note to p. 377.

the iris at will, without changing the position of his eye, and without an effort of adaptation to distance.

To move the ears is impossible to most men. Yet some do it with ease, and all could learn to do it. Some men have learned to "ruminate" their food; others to vomit with ease; and some are said to have the power of perspiring at will.* Now, if once we recognise a link of sensation and motion, we recognise a possible source of control; and if the daily needs of life were such that to fulfil some purpose the action of the heart required control, we should learn to control it. Some men have, without such needs, learned how to control it. The eminent physiologist, E. F. Weber of Leipzig, found that he could completely check the beating of his heart. By suspending his breath and violently contracting his chest, he could retard the pulsations; and after three or five beats, unaccompanied by any of the usual sounds, it was completely still. On one occasion he carried the experiment too far, and fell into a syncope. Cheyne, in the last century, recorded the case of a patient of his own who could at will suspend the beating of his pulse, and always fainted when he did so.

65. It thus appears that even the actions which most distinctly bear the character recognised as involuntary—uncontrollable—are only so because the ordinary processes of life furnish no necessity for their control. We do not learn to control them, though we could do so, to some extent; nor do we learn to control the motions of our ears, although we could do so. And while it appears that the involuntary actions can become voluntary, it is familiar to all that the voluntary actions tend, by constant repetition, to become involuntary. Thus involuntary actions, under certain limitations, may be controlled; on the other hand, the voluntary are incapable of being controlled under the urgency of direct stimulation. Both are reflexes.

Inasmuch as almost all actions are the products of stimulated nerve-centres, it is obvious that these actions are

* MAYER: *Die Elementarorganisation des Seelenorgans*, p. 12, is the authority for the last statement.

reflex—reflected from those centres. It matters not whether I wink because a sensation of dryness, or because an idea of danger, causes the eyelid to close: the act is equally reflex. The nerve-centre which supplies the eyelid with its nerve has been stimulated; the stimuli may be various, the act is uniform. At one time the stimulus is a sensation of dryness, at another an idea of danger, at another the idea of communicating by means of a wink with some one present; in each case the stimulus is reflected in a muscular contraction. Sensations excite other sensations; ideas excite other ideas; and one of these ideas may issue in an action of control. But the restraining power is limited, and cannot resist a certain degree of urgency in the original stimulus. I can, for a time, restrain the act of winking, in spite of the sensation of dryness; but the reflex which sets going this restraining action will only last a few seconds; after which, the urgency of the external stimulus is stronger than that of the reflex feeling—the sensation of dryness is more imperious than the idea of resistance—and the eyelid drops.

If a knife be brought near the arm of a man who has little confidence in the friendly intentions of him that holds it, he shrinks, and the shrinking is "involuntary," *i.e.*, in spite of his will. Let him have confidence, and he does not shrink, even when the knife touches his skin. The idea of danger is not excited in the second case, or if excited, is at once banished by another idea. Yet this very man, who can thus repress the involuntary shrinking when the knife approaches his arm, cannot repress the involuntary winking when the same friend approaches a finger to his eye. In vain he prepares himself to resist that reflex action; in vain he resolves to resist the impulse; no sooner does the finger approach, than down flashes the eyelid. Many men, and most women, would be equally unable to resist shrinking on the approach of a knife: the association of the idea of danger with the knife would bear down any previous resolution not to shrink. It is from this cause that timorous women tremble at the approach of firearms. An association is established in their minds which no idea is powerful enough to loosen. You may assure them the gun is not loaded; "*that* makes very little difference," said a naïve old lady to a friend of mine. They tremble, as the child trembles when he sees you put on the mask. These illustrations show that the urgency of any one idea may, like the urgency of a sensation, bear down the resistance offered by some other idea; as the previous illustrations showed that an idea could restrain or control the action which a sensation or idea would otherwise have produced. According to the doctrines current, the Will is said to be operative when an idea determines an action; and yet all would agree that the winking which was involuntary when the idea of danger determined it, was voluntary when the idea of communicating with an accomplice in some mystification determined it.

66. There is no real and essential distinction between voluntary and involuntary actions. They all spring from Sensibility. They are all determined by feeling. It is convenient, for common purposes, to designate some actions as voluntary; but this is merely a convenience; no psychological nor physiological insight is gained by it; an analysis of the process discloses no element in a voluntary action which is not to be found in an involuntary action—except in the origin or degree of stimulation. In ordinary language it is convenient to mark a distinction between my raising my arm because I will to raise it for some definite purpose, and my raising it because a bee has stung me; it is convenient to say, "I *will* to write this letter," and "this letter is written against my will—I have no will in the matter." But Science is more exacting when it aims at being exact; and the philosopher, analysing these complex actions, will find that in each case certain muscular groups have been set in action by different sensational or ideational stimuli. The action itself is that of a neuro-muscular mechanism, which mechanism works in the same way, whatever be the source of the original impulse. The stimulation may be incited directly from the periphery, or indirectly from a remote centre; and the action may be arrested by a peripheral or central stimulation: the reflex which ordinarily follows

the excitation of a sensory nerve will be modified, or arrested, if some other nerve be at the same time stimulated. (See Law of Arrest, *Prob.* II. § 190.)

67. All actions are reflex, all are the operations of a mechanism, all are sentient, because the mechanism has Sensibility as its vital property. In thus preserving the integrity of the order of vital phenomena, and keeping them classified apart from physical and chemical phenomena, we by no means set aside the useful distinctions expressed in the terms voluntary and involuntary; any more than we set aside the distinction of vertebrate and invertebrate when both are classed under Animal, and separated from Plant, or Planet.

The mechanisms of the special Senses respond in special reactions; the mechanisms of special actions have also their several responses. The tail responds to stimulation with lateral movements, the chest with inspiration and expiration, and so on. These responses are called automatic, and have this in common with the actions of automata that they are uniform, and do not need the co-operation of Consciousness, though they do need the operation of Sensibility, and are thereby distinguished from the actions of automata. The facial muscles, and the limbs, also respond to stimulation in uniform ways, but owing to the varieties of stimulation the actions are more variable, and have more the character of volitional movements. With this greater freedom of possible action comes the eminently mental character of *choice*. In the cerebral rehearsal of an act not yet performed—its mental prevision—as when we intend to do something, yet for the moment arrest the act, so that there is only a nascent excitation of the motor process, there is a peculiar state of Consciousness expressive of this state of the mechanism: we call the prevision a *motive*—and it becomes a *motor* when the intention is realised, the nascent excitation becomes an unchecked impulse. The abstract of all motives we call Will. A motive is a volition in the sphere of the Intellect. In the sphere of Emotion it is a motor. Hence we never speak of the Will of a mollusc, or the motives of an insect, only of their sensations and motors. Yet it is obvious that the reflex in operation when a snail shrinks at the approach of an object is essentially similar to the reflex in operation when the baby shrinks, and this again is still more similar to that in operation when the boy shrinks: the boy has the idea of danger, which neither baby nor snail can have; the idea is a motive, which can be controlled by another idea; the baby and the snail can have no such motive, no such control—are they therefore automata?

68. If I see that a donkey has wandered into my garden, the motive which determines me to take a stick and with it drive the donkey away is a cerebral rehearsal of the effects which will follow my act. The sight of the donkey has roused disagreeable feelings, and these suggest possible means of alleviation; out of these possibilities — reproductions of former experiences—I choose one. But if I seize the stick with which some one is threatening me, I do not pause to choose, I snatch automatically without hesitation. Yet this unreflecting automatic act is itself as truly volitional as my seizing the stick to drive away the donkey—it is the motor which has been organised in me by previous experiences—it is the consequence of an emotion, not of a deliberation; and it has not been determined by any clear prevision of consequences. Feeling inspires, and feeling guides my movements, so that if my snatch has missed the stick, I snatch again, or duck under. This is the kind of Volition we ascribe to animals. It is a great part of our own. By insensible degrees, acts which originally were prompted by motives sink into the automatic class prompted by motors. When an angry man snatches up a knife, doffs bystanders aside, and rushes on his enemy to stab him, he does not distinctly prefigure the final result, he only obeys each motor, and is conscious of each step; but had he planned the murder he would have foreseen the end, and this prevision would have been the motive. The angry man is struck with horror at the sight of the bleeding corpse, and passionately declares he did not *mean* to kill. Nor did he will the consequences of his act, yet he certainly willed each separate step—he recog-

nised the knife, saw the bystanders, knew they would interfere with him, willed to push them aside. He may be right in declaring that the act was involuntary; but assuredly it was not purely mechanical.

69. Again: We are not conscious of the separate sensations which guide speech or writing; we cannot properly be said to will the utterance of each tone, or the formation of each letter. Are these processes mechanical and not volitional? By no means. We know that they were laboriously learned by long tentative efforts, each of which was accompanied by distinct consciousness. We also know that now when the mechanism is so easy in its adjustment as to suggest automatism, there needs but a slight alteration in the conditions to make us distinctly conscious of the processes—the wrong word spoken, or one letter ill formed, suffices to arrest the easy working of the mechanism. A similar mechanism operates in thinking, which also lapses from the conscious and voluntary to the unconscious and involuntary state. The logical process of Judgment is as purely a reflex from one neural group to another, as the physiological process of coordination. In ordinary thinking we are as little conscious of the particular steps—our interest being concentrated on the result—as we are of the particular stages of an action. The adjustments of the mechanism of Reproduction and Association are *set* going by a motive, and *kept* going by psychological motors. And here—as in bodily actions—there is often a conflict between motive and motors—between the foreseen result, and the available means of reaching it—the motors usually prevailing because they represent the active side of the mechanism. Thus when an oculist wishes to examine a patient's eye, he does not tell him to give a particular direction to his eye, knowing that the *motive* to do so will not suffice; instead of this he simply moves his own hand in the desired direction, certain that the eye will by reflex irresistibly follow it. Nay, there are sometimes such anomalies of innervation that the eye instead of obeying the motive, moves in a contrary direction. Meschede mentions a patient whose movements were mostly of this anomalous kind: when he

willed to move the eyes to the right, they moved to the left; when he willed to move them up, they moved down. It was thus also with his hands and feet. Yet he was distinctly conscious that his intention had been frustrated, and that he acted "because he could not help it." * How insensibly a motive sinks into a motor, that is to say, a voluntary into an involuntary act, may be recognised in speech, writing, singing, walking, &c., and in the incessant movements of the eye in fixing objects. Aubert has well remarked that we only give definite movements to the eye when we wish to see an object distinctly. Whenever the indistinct vision suffices—as in walking through the streets occupied in conversation or thought—we make no such movements; but no sooner does any object excite our attention, than the effort to fix that object at once excites the necessary reflex.†

70. By the Will, then, we must understand the abstract generalised expression of the impulses which determine actions, when those impulses have an ideal origin; by Volition the still more generalised expression of all impulses which determine actions. The one class is that of *motives*

* *Allgemeine Zeitschrift für Psychiatrie*, Bd. 31, p. 711.

† AUBERT: *Grundzüge der physiol. Optik*, 1876, p. 633. "The accommodative movement of the eye is to be considered voluntary. It is true we contract the pupil without being conscious of the contraction of muscular fibres, *but this holds good for every voluntary movement.* When a person raises the tone of his voice he is not conscious that by muscular contraction he makes his chordæ vocales more tense; he attains his object without being aware of the means by which he does so. The same is applicable to accommodation for near objects and to the contraction of the pupil accompanying it. The fact that *this last is only an associated movement does not deprive it of its voluntary character*, for there is perhaps no single muscle which can contract entirely by itself." DONDERS: *On the Anomalies of Accommodation*, 1864, p. 574. Professor BEER of Bonn has the rare power of contracting or dilating the pupils of his eye at will; here ideas act as motors. When he thinks of a very dark space the pupil dilates, when of a very bright spot the pupil contracts. (NOBLE: *The Human Mind*, 1858, p. 124.) I believe this to be only an exaggerated form of the normal tendency. In all of us the mechanism is so disposed that the feelings of dilatation are associated with feelings (and consequently ideas) of darkness; and by this association a reversal of the process obtains, so that the idea of darkness calls up the feeling it symbolises.

with ideal elements; the other that of *motors* with sensational or emotional elements. But both are mental states, both are neural processes in a sentient organism; neither is mechanical, except in so far as all actions are expressible in mechanical terms. For convenience we class actions as reflex, automatic, involuntary, unconscious, voluntary, and conscious. If we separate the reflex from the voluntary, we need not therefore dissociate the former from Sensibility; and the reason why we ought not to separate it is that we know it to be sense-guided from first to last, although the sensations may escape discrimination. The feeling of Effort, which was formerly felt when an action was performed, may have become so minimised that it is too faint for more than a momentary consciousness, too evanescent for the memory to retain it; yet the feeling must always be operant when its mechanism is in action. The ease with which the mechanism works does not change the adjustment of its elements, nor alter its character. The facile unobtrusive performance of a vital function does not change it from a vital to a mechanical act. Mr. Spencer seems to me to express himself ambiguously when he says: "Just as any set of psychical changes originally displaying Memory, Reason, and Feeling cease to be conscious, rational, and emotional as fast as they by repetition grow closely organised, so do they at the same time pass beyond the sphere of Volition. Memory, Reason, Feeling, and Will disappear in proportion as psychical changes become automatic" *—for while it is perfectly true that we only call those psychical changes "automatic" which have lost the special qualities called "conscious, rational, and emotional," it is not less true that they remain from first to last *psychical* changes, and are thereby distinguished from *physical* changes. To suppose that they pass from the psychical to the physical by frequent repetition would lead to the monstrous conclusion that when a naturalist has by laborious study become so familiarised with the specific marks of an animal or plant that he can recognise at a glance a particular species, or recognise from a

* SPENCER: *Principles of Psychology*, i. 499.

single character the nature of the rest, the rapidity and certainty of this judgment proves it to be a mechanical, not a mental act. The intuition with which a mathematician sees the solution of a problem would then be a mechanical process, while the slow and bungling hesitation of the tyro in presence of the same problem would be a mental process: the perfection of the organism would thus result in its degradation to the level of a machine!

The operations of the intellect may furnish us with an illustration. Ideas are symbols of sensations. The idea of a horse is an abstraction easily traceable to concrete sensations, yet as an abstraction is so different a state of feeling that we only identify it with its concretes by a careful study of its stages of evolution, namely, sensation, image, reproduced images resembling yet differing from the original sensation, a coalescence of their resemblances, and finally the substitution of a verbal symbol for these images. With this symbol the intellect operates, and sometimes operates so exclusively with it that not the faintest trace of image or sensation is appreciable—the word horse takes the place of the image in the sequence of sensorial processes, just as the image takes the place of the sensation. It does this as a neural equivalent. In the same way we substitute verbal symbols for a bag of sovereigns when we pay a creditor with a cheque; he pays the cheque away to another; and this monetary equivalent passes from hand to hand without a single coin making its appearance. Does the transaction cease to be commercial, monetary, in this substitution of signs? No; nor does a process cease to be psychical when an image is substituted for a sensation, and a verbal symbol for an image. This every one will admit. Must we not go further, and extend the admission to automatic actions which originally were voluntary, and have now lost all trace of ideal prevision, and almost all traces of accompanying consciousness? *The motor mechanism has its symbols also;* in this sense, that whereas the action which at first needed complex sensorial processes to set it going and keep it going, is now determined by a single one of those processes taking the place of their resultant. When a practised accountant runs his eye up a column of figures, he does not pause to realise the values of those figures by decomposing the symbols into their numerical units, he simply groups one symbol with another according to their intuited relations, and the final result is reached with a certainty not less, and a rapidity far greater, than if it had been reached by step-by-step verification. It is thus with the pianoforte-player. It is thus with all automatic performances, except those dependent on the connate adjustments of the mechanism.

CHAPTER VI.

THE PROBLEM STATED.

71. If the preceding attempt to disengage the question from the ambiguities of its terms has been successful, we shall find little difficulty in rationally interpreting all the facts adduced in favour of Animal Automatism, without having recourse to a mechanical theory of biological phenomena. The objections to that theory are that it employs terms which have very misleading *connotations* even when they do not *denote* phenomena of widely different orders; so that the moral repugnance commonly felt at the attempt to treat the animal organism as if it were a machine, is sustained by the intellectual repugnance at the attempt to explain biological phenomena on principles derived from phenomena of a simpler order.

Remark, in passing, this piquant contradiction: the Automaton theory of Descartes, when applied to the animals, generally excited ridicule or repulsion; whereas the far more inconsistent and mechanical theory of Reflex Action has been almost universally welcomed as a great discovery, though it banishes the Sensibility which Descartes preserved. And further, the philosophers who most loudly protested against the idea that animals were machines, were the philosophers who most insisted that these animals were made, not evolved —planned by their maker, as a watch is planned by its maker, with a distinct purpose and prevision in the disposition of every part; whereas the philosophers who most emphatically reject this notion of organisms being made, are often those who liken organisms to machines.

72. The paradox propounded by Descartes loses much of its strangeness when we understand his meaning. Its terms are infelicitous because of their misleading connotations. When he says that all the actions of animals which seem to be due to Consciousness are in fact produced on the same principles as those of a machine, he means that animals have not souls to direct their actions; but since, on being questioned, he is ready to admit that animals have sensation, perception, emotion, and memory, his denial of their souls practically comes to much the same as the ordinary position that animals have not Thought nor Consciousness of Self.* The admission of sensation is, however, quite enough to mark the essential difference between an organism and a machine.

73. It was really a great step taken by Descartes when he directed attention to the fact that all animal actions were executed in strict conformity with mechanical principles, because both before his time, and since, we may observe a great disregard of the animal mechanism, and a disposition to interpret the phenomena on metaphysical principles. But the connotations of the term "machine" were such as to lead the mind away from the special conditions of the vital mechanism, and fix it exclusively on the general conditions of machinery. Hence his opponents misunderstood him, and some of his followers made the same oversight, and ended by eliminating sensation altogether. In pursuance of this mechanical point of view, to the exclusion of the biological, Thought and even Consciousness have been eliminated from

* DESCARTES expressly calls them sensitive machines. He refuses them Thought, but neither "la vie ou le sentiment." He adds, "Mon opinion n'est pas que les bêtes voient comme nous lorsque nous sentons que nous voyons."—*Œuvres*, iv. p. 339. This example is cited by him in proof of human automatism: "Que ce n'est point par l'entremise de notre âme que les yeux se ferment, puisque c'est contre notre volonté, laquelle est sa seule ou du moins sa principale action; mais c'est à cause que la machine de notre corps est tellement composée que le mouvement de cette main vers nos yeux excite un autre mouvement en notre cerveau qui conduit les esprits animaux dans les muscles qui font abaisser les paupières." All indeed that we assign to Sensibility, he assigns to these hypothetical animal spirits, and thence he concludes, "Qu'il ne reste rien en nous que nous devions attribuer à notre âme sinon nos pensées."—*Les Passions de l'Âme*, art. 13 and 17. Comp. *Discours de la Méthode*, partie iv.

among the organic agencies, and are said to have no more influence in determining even human actions than the whistle of the steam-engine has in directing the locomotive. There are thus two *meta*physiological theories. According to the one, Consciousness directs indeed the actions of the organism, but is not itself an organic process—it sits apart, like a musical performer playing on an instrument. According to the other, it is not a directing agency, but an accessory product of certain organic processes, which processes may go on quite as well without any accompaniment and interference of Consciousness.

74. Two observations arise here. First, we observe a want of due recognition of the objective and subjective aspects, and their respective criteria. Secondly, we observe mental facts of irresistible certainty interpreted by material hypotheses of questionable value; and not only so, but a higher validity is assigned to the material hypotheses than to the mental facts they are invented to explain. That we are conscious, and that our actions are determined by sensations, emotions, and ideas, are facts which may or may not be explained by reference to material conditions, but which no material explanation can render more certain. That animals resemble us in this as in other respects is an induction of the highest probability. It is also a fact that many actions take place, as we say, unconsciously and involuntarily; and that some take place now consciously, now unconsciously. These facts also we endeavour to explain; and when we find that some of the unconscious and involuntary actions take place after the brain has been removed, this is interpreted on the material hypothesis of the brain being the sole seat of sensation and consciousness; and is urged in favour of the hypothesis that consciousness cannot be an agent in the mechanism. Here the confusion of objective and subjective aspects is patent. Consciousness as a subjective fact cannot be a material or objective fact. But may it not be another aspect of that which is objective? So long as we are dealing with the objective aspect, we have nothing but material processes in a material mechanism before us.

A change within the organism is caused by a neural stimulation, and the resulting action is a reflex on the muscles. Here there is simply a transference of motion by a material mechanism. There is in this no evidence of a subjective agency; there could be none. But when we come to investigate the process, we find that it differs from similar processes in anorganisms, by the necessary co-operation of special conditions, and among these—the vital conditions—there are those which in their subjective aspect we express not in terms of Matter and Motion, but in terms of Feeling, *i.e.*, not in objective but in subjective terms. I see a stone move on being struck; I also see a man shrink on being struck, and hear a dog howl on being kicked. I do not infer that the stone feels as the man and dog feel, because I know the stone and the dog to be differently constituted, and infer a corresponding difference in their reactions. I infer that the man and dog feel, because I know they are like myself, and conclude that what I feel they feel, under like conditions.

75. Descartes says that animals are sensitive automata. They *always* act as we *sometimes* act, *i.e.*, when we are not conscious of what we do, as in singing, walking, playing the piano, &c. We are said to do these things mechanically, automatically, and hence the conclusion that these actions are those of a pure mechanism. But it would be truer to say that we never act mechanically, we always act organically. "When one who falls from a height throws his hands forwards to save his head," says Descartes, "it is in virtue of no ratiocination that he performs this action" (that depends on the definition: in the Logic of Feeling there is a process of ratiocination identical with that in the Logic of Signs). "It does not depend upon his *mind*" (again a question of definition), "but takes place merely because his senses being affected by *present danger*" (senses, then, have a perception of danger?) "some change arises in his brain which determines the animal spirits to pass thence into the nerves in such a manner as is required to produce this motion, in the same way as in a machine, and without his mind being able

to hinder it. Now since we observe this in ourselves, why should we be so much astonished if the light reflected from the body of a wolf into the eye of a sheep has the same force to excite in it the motion of flight?"

Here, both in the case of the man and the sheep, there is presupposed the very mental experience which is denied. The young child will not throw out its arm to protect itself; but after many experiences of falling and stumbling, there is an organised perception of the impending danger, and the means of averting it, and it is this which determines the throwing out of the arms. If this is not a mental fact—a process of judgment—then the logical conclusion by which a financier on hearing a war-rumour orders his broker to sell stock, is not a mental fact. The light reflected from the body of a wolf would not disturb the sheep unless its own, or its *inherited* organised experience were ready there to respond. But this organised experience, you say, enters into the mechanism? Yes: but it cannot be made to enter into the mechanism of an automaton, because however complex that mechanism may be, and however capable of variety of action, it is constructed solely for definite actions on calculated lines: all its readjustments must have been foreseen, it is incapable of adjusting itself to unforeseen circumstances. Hence every interruption in the prearranged order either throws it out of gear, or brings it to a standstill. It is regulated, not self-regulating. The organism, on the contrary—conspicuously so in its more complex forms—is variable, self-regulating, incalculable. It has *selective adaptation* (p. 197) responding readily and efficiently to novel and unforeseen circumstances; *acquiring* new modes of combination and reaction. An automaton that will learn by experience, and adapt itself to conditions not calculated for in its construction, has yet to be made; till it is made, we must deny that organisms are machines. Automatism in the organism implies Memory and Perception. A sudden contact—a sudden noise—a vague form seen in the twilight will excite the mechanism according to its organised experiences. We start automatically, before we automatically interpret the cause; we start first, and then ask, What is that? But we do not always start at sounds or sights which have no association with previous experiences. The child and the man both see the falling glass, but the child does not automatically stretch out a hand to save the glass. Having once learned the action of swimming or billiard-playing, we automatically execute these; without consciously remembering the rules, we unconsciously obey them; each feeling as it rises is linked on to another, each muscle is combined with others in a remembered synthesis.

76. Kempelen's chess-player surprised the public, but every instructed physiologist present knew that in some way or other its movements were directed by a human mind; simply because no machine could possibly have responded to the unforeseen fluctuations of the human mind opposed to it. Even the mind of a dog or a savage would be incompetent to pass beyond the range of its previous experiences, incompetent to seize the significance of an adversary's moves on the chessboard. Now just as we conclude that mental agency is essential to a game of chess, so we conclude that Sensibility is essential to the fluctuating responses of an organism under unforeseen circumstances. We can conceive an automaton dog that would bark at the presence of a beggar; but not of an automaton dog that would bark one day at the beggar and the next day wag his tail, remembering the food and patting that beggar had bestowed. Since all we know of machines forbids the idea of their being capable of adjusting their actions to new circumstances, or of evoking through experience new powers of combination, we conclude that wherever this capability of adaptation is present there is an agency in operation which does not belong to the class of mechanical agencies. Goltz has shown that a frog deprived of its brain manifests so much of vision as enables it to avoid obstacles—leaping to the right or to the left of a book placed in its path. This Professor Huxley regards as purely mechanical:—"Although the frog appears to have no sensation of light, visible objects act upon the motor mechanism of its body." Should we not rather conclude that if the frog had no sensation, no such effect would follow? because

although a machine *might* be constructed to respond to variations of light and shadows, none could be constructed (without Sensibility) to respond to the fluctuating conditions as an organism responds.* Were the reflex actions of the organism purely mechanical—*i.e.*, involving none of those fluctuating adjustments which characterise Sensibility—the effect would be uniform, and proportional to the impact; but it is variable, and proportional to the static condition of the nervous centres at the moment. Exaggerate this—by strychnine, for instance—and the slightest touch on the skin will produce general convulsions. Lower it—by an anæsthetic—and no reflex at all will follow a stimulus. In anæsthesia of the mucous membrane, no reflex of the eyelid, no secretion of tears, follows on the irritation of the mem-

* DESCARTES compares the animal mechanism to that of the grottos and fountains at Versailles, the nerves to the water-tubes :—"Les objets extérieurs qui par leur seul présence, agissent contre les organes des sens, et qui par ce moyen, la déterminent à se mouvoir en plusieurs diverses façons, selon comme les parties du cerveau sont disposées, sont comme les étrangers, qui entrant dans quelques unes des grottes de ces fontaines causent euxmêmes sans y penser les mouvements qui s'y font en leur présence : car ils n'y peuvent entrer qu'en marchant sur certains carreaux tellement disposés, que s'ils approchent d'une Diane qui se baigne, ils la font cacher dans les roseaux ; et s'ils passent outre pour la poursuivre, ils feront venir vers eux un Neptune qui les menacera de son trident ; ou s'ils vont de quelque autre costé, ils en feront sortir un monstre marin qui leur vomira de l'eau contre la face."—*Traité de l'Homme*, 1664, p. 12. Ingenious as the comparison is, it only illustrates how machines may be constructed to imitate animal actions. Diana always hides herself when a certain spot is trodden upon; and Neptune always appears when another spot is trodden upon. There is no fluctuation, no sensibility discerning differences and determining variations. Compare the following experiment: A monkey was placed on the table and a shrill whistle made close to its ear: "Immediately the ear was pricked and the animal turned with an air of intense surprise, with eyes widely opened and pupils dilated, to the direction whence the sound proceeded. On repetition of the experiment several times, though the pricking of the ear and the turning of the head and eyes constantly occurred, the look of surprise and dilatation of the pupils ceased to be manifested."—FERRIER : *The Functions of the Brain*, 1876, p. 171. A mechanical monkey would always have reacted in precisely the same way on each stimulus.

brane; no sneezing follows irritation of the inside of the nose; no vomiting follows irritation of the fauces.

77. The question has long ceased to be whether the organism is a mechanism. To the physiologist it is this before all things. To the psychologist also it has of late years more and more assumed this character; because even when he postulates the existence of a spiritual entity *in* the organism but not *of* it, he still recognises the necessity of a mechanism for the execution of the acts determined by the spirit; and when the psychologist adopts the theory of spiritual phenomena as the subjective aspect of what objectively are material phenomena, he of course regards the bodily mechanism and the mental mechanism as one and the same real.

This settled, the problem of Automatism may be thus stated: Granting the animal organism to be a material mechanism, and all its actions due to the operation of that mechanism, are we to conclude that it is an automaton essentially resembling the automata we construct, the movements of which may, or may not, be *accompanied* by Feeling, but are in no case *determined* by Feeling?

Descartes says that animals are sensitive automata. Professor Huxley says that both animals and men are sensitive and conscious automata; so that misleading as the language of Descartes and Professor Huxley often is in what its terms connote, we do them great injustice if we suppose them to have overlooked the points of difference between organisms and machines which have been set forth with so much emphasis in a preceding chapter; and the reader is requested to understand that without pretending to say how much the inevitable connotation of their language expresses their opinions, and how much it may have only led to their being misunderstood, my criticisms are directed against this connotation and this interpretation.

CHAPTER VII.

IS FEELING AN AGENT?

78. DESCARTES having attributed all animal actions to a sensitive mechanism, and indeed all human actions to a similar mechanism, endeavoured to reconcile this hypothesis with the irresistible facts of Consciousness—which assured us that *our* actions, at least, were determined by Feeling. To this end he assumed that man had a spiritual principle over and above the sentient principle. The operation of this principle was, however, limited to Thought; the actions themselves were all performed by the automatic mechanism; so that, in strict logic, the conclusion from his premisses was the same for man as for animals.

This conclusion Professor Huxley announced in his Address before the British Association, 1874*—to the great scandal of the general public, which did not understand him aright; and to the scandal also of a physiological public, which, strangely enough, failed to see that it was the legitimate expression of one of their favourite theories—the celebrated Reflex Theory. Now although it is quite open to any one to reject the premisses which lead to such a conclusion, if he sees greater evidence against the conclusion than for the premisses, it is surely irrational to accept the premisses as those of scientific induction, and yet reject the conclusion because it endangers the stability of other opinions? For my own part, I do not accept the premisses, and my polemic will have reference to them.

79. Professor Huxley adopts certain Theses which represent the views generally adopted by physiologists; to which he adds a Thesis which is adopted by few, and which he only puts forward hypothetically. Against these positions I place

* Printed in the *Fortnightly Review*, November 1874, from which all my citations are made.

Antitheses, less generally adopted, but which in my belief approximate more nearly to the inductions of experience.

Theses.	*Antitheses.*
I. There can be no sensation without consciousness.	I. There is sensation without consciousness, if consciousness means a special mode of Sentience.
II. There can be no consciousness without the co-operation of the brain.	II. The co-operation of the brain is only necessary for a special mode of Sentience; other modes are active when the brain is inactive.
III. Sensation and Consciousness are in some inexplicable way caused by molecular changes in the brain, following upon these as one event follows another, the causal link between motion and sensation being a mystery.	III. Unless the molecular changes be limited to the brain as the *occasional* cause, there is no *following* of sensation or motion, no causal link between the two; but the neural process *is* the sensation, viewed objectively, the sensation is the neural process, viewed subjectively. In this antithesis, Neural Process is not limited to the brain, but comprises the whole sensitive organism as the *efficient* cause.
IV. All actions which take place unconsciously are reflex, and reflex actions are the operation of an insentient mechanism; they are therefore as purely mechanical as those of automata.	IV. All actions are the actions of a reflex mechanism, and all are sentient, even when unconscious; they are therefore never purely mechanical, but always organical.
V. The animal body is a reflex mechanism; even when the brain co-operates with the other centres, and produces consciousness, this product is not an agent in determining action, it is a collateral result of the operation.	V. Sentience being necessary to reflex action, it is necessarily an agent.

80. The first four Theses are those current in our text-books, so that it is only the fifth which will have the air of a paradox. Nor, as a paradox, is it without advocates. Schiff long ago suggested it hypothetically. Hermann mentions it as entertained by physiologists, whom he does not name.* Laycock, and, if I remember rightly, Dr. Drysdale, have in-

* SCHIFF: *Lehrbuch der Physiol.*, 1858, p. 212. HERMANN: *Physiology*, translated by GAMGEE, 1875, p. 511.

sisted on it; and Mr. Spalding has proclaimed it with iterated emphasis. Of the Antitheses nothing need be said here, since the whole of this volume is meant to furnish their evidence.

I have already stated that my polemic is against the views that Professor Huxley is *supposed* to hold by those whom his expressions mislead, rather than against the views I imagine him really to hold. I have little doubt that he would disavow much that I am forced to combat, although his language is naturally interpreted in that sense. But I do not know in how far he would agree with me, and in the following remarks I shall confine myself to what seems to be the plain interpretation of his words, since *that* is the interpretation which has been generally adopted, and which I most earnestly desire to refute.

81. To begin with this passage. After stating the views of Descartes, he says: "As actions of a certain degree of complexity are brought about by mere mechanism, why may not actions of still greater complexity be the result of a more refined mechanism? What proof is there that brutes are other than a superior race of marionnettes, which eat without pleasure, cry without pain, desire nothing, know nothing, and only simulate intelligence as a bee simulates a mathematician?" What proof? Why, in the first place, the proof which is implied in the "more refined mechanism" required for the greater complexity of actions. In the next place, the proof that the organism of the brute is very different from the mechanism of a marionnette, and is so much more like the organism of man, that since we know man to eat with pleasure and cry with pain, there is a strong presumption that the brute eats and cries with somewhat similar feelings.

82. Having stated the hypothesis, Professor Huxley says he is not disposed to accept it, though he thinks it cannot be refuted. His chief reason for not accepting it is that the law of continuity forbids the supposition of any complex phenomenon suddenly appearing; the community between animals and men is too close for us to admit that Consciousness could appear in man without having its beginnings in ani-

mals. Finding that animals have brains, he justly concludes that they also must have brain functions; and they also therefore must be credited with Consciousness. This argument seems to me to have irresistible cogency; and to be destructive not only of the automaton hypothesis, but equally of the hypothesis on which the Reflex Theory is founded. If the law of continuity forbids the sudden appearance of Consciousness, the law of similarity of property with similarity of structure forbids the supposition that central nerve-tissue in one part of the system can suddenly assume a totally different property in another part. If the brain of an animal, a bird, a reptile, or a fish—and *a fortiori* if the œsophageal ganglia of an insect or a mollusc—may be credited with Sensibility, because of the fundamental similarity of these structures with the structures of the human brain, then surely the spinal cord must be credited with Sensibility; for the tissue of the spinal cord is more like that of the brain, than the brain of a reptile is like the brain of a man. The sudden disappearance of all Sensibility, on the removal of one portion of the central nervous system, would be a violation of the law of continuity. And if it be said that Consciousness is not the same as Sensibility, but is a specially evolved function of a specially developed organ, the answer will be that this is only a difference of mode, and that the existence of Sensibility is that which renders the automaton and reflex theories untenable.

83. Professor Huxley would probably admit this; for however his language may at times seem to point to another conclusion, and is so far ambiguous, he has expressed the view here maintained with tolerable distinctness in the following passage, to which particular attention is called:—

"But though we may see reason to disagree with Descartes' hypothesis, that brutes are unconscious machines, it does not follow that he was wrong in regarding them as automata. *They may be more or less conscious sensitive automata;* and the view that they are such conscious machines is that which is implicitly or explicitly adopted by most persons. When we speak of the actions of the lower animals being guided by instinct and not by reason, what we really mean is that though they feel as we do, yet their actions are the results of their physical organisation. We believe, in short, that they are machines, one part of which (the nervous system) not only sets the rest in motion and co-ordinates its movements in relation with changes in surrounding bodies, but is provided with a special apparatus the function of which is the calling into existence of those states of consciousness which are termed sensations, emotions, and ideas."

84. To say that they are "conscious automata" seems granting all that I demand; but there are two objectionable positions which the phrase conceals: first, that Consciousness is not a coefficient; and secondly, that Reflex Action is purely mechanical.

Professor Huxley nowhere, I think, establishes the distinction between Consciousness as a term for a special mode of Feeling, and Consciousness as the all-embracing term for sentient phenomena. His language always implies that an action performed unconsciously is performed mechanically; which may be acceptable if by unconsciously be meant insentiently. I hold that whether consciously or unconsciously performed, the action is equally vital and sentient. In the case he has cited of a soldier now living who is subject to periodic alternations of normal and abnormal states, in the latter states all the actions being said to be "unconscious," we have only to read the account to recognise ample evidence of Sentience. Here is a descriptive passage:—

85. "His [the soldier's in the abnormal state] movements remain free, and his expression calm, except for a contraction of the brow, an incessant movement of the eyeballs, and a chewing motion of the jaws. The eyes are wide open, and their pupils dilated. If the man happens to be in a place to which he is accustomed he walks about as usual; but if he is in a new place, or if obstacles are intentionally placed in his way, he stumbles against them, *stops, and then feeling over the objects with his hands, passes on one side of them.* He offers no resistance to any change of direction which may be impressed upon him, or to the forcible acceleration or retardation of his movements. He eats, drinks, smokes, walks about,

dresses and undresses himself, rises and goes to bed at the accustomed hours. Nevertheless pins may be run into his body, or strong electric shocks sent through it, without causing the least indication of pain; no odorous substance, pleasant or unpleasant, makes the least impression; he eats and drinks with avidity whatever is offered, and takes asafœtida or vinegar or quinine as readily as water; no noise affects him; and light influences him only under certain conditions."

There is no one of these phenomena that is unfamiliar to students of mental disease. The case is chiefly remarkable from the periodicity of the recurrence of the abnormal state. I have collected other cases of the kind, and may hereafter find a fitting occasion to quote them.* The anæsthesia and "unconsciousness" noted, no more prove the actions performed by this soldier to have been purely mechanical, *i.e.*, undetermined by sensation, than anæsthesia and unconsciousness prove somnambulists and madmen to be machines. In the pathological state called "ecstasy" there is a considerable diminution of sensibility to external stimuli; with a concentration on certain feelings, images, trains of thought, exhibiting itself in expressions of emotion. "Les malades," says a master, "paraissent entièrement absorbés par leurs mouvements intérieurs, ils refusent généralement de manger, et spécialement la volonté de l'âme semble complètement enchainée." †

86. Observe that while this soldier exhibits such insensibility to certain stimuli, he unequivocally exhibits sensibility to other stimuli. All his acts show sense-guidance. Sight and Touch obviously regulate his movements. And when he feels objects placed in his way, and then passes beside them, wherein does this differ from the normal procedure of sensitive organisms? wherein does it resemble automata? Dr. Mesmet—from whose narrative the case is

* Meanwhile the reader is referred to SCHRÖDER VAN DER KOLK: *Pathologie der Geisteskrankheiten*, 1863, p. 51; or JESSEN: *Physiologie des menschlichen Denkens*, 1872, p. 66.

† GRIESINGER: *Les Maladies Mentales*, p. 96.

cited—remarks that the sense of Touch seems to persist "and indeed to be more acute and delicate than in the normal state;" upon which Professor Huxley has this comment:—"Here a difficulty arises. It is clear from the facts detailed that the nervous apparatus by which in the normal state sensations of touch are excited is that by which external influences determine the movements of the body in the abnormal state. But does the state of consciousness, which we term a tactile sensation, accompany the operation of this nervous apparatus in the abnormal state? or is consciousness utterly absent, the man being reduced to a pure mechanism? It is impossible to obtain direct evidence in favour of the one conclusion or the other; all that can be said is that the case of the frog shows that the man may be devoid of any kind of consciousness."

87. It is here we are made vividly aware of the absolute need there is to disengage the terms employed from their common ambiguities. All the evidence of a tactile sensation which can possibly be furnished, on the objective side, is furnished by the actions of this soldier; to doubt it would be to throw a doubt on the sensibility of any animal unable to *tell* us what it felt; nay, even a man if he were dumb, or spoke a language we could not understand, could give us no other proof. We conclude that the soldier had tactile sensations, because we see him guided by them as we ourselves are guided by tactile sensations; we know that he is an organism, not a machine, and therefore reject the inference that he has become reduced to a "pure mechanism" because it is inferred that his consciousness is absent. And on what is this inference grounded? 1°, The belief that the brain is the sole organ of consciousness (Sentience)—a belief flatly disproved by the facts, which show Sentience when the brain has been removed; and 2°, the belief that the decapitated frog, because it avoids obstacles and redirects its leaps to avoid them, does so without Sentience. According to the definition we adopt, we may either say that the decapitated frog, and the soldier in his abnormal state, act without consciousness, or with it. But what does not seem permissible is to deny that their actions exhibit the clearest evidence of *sense-guidance*, and the kind of volition which this sense-guidance implies; and this is quite enough to separate them from actions of automata. When a man ducks his head to avoid a stone which he sees falling towards him, he assuredly has a sensation, *i.e.*, there is a grouping of neural elements, which subjectively is a sensation, and this originates a grouping of other neural elements, the outcome of which is a muscular movement, which subjectively is a motor sensation: *this* grouping would not have been originated unless the particular grouping had preceded it; nor would the simple retinal stimulus have excited this sensation unless the nerve-centres had been attuned to such response by many previous experiences: the ignorant child would not duck its head on seeing the stone approach. In our familiar use of the word Consciousness it would be correct to say that the man ducks his head "unconsciously;" and yet expressing the fact in psychological language, we also say: He ducks his head because *remembering* the pain of former similar experiences, he *knows* that if the stone strikes him he will again be hurt as before, therefore he *wills* to avoid it; expressing it in physiological language we may say: The man acts thus because he is so organised that a particular neural process is the stimulus of a particular central discharge; and he became thus organised through a long series of anterior adjustments responding to stimuli, each adjustment being the activity of the vital organism.

88. There can be no doubt that the soldier had perceptions, and that these perceptions guided his movements; whether these shall be called "states of consciousness" or not, is a question of terms. Now since we know that *certain actions are uniformly consequent on certain perceptions*, we are justified in inferring that *whenever the actions are performed, the perceptions preceded them:* this inference may be erroneous, but in the absence of positive evidence to the contrary it is that which claims our first assent. Is it evidence to the contrary that the perception may have stimulated the action, yet been unaccompanied by the special mode named

consciousness? Not in the least. We learn to read with conscious effort; each letter has to be apprehended separately, its form distinguished from all other forms, its value as a sign definitely fixed, yet how very rarely are we "conscious" of the letters when we read a book? Each letter is perceived; and yet this process passes so rapidly and smoothly, that unless there be some defect in a letter, or the word be misspelled, we are not "conscious" of the perceptions. Are we therefore reading automata? *

We are said to walk unconsciously at times; and the continuance of the movement is said to be due to reflex action. But it is demonstrable that the cutaneous sensibility of the soles of the feet is a primary condition. If the skin be insensible, the walking becomes a stumble. In learning to walk, or dance, the child fixes his eyes on his feet, as he fixes them on his fingers in learning to play the piano. After awhile these registered sensations *connected* with the muscular sense, suffice to guide his feet or his fingers; but not if feet or fingers lose their sensibility.

89. With these explanations let us follow the further details of this soldier's abnormal actions:—

"The man is insensible to sensory impressions made through the ear, the nose, the tongue, and to a great extent, the eye; nor is he susceptible to pain from causes operating during his abnormal state. Nevertheless it is possible *so to act upon his tactile apparatus as to give rise to those molecular changes in his sensorium which are ordinarily the causes of associated trains of ideas.* I give a striking example of this process in Dr. Mesmet's words: 'Il se promenait dans le jardin, on lui remet sa canne qu'il avait laissé tomber. Il la palpe, promène à plusieurs reprises la main sur la poignée

* M. Luys cites the case of a patient who conversed quite rationally with a visitor "sans en avoir conscience, et ne se souvenait de rien;" and he draws the extraordinary conclusion that the conversation "s'opérait en vertu des forces réflexes:" *Etudes de Physiologie et de Pathologie Cérébrales*, 1874, p. 117. Is it not obvious that the patient must have been conscious at the time, though the consciousness vanished like that in a dream? The persistent consciousness is the continuous linking on of one state with previous states—the apperception of the past.

coudée de sa canne—devient attentif—semble prêter l'oreille —et tout à coup appelle, "Henri! les voilà!" Et alors portant la main derrière son dos comme pour prendre une cartouche, il fait le mouvement de charger son arme, se couche dans l'herbe à plat ventre dans la position d'un tirailleur, et suit avec l'arme épaulée tous les mouvements de l'ennemi qu'il croit voir à courte distance.' In a subsequent abnormal period Dr. Mesmet caused the patient to repeat this scene by placing him in the same conditions. Now in this case the question arises whether the series of actions constituting this singular pantomime was accompanied by the ordinary states of consciousness, the appropriate trains of ideas, or not? Did the man dream that he was skirmishing? or was he in the condition of one of Vaucanson's automata—*a mechanism worked by molecular changes in the nervous system?* The analogy of the frog shows that the latter assumption is perfectly justifiable."

90. Before criticising this conclusion let me adduce other illustrations of this dreamlike activity. "A gentleman whom I attended in a state of perfect apoplexy," says Abercrombie, "was frequently observed to adjust his nightcap with the utmost care when it got into an uncomfortable state: first pulling it down over his eyes, and then turning up the front of it in the most exact manner." According to the current teaching, these actions, which seem like evidence of sensation, are nothing of the kind, because—the patient was "unconscious;" that is to say, because he did not exhibit one complex kind of Sensibility, it is denied that he exhibited another kind! he did not feel discomfort, nor feel the movements by which it was rectified—because he could not speak, discuss impersonal questions, nor attend to what was said to him! Abercrombie cites other cases:—"A gentleman who was lying in a *state of perfect insensibility* from disease of the brain" (note the phrase, which really only expresses the fact that external stimuli did not create their normal reactions) "was frequently observed even the day before his death to take down a repeating watch from a little bag at the head of his bed, put it close to his ear and make it strike the hour,

and then replace it in the bag with the greatest precision. Another whom I saw in a state of profound apoplexy, from which he recovered, had a perfect recollection of what took place during the attack, and mentioned many things which had been said in his hearing when he was supposed to be in a state of perfect unconsciousness." Dr. Wigan also tells of a lady whom he knew, and who was actually put in a coffin, under the belief that she was dead when in a trance. Her sense of hearing was then preternaturally acute. In her second-floor bedroom she heard what the servants said in her kitchen. When her brother came to see her and he declared she should not be buried until putrefaction set in, she felt intense gratitude and a gush of tenderness, but was unable to move even an eyelid as a manifestation of her feeling. Suddenly all her faculties returned. Dr. Wigan adds that he visited the Countess Escalante, one of the Spanish refugees, who remained in a similar state for a short period, during which she saw her husband and children, and was quite conscious of all they did and said—but did not recognise them as her own. She was absolutely without the power of moving a finger or of opening her mouth. Dr. Neil Arnott told me of a similar case in his practice. In these last cases we learn that consciousness—in its ordinary acceptation—was present, though bystanders could see no trace of it. And very often in cases where Consciousness, or at any rate Sensibility, is clearly manifested, its presence is denied, because the patient on recovering his normal condition is quite unable to remember anything that he felt and did. Under anæsthetics patients manifest sensation, but on awaking they declare that they felt nothing—of what value is their declaration? M. Despine tells us of a patient who under chloroform struggled, swore, and cried out, "*Mon Dieu! que je souffre!*" yet when the operation was over, and he emerged from the effects of the chloroform, he remembered nothing of what he had felt.*

* ABERCROMBIE: *Inquiries concerning the Intellectual Powers*, 1840, p. 151. WIGAN: *The Duality of the Mind*, 1844, p. 270. DESPINE: *La Psychologie Naturelle*, 1868, i. 54.

91. Returning now to Dr. Mesmet's soldier, and to the conclusion that his dreamlike acts were no more than the actions of one of Vaucanson's automata, surely we are justified in concluding, first, that these actions were not of the same kind as those of an automaton, since they were those of a living organism; secondly, that they present all the evidence positive and inferential which Sensibility can present in the actions we observe in another, and do not feel in ourselves; and thirdly, if with physiologists we agree that the mechanism of these actions is "worked by molecular changes in the nervous system," there is some difficulty in understanding how Consciousness, which is said to be caused by such changes, could have been absent—how the *cause could operate yet no effect be produced.*

92. What automata can be made to perform is surprising enough, but they can *never* be made to display the fluctuations of sense-guided actions, such as we see in the report of Dr. Mesmet's soldier:—

"The ex-sergeant has a good voice, and had at one time been employed as a singer at a café. In one of his abnormal states he was observed to begin humming a tune. He then went to his room, dressed himself carefully, and took up some parts of a periodical novel which lay on the bed, as *if he were trying to find something.* Dr. Mesmet suspecting that he was seeking his music, made up one of these into a roll and put it into his hand. *He appeared* satisfied, took up his cane, and went downstairs to the door. Here Dr. Mesmet turned him round, and he walked quite contentedly in the opposite direction. The *light of the sun* shining through a window happened to fall upon him, and *seemed to suggest the footlights of the stage* on which he was accustomed to make his appearance. He stopped, opened his roll of imaginary music, put himself in the attitude of a singer, and sang with perfect execution three songs one after the other. After which he wiped his face with his handkerchief and drank without a grimace a tumbler of strong vinegar-and-water."

93. Epileptic patients have frequently been observed going through similar dreamlike actions in which only those ex-

ternal stimuli which have a relation to the dream seem to take effect.* We interpret these as phenomena of *disordered* mental action, the burden of proof lies on him who says they are phenomena of pure mechanism. A mail-coach does not suddenly cease to be a mail-coach and become a wheel-barrow because the coachman is drunk, or has fallen from the box. The horses, no longer guided by the reins, may dash off the highroad into gardens or ditches; but it is their muscular exertions which still move the coach.

Can any one conceive an automaton acting as the sergeant is described to be in the following passage?—

"Sitting at a table he took up a pen, felt for paper and ink, and began to write a letter to his general, in which he *recommended himself for a medal* on account of his good conduct and courage. It occurred to Dr. Mesmet to ascertain experimentally how far vision was concerned in this act of writing. He therefore interposed a screen between the man's eyes and his hands; under these circumstances he *went on writing for a short time, but the words became illegible, and he finally stopped.* On the withdrawal of the screen, he *began to write again where he had left off.* The substitution of water for ink in the inkstand had a similar result. He stopped, *looked at his pen, wiped it on his coat,* dipped it in the water, and began again, with the same effect. On one occasion he began to write upon the topmost of ten superposed sheets of paper. After he had written a line or two, this sheet was suddenly drawn away. *There was a slight expression of surprise,* but he continued his letter on the second sheet exactly as if it had been the first. This operation was repeated five times, so that the fifth sheet contained nothing but the writer's signature at the bottom of the page. Nevertheless, when the signature was finished, his eyes turned to the top of the blank sheet, and he went through the form of reading over what he had written, a movement of the lips

* Dr. HUGHLINGS JACKSON has quite recently cited some curious examples in his own practice. See *West Riding Lunatic Asylum Reports for* 1875.

accompanying each word; moreover, with his pen *he put in such corrections as were needed.*"

94. Dr. Mesmet concludes that "his patient sees some things and not others; that the sense of sight is accessible to all things which are brought into relation with him by the sense of touch, and, on the contrary, is insensible to things which lie outside this relation." In other words, the sensitive mechanism acts, but acts abnormally. This is precisely what is observed in somnambulists. Yet Professor Huxley, who makes the comparison, appears to regard both states as those in which the organism is reduced to a mere mechanism, because on recovering their normal state the patients are unconscious of what has passed; and because the frog, without its brain, also manifests analogous phenomena. Neither premiss warrants the conclusion. I have already touched on the unconsciousness of past actions; let me add the case of Faraday, who was assuredly not an automaton when he prepared and delivered a course of lectures which were nevertheless so entirely obliterated from his memory that the next year he prepared and delivered the same course once more, without a suspicion that it was not a new one. As to the frog, I must leave that case till I come to examine the evidence on which the hypothesis of the purely mechanical nature of spinal action rests.

95. The point never to be left out of sight is that actions which are known to be preceded and accompanied by sensations do not lose their special character of Sentience, as actions of a sentient mechanism, because they are not also preceded and accompanied by that peculiar state which is specially called Consciousness, *i.e.*, attention to the passing changes (comp. p. 356). When we see a man playing the piano, and at the same time talking of something far removed from the music, we say his fingers move unconsciously; but we do not conclude that he is a musical machine—muscular sensations and musical sensations regulate every movement of his fingers; and if he strikes a false note, or if one of the notes jangles, he is instantly conscious of the fact. Either we must admit that his brain is an essential part of the mechanism by which the piano was played, and its function an

essential agent in the playing; or else we must admit that the brain and its function were not essential, and therefore the playing would continue if the brain were removed. In the latter case, we should have a musical automaton. That a particular group of sensations, such as musical tones, will set going a particular group of muscular movements, without the intervention of any *conscious* effort, is not more to be interpreted on purely mechanical principles, than that a particular phrase will cause a story-teller to repeat a familiar anecdote, or an old soldier "to fight his battles o'er again."

96. Let us now pass to another consideration, namely, whether Consciousness—however interpreted—is legitimately conceived as a factor in the so-called conscious and voluntary actions; or is merely a *collateral result* of certain organic activities? To answer this, we must first remember that Consciousness is a purely subjective process; although we may believe it to be objectively a neural process, we are nevertheless passing out of the region of Physiology when we speak of Feeling determining Action. Motion may determine Motion; but Feeling can only determine Feeling. Yet we do so speak, and are justified. For thereby we implicitly declare, what Psychology explicitly teaches, namely, that these two widely different aspects, objective and subjective, are but the two faces of one and the same reality. It is thus indifferent whether we say a sensation is a neural process, or a mental process: a molecular change in the nervous system, or a change in Feeling. It is either, and it is both, as I have elsewhere explained.* There it was argued that the current hypothesis of a neural process *causing* the mental process—molecular movement being in some mysterious way *transformed* into sensation—is not only inconceivable, but altogether unnecessary; whereas the hypothesis that the two aspects of the one phenomenon are simply two different expressions, now in terms of Matter and Motion, and now in terms of Consciousness, is in harmony with all the inductive evidence.

* PROBLEMS, vol. ii. p. 457, *sq.*

97. "It may be assumed," says Professor Huxley, "that molecular changes in the brain are the causes of all the states of consciousness of brutes. Is there any evidence that these states of consciousness may conversely cause those molecular changes which give rise to muscular motion? I see no such evidence. The frog walks, hops, swims, and goes through his gymnastic performances, quite as well without consciousness, and consequently without volition, as with it; and if a frog in his natural state possesses anything corresponding with what we call volition, there is no reason to think that *it is anything but a concomitant of the molecular changes in the brain,* which *form part of the series involved in the production of motion.* The consciousness of brutes would appear to be related to the mechanism of their body simply as a collateral product of its working, and to be *as completely without any power of modifying that working as the steam-whistle which accompanies the work of a locomotive engine is without influence upon its machinery.* Their volition, if they have any, is an emotion *indicative* of physical changes, not a *cause* of such changes." Particular attention is called to the passages in italics. In the first is expressed a view which seems not unlike the one I am advocating, but which is contradicted by the second. Let us consider what is implied.

98. When Consciousness is regarded solely under its subjective aspect there is obviously no place for it among material agencies, regarded as objective. So long as we have the material mechanism in view we have nothing but material changes. This applies to the frog, with or without its brain; to man, supposed to be moved by volition, or supposed to move automatically. The introduction of Consciousness is not the introduction of another agent in the series, but of a new aspect; the neural process drops out of sight, the mental process replaces it. The question whether we have any ground for inferring that in the series there is included the particular neural state which subjectively is a state of Consciousness, must be answered according to the evidence. Well, the evidence shows that the actions do involve the co-operation; and this Professor Huxley expresses when he says that the molecular changes in the brain form part of the series involved in the production of motion. Whether we regard the process objectively as a series of molecular changes, or subjectively as a succession of sentient changes, the sum of which is on the one side a motor impulse, on the other a state of consciousness, we must declare Consciousness to be an agent, *in the same sense that we declare one change in the organism to be an agent in some other change.* The facts are the same, whether we express them in physiological or in psychological terms. The physiologist, having only the material aspect of the organism in view, says, "A cerebral process initiates a motor process;" the psychologist says, "A sensation determines an action." Unless the two processes have been linked together by an organic disposition, native or acquired, there will be no such motor process following the cerebral process. A dog standing outside the gate is unable to ring the bell, though having seen another dog ring it, he may wish to do so; but the cerebral process (his wish) is not linked on to the needful motor process—he has not learned to realise the wish; whereas the other dog, having by trial hit upon the right mode of directing his muscles, has registered this experience, and can ring the bell. The organised disposition which enables the dog to do this may truly enough be called a modification of the mechanism; but what we have here to note is that a sensation originally determined the movement, and always determines it.

99. It is the unfortunate ambiguity of the word Consciousness, and the questionable hypothesis of the brain being the sole seat of Sensibility, which darken this investigation. Because animals, after the brain has been removed, are seen to perform certain actions as deftly as before, they are said to perform these without the intervention of Consciousness; when all that is proved by the facts is that these actions are performed without the intervention of the brain. In support of this explanation, examples are cited of unconscious actions performed by human beings. But if we assign Sensibility not to one part of the nervous system exclusively, but to the whole, we can readily understand how the loss of a part will be

manifested by very marked changes in the reactions of the whole, and yet not altogether prevent the reactions of the parts remaining intact. An animal must respond somewhat differently with and without a brain. One marked difference is the spontaneity of the actions when the brain is intact, and the loss of much spontaneity when the brain is injured or removed. Cerebral processes prompt and regulate actions, as the pressure of the driver on the reins prompts and regulates the movements of the horses; but the carriage is moved by the horses and not by the driver; and the action is executed by the motor mechanism, whether the incitation arise in a cerebral process or a peripheral stimulation.

100. If we admit that Consciousness is itself an organic process, accompanying the molecular changes as a convex surface accompanies a concave, we must also admit that its fluctuations are adjustments and readjustments of the organic mechanism, and that the actions are the effects of these—their resultants. The loss of the brain must obviously cause a great disturbance in these adjustments. We may call that a loss of Consciousness, if we choose to limit the term to one *mode* of sentient reaction. But this loss of a mode does not change those reactions which persist so as to convert them into purely mechanical reactions. A troop of soldiers may have lost its directing officer, but will fight with the old weapons and the old intelligence, though not with the same convergence of individual efforts. A frog or a pigeon no more acts *as well* without a brain as with a brain, than the troop of soldiers fights as well without an officer.

101. Having thus claimed a place for Consciousness in the series of organic processes, let us now see whether it has a place among the active agencies. According to Professor Huxley it is not itself an agent, but only the "collateral product of the working of the machine." It accompanies actions, it does not direct them. It is an index, not a cause.

Surely it seems more accurate to say that it accompanies *and* directs the working? It accompanies the working in two senses: first, as the subjective aspect of the objective process; secondly, as the change which produces a subsequent change, that is to say, the movements initiated by a feeling are themselves also *felt as they pass;* and this feeling enters into the general stream of simultaneous excitations out of which new movements and feelings arise; or to express it physiologically, the sensory impressions determine muscular movements, which in turn react on the nerve-centres, and these reactions blend with the general excitation of reflected and re-reflected processes.* Since every change in Consciousness is a change in the sentient organism, which objectively is a change in the nervous centres, the working of the mechanism being itself a dependent series of such changes, each movement must have a reflected influence on the general state. This reflected influence may be viewed as a collateral product of the working; but there is no real analogy between it and the whistle of the steam-engine, because this reflected influence demonstrably *does* intervene in the *subsequent* movements. The feeling which accompanies or follows a particular movement cannot indeed modify *that* movement, since that is already set going, or has passed; here there is some analogy to the steam-whistle; but the analogy fails in the subsequent history: no movements whatever of the steam-engine are modified by the whistle which accompanies the working of that engine; yet how the reflected influence modifies the working of the organism! If the hand be passing over a surface, there is, accompanying this movement, a succession of muscular and tactile feelings which may be said to be collateral products. But the feeling which *accompanies* one muscular contraction *is itself the stimulus* of the next contraction; if anywhere during the passage the hand comes upon a spot on the surface which is wet, or rough, the change in feeling thus produced, although a collateral product of the movement, instantly changes the direction of the hand, suspends or alters the course—that is to say, the *collateral product of one movement becomes a directing factor in the succeeding movement.* Now this is precisely what no automaton can

* "Le sentiment fait naître le mouvement, et le mouvement donne naissance au sentiment."—VAN DEEN: *Traités et Découvertes sur la Moëlle Épinière,* 1841, p. 102.

effect, unless for changes that are prearranged. A steam-engine drives its locomotive over the rails, be they smooth or rough, entire or broken; it whistles as it goes, but no whistling directs and redirects its path.

102. Volition is said to be an "emotion indicative of physical changes, not a cause of such changes." Here it is necessary to understand in what sense the term cause is employed. I should prefer stating the proposition thus: a volition is a state of the sentient organism, indicative of physical changes which have taken place, and of changes which will take place. Because it is the *expression* of the first group of changes, it cannot be their *origin;* but it can be, and is the origin of the second group, which it initiates. The indignation excited by an insult or a blow is not the origin of the emotion or the pain, but it is the origin of the actions which are prompted by this sentient state. In fact no sooner do we admit that the organism is a sentient mechanism, than the conclusion is irresistible that Sensibility is a factor in the working of that mechanism.

103. "Much ingenious argument," says Professor Huxley, "has at various times been bestowed upon the question: How is it possible to imagine that volition which is a state of consciousness, and as such has not the slightest community of nature with matter and motion, can act upon the moving matter of which the body is composed, as it is assumed to do in voluntary acts? But if, as is here suggested, the voluntary acts of brutes—or in other words, the acts which they desire to perform—are as purely mechanical as the rest of their actions, and are simply accompanied by the state of consciousness called volition, the inquiry, so far as they are concerned, becomes superfluous. Their volitions do not enter into the chain of causation of their actions at all. . . . As consciousness is brought into existence only as the consequence of molecular motion in the brain, it follows that it is an indirect product of material changes. The soul stands related to the body as the bell of a clock to the works, and consciousness answers to the sound which the bell gives out when it is struck." This has been answered in the foregoing

pages; nor do I think the reader who has recognised the ambiguity of the term Consciousness, and the desirability of replacing it in this discussion by the less equivocal term Sentience, will need more to be said.

104. The important question whether reflex actions are insentient, and therefore mechanical, will occupy us in the next problem. The question of Automatism which has been argued in the preceding chapters, may, I think, be summarily disposed of by a reference to the irresistible evidence each man carries in his own consciousness that his actions are frequently—even if not always—determined by feelings. He is quite certain that he is not an automaton, and that his feelings are not simply collateral products of his actions, without the power of modifying and originating them. Now this fundamental fact cannot be displaced by any theoretical explanation of its factors. Nor would this fundamental truth be rendered doubtful, even supposing we were to grant to the full all that is adduced as evidence that *some* actions were the result of purely mechanical processes without sentience at all. I am a conscious organism, even if it be true that I sometimes act unconsciously. I am not a machine, even if it be true that I sometimes act mechanically.

PROBLEM IV.

THE REFLEX THEORY.

"Si omnes patres sic, at Ego non sic."

ABELARD: *Sic et Non.*

"Will man bestimmen wo der Mechanismus aufhört und wo der Wille anfängt so ist die Frage überhaupt falsch gestellt. Denn man setzt hier Begriffe einander gegenüber die gar keine Gegensätze sind. Vorgebildet in den mechanischen Bedingungen des Nervensystems sind *alle* Bewegungen."

WUNDT: *Physiologische Psychologie.*

"Sollte die so durchsichtige Homologie zwischen Hirn und Rückenmark, wie solche sich schlagend in Bau und Entwicklung darthut, wesentlich andere physiologische Qualitäten bedingen?"

LUSCHINGER in *Pflüger's Archiv*, Bd. xiv. 384.

THE REFLEX THEORY.

CHAPTER I.

THE PROBLEM STATED.

1. The peculiarity of the Reflex Theory is its exclusion of Sensibility from the actions classed as reflex; in consequence of which, the actions are considered to be "purely mechanical."

No one denies that most of the reflex actions often have conscious sensations preceding and accompanying them, but these are said not to be essential to the performance of the actions, because they may be absent and the actions still take place. It is notorious that we breathe, wink, swallow, &c., whether we are conscious of these actions or not. Our conclusion therefore is that these peculiar states of Consciousness are *accessory*, not essential to the performance of these actions. The fact is patent, the conclusion irresistible. But now consider the equivoque: because an action takes place without our being conscious of it, the action is said to have had no sensation determining it. This which is a truism when we limit Consciousness to one of the special modes of Sensibility, or limit Sensation to this limited Consciousness, is a falsism when we accept Consciousness as the total of all combined sensibilities, or Sensation as the reaction of the sensory mechanism. That a reflex action is determined by the sensory mechanism, no one disputes; whether the reaction of a sensory mechanism shall be called a sensation or not, is a question of terms. I have shown why it must be so called if anything like coherence is to be preserved in physiological investigations; and I have more than once suggested that the fact of intellectual processes taking place at times with no more consciousness than reflex actions, is itself sufficient to show that a process does not lapse from the mental to the mechanical sphere simply by passing unconsciously.

Inasmuch as an organism is a complex of organs, its total function must be a complex of particular functions, each of which may analytically be treated apart. Vitality is the total of all its physiological functions, and Consciousness the total of all its psychological functions. But inasmuch as it is only in its relation to the whole that each part has functional significance, and cannot therefore be isolated in reality, as it is in theory—cannot live by itself, act by itself, independently of the organism of which it is an organ, there is strict accuracy in saying that no particular sensation can exist without involving Consciousness; for this is only saying that no sensory organ can react without at the same time involving a reaction of the general sensorium. But since this general sensorium is simultaneously affected by various excitations each of which is a force, every sensation, perception, emotion, or volition is a *resultant* of the composition of these forces; and as there can be only one resultant at a time, to be replaced by another in swift succession, this one represents the *state* of Consciousness, and this state may or may not be felt under the peculiar *mode* named "Consciousness," in its special meaning. In other words, the reaction of a sensory organ is always sentient, but not always consentient.

2. Let us illustrate this by the sensation of musical tone. When we hear a tone we are affected not only by the fundamental tone, representing the vibrations of the sounding body as a whole, but also by the harmonics or overtones, representing the vibrations of the several parts of that whole. It is these latter vibrations which give the tone its timbre, or peculiar *quality;* and as the harmonics are variable with the variable structure of the vibrating parts, two bodies which have the same fundamental tone may have markedly different

qualities. There are some tones which are almost entirely free from harmonics; that is to say, their harmonics are too faint for our ear to appreciate them, though we know that the vibrations must be present. Apply this to the excitations of the sensorium. Each excitation will have its fundamental feeling, and more or less accompanying thrills of other feelings: it is these thrills which are the harmonics, giving to each excitation its specific quality; but they may be so faint that no specific quality is discriminated. A fly settles on your hand while you are writing, the faint thrill which accompanies this excitation of your sensory nerve gives the specific sensation of tickling, and this causes you to move your hand with a jerk. If your attention is preoccupied, you are said to be unconscious of the sensation, and the jerk of your hand is called a reflex action; but if your attention is not preoccupied, or if the thrill is vivid, you are said to be conscious of the sensation, and the action is no longer reflex, but volitional. Obviously here the difference depends not on the sentient excitation by an impression on the nerve, but on the state of the general sensorium and its consequent reaction. Had not the impression been carried to the sensorium, no movement would have followed the fly's alighting on your hand, because no sensation (sensory reaction) would have been excited; the hypothesis of a purely mechanical reflex is quite inadmissible.

3. Or take another case. It sometimes happens that we fall asleep while some one is reading to us aloud. The sounds of the reader's voice at first awaken the familiar thrills which give the tones their quality, and the words their significance; but gradually as sleep steals over us, the organism ceases to react thus; the words lose more and more of their significance, the tones lose more and more of their harmonics; at last we pass into the state of unconsciousness —we cease to hear what is read. But do we cease to feel? We have not *heard*, but we have been *affected* by the sounds. Not by distinguishable sensations; nevertheless a state of the general Sensibility has been induced. To prove that we have been affected is easy. Let the reader suddenly cease, and if our

sleep be not too profound, we at once awake. Now, unless the sound of his voice had affected us, it is clear that the cessation of that could not have affected us. Or let us suppose our sleep to be unbroken by the cessation of the sound; even this will not prove that we have been unaffected by the sounds, it will merely prove that those sounds, or their cessation, did not excite a conscious state. For let the reader, in no louder tone, ask, "Are you asleep?" and we start up, with round eyes, declaring, "Not at all." Nay, should even this question fail to awaken us, the speaker need only utter some phrase likely to excite a thrill—such as, "There's the postman!" or, "I smell fire!" and we start up.

I remember once trying the experiment on a wearied waiter, who had fallen asleep in one of the unoccupied boxes of a tavern. His arm rested on the table, and his head rested on his arm: he snored the snore of the weary, in spite of the noisy laughter and talk of the guests. I called out "Johnson," in a loud tone. It never moved him. I then called "Wilson," but he snored on. No sooner did I call "waiter," than he raised his head with a sleepy "*yessir*." Now, to suppose, in this case, that he had *no* sensation when the words "Johnson" and "Wilson" reached his ears, but had a sensation when the word "waiter" reached his ears, is to suppose that two similar causes will not produce a similar effect. The dissyllable "Johnson" would excite as potent a reaction of his sensory organ as the dissyllable "waiter;" but the thrills—the reflex feelings—were different, because the word "Johnson" was not associated in his mind with any definite actions, whereas the word "waiter" was so associated as to become an automatic impulse.*

4. Two sisters are asleep in the same bed, and a child cries in the next room. The sounds of these cries will give a similar stimulus to the auditory nerve of each sister, and excite a similar sensory reaction in each. Nevertheless, the

* Dr. CARPENTER tells a similar story of Admiral CODRINGTON, who, when a midshipman, could always be awakened from the profoundest slumber if the word "signal" were uttered; whereas no other word disturbed him.

one sister sleeps on undisturbed, and is said not to hear the cry. The other springs out of bed, and attends to the child, because she being accustomed to attend on the child and soothe it when crying, the primary sensation has excited secondary sensations, thrills which lead to accustomed actions. Could we look into the mind of the sleeping sister, we should doubtless find that the sensation excited by the child's cry had merged itself in the general stream, and perhaps modified her dreams. Let her become a mother, or take on the tender duties of a mother, and her vigilance will equal that of her sister; because the cry will *then* excite a definite reflex feeling, and a definite course of action. But this very sister, who is so sensitive to the cry of a child, will be undisturbed by a much louder noise; a dog may bark, or a heavy waggon thunder along the street, without causing her to turn in bed.*

Although during sleep the nervous centres have by no means their full activity, they are always capable of responding to a stimulus, and sensation will always be produced. When the servant taps at your bedroom door in the morning, you are said not to hear the tap, if asleep; you do not perceive it; but the sound reaches and rouses you nevertheless, since when the second tap comes, although no louder, you distinctly recognise it. In etherised patients, sensation is constantly observed returning before any consciousness of what is going on returns. "I was called," says Mr. Potter, "to give chloroform to a lady for the extraction of ten teeth. The first five were extracted without the slightest movement, but as the operation proceeded, sensation returned, and I was obliged to use considerable force to keep her in the chair during the extraction of the last tooth. She came to herself very shortly after, and was delighted to find she had got over all her troubles without having felt it the least in the world." †

5. We do not see the stars at noonday, yet they shine.

* Compare an interesting personal example given by JOUFFROY, quoted in Sir W. HAMILTON'S *Lectures*, i. 331.

† *Lancet*, 10th July 1858.

We do not see the sunbeams playing among the leaves on a cloudy day, yet it is by these beams that the leaves and all other objects are visible. There is a general illumination from the sun and stars, but of this we are seldom aware, because our attention falls upon the illumined objects, brighter or darker than this general tone. There is a sort of analogy to this in the general Consciousness, which is composed of the sum of sensations excited by the incessant simultaneous action of internal and external stimuli. This forms, as it were, the daylight of our existence. We do not habitually attend to it, because attention falls on those particular sensations of pleasure or of pain, of greater or of less intensity, which usurp a prominence among the objects of the sensitive panorama. But just as we need the daylight to see the brilliant and the sombre forms of things, we need this living Consciousness to feel the pleasures and the pains of life. It is therefore as erroneous to imagine that we have no other sensations than those which we distinctly recognise—as to imagine that we see no other light than what is reflected from the shops and equipages, the colours and splendours which arrest the eye.

The amount of light received from the stars may be small, but it is present. The greater glory of the sunlight may render this starlight inappreciable, but it does not render it inoperative. In like manner the amount of sensation received from some of the centres may be inappreciable in the presence of more massive influences from other centres; but though inappreciable it cannot be inoperative—it must form an integer in the sum.

6. The reader's daily experience will assure him that over and above all the particular sensations capable of being separately recognised, there is a general stream of Sensation which constitutes his feeling of existence—the Consciousness of himself as a sensitive being. The ebullient energy which one day exalts life, and the mournful depression which the next day renders life a burden almost intolerable, are feelings not referable to any of the particular sensations, but arise from the massive yet obscure sensibilities of the viscera,

which form so important a part of the general stream of Sensation. Some of these may emerge into distinct recognition. We may feel the heart beat, the intestines move, the glands secrete; anything *unusual* in their action will force itself on our attention.

"What we have been long used to," says Whytt, "we become scarcely sensible of; while things which are new, though much more trifling, and of weaker impression, affect us remarkably. Thus he who is wont to spend his time in the country is surprisingly affected, upon first coming into a populous city, with the noise and bustle which prevail there: of this, however, he becomes daily less sensible, till at length he regards it no more than they who have been used to it all their lifetime. The same seems to be the case also with what passes within our bodies. Few persons in health feel the beating of their heart, though it strikes against their ribs with considerable force every second; whereas the motion of a fly upon one's face or hands occasions a very sensible and uneasy titillation. The pulsation of the great *aorta* itself is wholly unobserved by us; yet the unusual beating of a small artery in any of the fingers becomes very remarkable."

7. A large amount of sensation is derived from the muscular sense, yet we are not aware of the nice adjustments of the muscles, regulated by this sensibility, when we sit or walk. No sooner are we placed in an exceptional position, as in walking on a narrow ledge, than we become distinctly aware of the effort required to preserve equilibrium. It is not the novelty of the position which has increased our sensibility; that has only caused us to attend to our sensations. In like manner, the various streams of sensation which make up our general sense of existence, separately escape notice until one of them becomes obstructed, or increases in impetuosity. When we are seated at a window, and look out at the trees and sky, we are so occupied with the aspects and the voices of external Nature, that no attention whatever is given to the fact of our own existence; yet all this while there has been a massive and diffusive feeling arising from

the organic processes; and of this we become distinctly aware if we close our eyes, shut off all sounds, and abstract the sensations of touch and temperature—it is then perceived as a vast and powerful stream of sensation, belonging to none of the special Senses, but to the System as a whole. It is on this general stream that depend those well-known but indescribable states named "feeling well" and "feeling ill"—the *bien être* and *malaise* of every day. Of two men looking from the same window, on the same landscape, one will be moved to unutterable sadness, yearning for the peace of death; the other will feel his soul suffused with serenity and content: the one has a gloomy background, into which the sensations excited by the landscape are merged; the other has a happy background, on which the sensations play like ripples on a sunny lake. The tone of each man's feeling is determined by the state of his general consciousness. Except in matters of pure demonstration, we are all determined towards certain conclusions as much by this general consciousness as by logic. Our philosophy, when not borrowed, is little more than the expression of our personality.

8. Having thus explained the relation of particular sensations to the general state of Consciousness considered as the function of the whole organism, we may henceforward speak of particular sentient states, as we speak of particular organs and functions, all the while presupposing that the organs and functions necessarily involve the organism, since *apart* from the organism they have no such significance. The reaction of a sensory organ is therefore always a sentient phenomenon. Apart from the living organism there can be no such vital reaction, but only a physical reaction. It is commonly supposed that sensation is simply the molecular excitation of the cerebrum; yet no one will maintain that if the cerebrum of a corpse be excited, by a galvanic current sent through the optic nerve, for instance, this excitation will be a sensation. Whence we may conclude that it is not the physical reaction or stimulus which constitutes sensation, but the physiological reaction of the living organism.

9. Now this is the point which the advocates of the Reflex

Theory, implicitly or explicitly, always deny. Let us trace the origin of the fallacy, if possible. When we remove the eye from a recently-killed animal, and let a beam of light fall on it, the pupil contracts. This is a purely mechanical action; no one would suggest that a sensation determined it. When we remove the leg, and irritate its nerve, the leg is jerked out. This is also a purely mechanical action. When we remove the brain from an animal, and pinch its toes, the leg is withdrawn or the pincers are pushed aside. Is this equally a purely mechanical action? And if not, why not?

The Reflex Theory would have us believe that all three cases were mechanical, at least in so far as they were all destitute of sentient co-operation. The ground for this conclusion being the hypothesis that the brain is the exclusive seat of sensation. The Reflex Theory further concludes that since these, and analogous actions, are performed when the brain is removed, they, being thus independent of sentience, may be performed when the brain is present without any co-operation of sentience. The grounds for this conclusion being the facts that in the normal state of the organism there are many actions of which we are sometimes conscious, and at other times unconscious; and some actions—such as the dilatation and contraction of the pupil—of which we are never conscious. This observation of parts detached from the organism seems confirmed by observation of actions passing in our own organisms, both converging to the conclusion that the actions in question are purely mechanical, involving no sentience whatever. We are taught, therefore, that there is besides the sentient mechanism, to which all conscious actions are referred, a reflex mechanism, to which all unconscious actions are referred. The cerebro-spinal axis, acting as a whole, constitutes the first; the spinal axis, acting without the co-operation of the cerebrum, constitutes the second.

10. Before proceeding with our exposition of the theory it may be well to state two considerations which must be constantly in view. If it should appear that there is any reasonable evidence for refusing to limit Sensibility to the cerebrum—and this evidence I shall adduce—the Reflex Theory must

obviously be remodelled. Nor is this all. We might see overwhelming evidence in favour of the hypothesis that the cerebrum is the exclusive seat of Sensibility, and still reject as a fallacy the conclusion that because certain actions can be performed in the absence of the cerebrum, therefore those actions in the normal organism are likewise performed without cerebral co-operation. I mean that it is a fallacy to conclude from the contractions of the pupil, and the jerking of the leg, when eye and leg are detached from the organism, that therefore when eye and leg form integral parts of the organism, such contractions and jerkings are mechanical reflexes without sentient conditions. And the fallacy is analogous to that which would conclude from the observations of a mechanical automaton, that similar appearances in a vital organism were equally automatic and mechanical. So long as both sets of phenomena are apprehended simply as they appear to the sense of sight, they may be indistinguishable; but no sooner do we apprehend them through other modes, and examine the *modes of production* of the phenomena, than we come upon cardinal differences. A limb detached from the organism is like a phrase detached from a sentence: it has lost its vital significance, its functional value, in losing its connection with the other parts. The whole sentence is necessary for the slightest meaning of its constituent words, and each word is a language-element only when ideally or verbally connected with the other words required to form a sentence; without subject, predicate, and copula, no sentence can be formed. So the organic connexus of parts with a living whole is necessary for the simplest function of each organ; and a limb, or any other part, is a physiological element only when (ideally or really) an integral of a vital whole. The organism may be truncated by the removal of certain parts, as the sentence may be abbreviated by the removal of certain phrases; but so long as subject, predicate, and copula remain, there is a meaning in the sentence; and so long as the organic connexus needful for vitality remains, there will be vital function. The eye detached from the organism is no longer a part of the living whole, it no longer lives, its phenomena cease to be vital, its movements cease to have sentient conditions. The movements of the pupil may seem to be the same as those of the living eye; but when we come to examine their modes of production, we learn that they are not the same. The stimulus of light falling on the eye in the two cases necessarily has a different effect, because the effect is the result of the co-operating causes, and the co-operation in the one case is that of a lifeless organ, in the other that of a living organism. So long as the eye forms an integral part of the organism, every stimulus acting on the eye necessarily acts on the organism, and every reaction of the organ is necessarily conditioned by the state of the organism. Further, every stimulation of a sensory nerve necessarily affects the general sensorium, since the whole nervous system is structurally continuous and functionally co-operant. (See Prob. II. § 16.) Therefore, the stimulation of the eye, although too faint to be discriminated as a conscious sensation, must enter as a sentient tremor into the general stream of Sentience; and although we have no test delicate enough to reveal this operation, we know the *obverse* operation of conscious sensation on the movements of the pupil—in surprise, for example, the pupil is dilated.

11. There are still stronger reasons for asserting that the spinal reflexes are necessarily conditioned by the general state of the sensorium, so that in the normal organism we cannot legitimately exclude them from Sentience; and the Reflex Theory is therefore unphysiological, even on the hypothesis that the cerebrum is the exclusive seat of Sensibility. This hypothesis, however, seems to me untenable; and all the observed facts which it is invented to explain admit of a far more consistent explanation. It is irrational to suppose that a limb, detached from the body, *felt* the stimulus which caused its muscles to contract. The limb is not a living organism, having a sentient mechanism in its nervous mechanism. Not less irrational is it to suppose that when the limb forms an integral part of a living organism, with a sentient mechanism of nerves and nerve-

centres, this organism does not react on the stimulus which excites the muscles of the limb to contract; nor, pursuing the same train of reasoning, is it irrational to suppose that when this living organism has been mutilated, and certain parts destroyed, which do not in their destruction prevent the connexus of the rest, but leave intact a sentient mechanism of nerves and nerve-centres, then also this truncated organism still reacts as a whole, still feels the stimulus which causes the muscles of the limb to contract. Hypothesis for hypothesis, we may at least say that the one is as reasonable as the other. And I shall be disappointed if, when the reader has gone through all the evidence hereafter to be adduced, he does not conclude that the hypothesis which assigns Sensibility to the nervous mechanism as a whole is not the more acceptable of the two.

12. Let us now pursue our exposition of the Reflex Theory. All that we have endeavoured to establish respecting the essential identity of the processes in conscious and unconscious states, and voluntary and involuntary actions,—an identity which does not exclude differences of degree corresponding with these different terms,—is ignored or denied in the Reflex Theory. Whereas I suppose all processes to be reflex processes, some of them having the voluntary, others the involuntary character, physiologists generally distinguish the involuntary as reflex, and invent for this class a special mechanism. According to Marshall Hall, who originated the modern form of this theory, actions are divisible into four distinct classes: the *voluntary*, dependent on the brain; the *involuntary*, dependent on the irritability of the muscular fibre; the *respiratory*, wherein "the motive influence passes in a *direct line* from one point of the nervous system to certain muscles;" and the *reflex*, dependent on the "true spinal system" of *incident-excitor* nerves, and of *reflex-motor* nerves. These last-named actions are produced when an *impression* on the sensitive surface is conveyed, by an excitor-nerve, to the spinal cord, and is there *reflected* back on the muscles by a corresponding motor-nerve. In this process *no* sensa-

tion whatever occurs. The action is purely reflex, purely *excito-motor*—like the action of an ordinary mechanism.*

Müller, who shares with Marshall Hall the glory of having established this classification, thinks that although the absence of sensation is a characteristic of the reflex actions, these actions may be, and are at times, accompanied by sensation. "The view I take of the matter is the following: Irritation of sensitive fibres of a spinal nerve excites primarily a centripetal action of the nervous principle, conveying the impression to the spinal cord; if the centripetal action can then be continued to the *sensorium commune*, a true sensation is the result; if, on account of division of the cord, it cannot be communicated to the sensorium, it still exerts its whole influence upon the cord; in both cases a reflex motor action may be the result." †

13. It is needless nowadays to point out that the existence of a distinct system of excito-motor nerves belongs to Imaginary Anatomy; but it is not needless to point out that the Imaginary Physiology founded on it still survives. The hypothetical process seems to me not less at variance with observation and induction, than the hypothetical structure invented for its basis. We have already seen that what Anatomy positively teaches is totally unlike the reflex mechanism popularly imagined. The sensory nerve is not seen to enter the spinal cord at one point, and pass over to a corresponding point of exit; it is seen to enter the grey substance, which is continuous throughout the spinal cord; it is there lost to view, its course being untraceable. Nor does the physiological process present the aspect demanded by the theory: it is not that of a direct and uniform reflexion, such as would result from an impression on one spot transmitted across the spinal cord to a corresponding motor-nerve. The impression is sometimes followed by one movement, sometimes by another very different movement, each determined

* Marshall Hall in *Philos. Trans.*, 1833. *Lectures on the Nervous System and its Diseases*, 1836. *New Memoir on the Nervous System*, 1843.

† Müller: *Physiology*, i. 721.

by the state of neural tension in the whole central system.

Even the facts on which the Reflex Theory is based are differently interpreted by different physiologists. Van Deen, for instance, considers that Reflexion takes place without Volition, but not without Sensation; and Budge, that it takes place without Perception (*Vorstellung*). And when it is remembered that most of the reflex actions will be accompanied by distinct consciousness whenever attention is directed to them, or the vividness of the stimulation is slightly increased, it becomes evident that the absence of Consciousness (discrimination) is not the differentia of Reflex action.

14. Nor can the absence of spontaneity be accepted as a differentia. *All* actions are excited by stimulation, internal or external. What are called the spontaneous actions are simply those which are prompted by internal, or by not recognisable stimuli; and could we see the process, we should see a neural change initiated by some stimulation, whether the change was conscious and volitional, or unconscious and automatic. The dog rising from sleep and restlessly moving about, is acting spontaneously, whether the stimulation which awakens him be a sensation of hunger, a sensation of sound, the sharp pain of a prick, or a dash of cold water. If he wags his tail at the sight of his master, or wags it when dreaming, the stimulation is said to be spontaneous; but if after his spinal cord has been divided the tail wags when his abdomen is tickled, the action is called reflex. In all three cases there has been a process of excitation and reflexion.

15. The advocates of the Reflex Theory insist that spontaneity is always absent in brainless animals; whence the conclusion that the brain is the exclusive organ of sensation. But the fact asserted is contradicted by the evidence. No experimenter can have failed to observe numberless examples of spontaneity in brainless animals. Many examples have already been incidentally noticed in previous pages. Let me add one more from my notes: I decapitated a toad and a triton, and divided the spinal cord of another triton and a frog. At first the movements of the decapitated animals

were insignificant; but on the second day the headless toad was quite as lively as the frog; and the headless triton little less so than his companion with cord divided but brain intact. I have, at the time of writing this, a frog whose cord was divided some weeks ago. He remains almost motionless unless when touched; he is generally found in the same spot, and in the same attitude to-day as yesterday, unless touched, or unless the table be shaken. He occasionally moves one of the forelegs; occasionally one of the hind-legs; but without changing his position. If he were brainless, this quiescence would be cited in proof of the absence of spontaneity in the absence of the brain; but this conclusion would be fallacious, and is seen to be so in the spontaneous movements of his companion who has *no* brain.

16. With spontaneity is associated the idea of volition, and with volition *choice.* Now I admit that it is complicating the question to ask any one to conceive a headless animal choosing one action rather than another; but it is equally difficult to reconcile ourselves to the idea of "choice" in contemplating the actions of a mollusc. In what sense we can speak of the volition of a mollusc or an insect has already been considered (p. 361). When a man in a fit of coughing seizes a glass of water to allay the tickling in his throat, we have no hesitation in declaring this to be volitional—and the remedy to be *chosen.* But when a brainless animal adopts some *unusual* means, after the failure of the usual means, to allay an irritation, we still hesitate to call the action volitional. I see, however, no objection to calling it the adaptation of a sensitive mechanism which is markedly unlike any inorganic mechanism.

Place a child of two or three years old upon his back, and tickle his right cheek with a feather. He will probably move his head away. Continue tickling, and he will rub the spot with his right hand, *never* using the left hand for the right cheek, so long as the right hand is free; but if you hold his right hand, he will use the left. Does any one dispute the voluntary character of these actions?

Now compare the actions of the sleeping child under similar circumstances, and their sequence will be precisely similar. This contrast is the more illustrative, because physiologists generally assume that in sleep consciousness and volition are *suspended*. They say: "The brain sleeps, the spinal cord never; volition and sensation may be suspended, but not reflex action." This proposition is extremely questionable; yet it is indispensable to the reflex theory; because unless sensation and volition *are* suspended during sleep, we must admit that they can act, without at the same time calling into activity that degree of sensibility which is supposed to constitute consciousness. The child moves in his sleep, defends himself in his sleep; but he is not "aware" of it.

"Children," says Pflüger, "sleep more soundly than adults, and seem to be more sensitive in sleep. I tickled the right nostril of a three-year-old boy. He at once raised his right hand to push me away, and then rubbed the place. When I tickled the left nostril he raised the left hand. I then softly drew both arms down, and laid them close to the body, embedding the left arm in the clothes, and placing on it a pillow, by gentle pressure on which I could keep the arm down without awakening him. Having done this I tickled his left nostril. He at once began to move the imprisoned arm, but could not reach his face with it, because I held it firmly though gently down. He now drew his head aside, and I continued tickling, whereupon he raised the *right* hand, and with it rubbed the *left* nostril—an action he never performed when the left hand was free."

17. This simple but ingenious experiment establishes one important point, namely, that the so-called reflex actions observed in sleep are determined by sensation and volition. The sleeping child behaves exactly as the waking child behaved; the only difference being in the energy and rapidity of the actions. If the waking child felt and willed, surely the sleeping child, when it performed precisely similar actions, cannot be said to have felt nothing, willed nothing? It is not at one moment a sentient organism, and at the next an insentient mechanism.

It is possible to meet this case by assuming that the child

was nearly awake, and that a dim consciousness was aroused by the tickling, so that the cerebral activity was in fact awakened. But, plausible as this explanation may be (and I am the more ready to admit it because I believe the brain always co-operates when it is present), it altogether fails when we come to experiments on decapitated animals. If any one will institute a series of such experiments, taking care to compare the actions of the animal before and after decapitation, he will perceive that there is no more difference between them than between those of the sleeping and the waking child.

18. Even more striking is the following experiment, devised by Pflüger, which I have verified, and varied, many times: A frog is decapitated, or its brain is removed.* When it has recovered from the effect of the ether, and manifests lively sensibility, we place it on its back, and touch, with acetic acid, the skin of its thigh just above the *condylus internus femoris*. (Let the reader imagine his own shoulder burnt at the point where it can be reached with the thumb of the same arm, and he will realise the operation.) No sooner does the acid begin to burn than the frog stretches out the *other* leg, so that its body is somewhat drawn towards it. The leg that has been burnt is now bent, and the back of the foot is applied to the spot, rubbing the acid away—just as your thumb might rub your shoulder. This is very like the action of the tickled child, who always uses the right hand to rub the right cheek, unless it be held; but when the child's right hand is prevented from rubbing, the left will be employed; and precisely this do we observe with the brainless frog: prevent it from using its right leg, and it will use its left!

This has been proved by decapitating another frog, and cut-

* It is better simply to remove the brain, than to remove the whole head, which causes a serious loss of blood. An etherised animal may be operated on with ease and accuracy. For many experiments, mere division of the spinal cord is better than decapitation. Great variations in the results must be expected, because the condition of the animal, its age and sex—whether fasting or digesting—whether the season be spring or summer—and a hundred other causes, complicate the experiment.

ting off the foot of the leg which is to be irritated. No sooner is the acid applied, than the leg is bent as before, and the stump is moved to and fro, as if to rub away the acid. But the acid is not rubbed away, and the animal becomes restless, as if trying to hit upon some other plan for freeing himself of the irritation. And it is worthy of remark that he often hits upon plans very similar to those which an intelligent human being adopts under similar circumstances. Thus, the irritation continuing, he will sometimes cease the vain efforts with his stump, and stretching that leg straight out, bends the *other* leg over towards the irritated spot, and rubs the acid away. But, to show how far this action is from one of "mere mechanism," how far it is from being a direct reflex of an impression on a group of muscles, the frog does not *always* hit even on this plan. Sometimes it bends its irritated leg more energetically, and likewise bends the body towards it, so as to permit the spot to be rubbed against the flank—just as the child, when both his hands are held, will bend his cheek towards his shoulder and rub it there.

19. It is difficult to resist such evidence as is here manifested. The brainless frog "chooses" a new plan when the old one fails, just as the waking child chooses. And an illustration of how sensations guide and determine movements, may be seen in another observation of the brainless frog, when, as often happens, it does not hit upon either of the plans just mentioned, but remains apparently restless and helpless; if under these circumstances we perform a part of the action for it, *it will complete what we have begun:* if we rub the irritated leg, at some distance from the spot where the acid is, with the foot of the other, the frog suddenly avails itself of this *guiding sensation,* and at once directs its foot to the irritated spot.

In these experiments on the triton and the frog, the evidence of sensation and volition is all the stronger, because the reactions produced by irritations are not uniform. If when a decapitated animal were stimulated it always reacted in *precisely the same way,* and never chose *new means* on the failure of the old, it would be conceivable to attribute the results to simple reflex action—*i.e.*, the mechanical transference of an impulse along a prescribed path. It is possible so to conceive the breathing, or the swallowing mechanism: the impression may be directly reflected on certain groups of muscles. But I cannot conceive a machine suddenly striking out new methods, when the old methods fail. I cannot conceive a machine thrown into disorder when its accustomed actions fail, and in this disorder suddenly lighting upon an action likely to succeed, and continuing *that;* but I can conceive this to be done by an organism, for my own experience and observation of animals assures me that this is always the way new lines of action are adopted. And this which is observed of the unmutilated animal, I have just shown to be observed of the brainless animal; wherefore the conclusion is, that if ever the frog is sentient, if ever its actions are guided by sensation, they are so when its brain is removed.

20. Schröder van der Kolk thinks that Pflüger was deceived in attributing sensation and volition to the frog, because the reflex actions are, he says, so nicely adapted to their ends, that they are undistinguishable from voluntary actions. The mechanism is such that, by means of the communications established between various groups of cells, all these actions adapted to an end may be excited by every stimulus. But I deny the fact. I deny that all the actions are awakened by every stimulus. Only some few are awakened, and those are not always the same, nor do they follow the same order of succession. One decapitated frog does not behave exactly like another under similar circumstances; does not behave exactly like himself at different seasons; unlike a machine, he manifests spontaneity in his actions, and volition in the direction of his actions.

21. The reader will notice that my illustrations show these actions of the brainless animal to have the same external characters as those of the unmutilated animals. I am therefore not here concerned to prove the psychical nature of these actions, unless it be granted that the unmutilated animal has sensation and volition. This of course can only be inferred, not proved. But the inference must not be allowed

in the one case and refused in the other. Young rabbits and puppies when taken from their mothers manifest discomfort by restless movement and whining. Do they feel the discomfort they thus express? If ever rabbits and puppies may be said to feel, we must answer, Yes. Well, if the brain be removed from rabbits and puppies, precisely similar phenomena are observed when these young animals are taken from their mothers. "I observed the motions, which seemed the result of discomfort, quickly cease when I warmed the young rabbit by breathing on it. After a while it was completely at rest, and seemed sunk in deep sleep; occasionally, however, it moved one of its legs without any external stimulus having been applied, and this not spasmodically, but in the manner of a sleeping animal."* Is this cessation of the restlessness, when warmth is restored, not evidence of sensation? We see an infant restless, struggling, and squalling; and we believe that it is hungry, or that some other sensations agitate it; it is put to the breast, and its squalls subside; or a finger is placed in its mouth, and it sucks that, in a peaceful lull, for a few moments, to recommence squalling when the finger yields no satisfaction. If we accept these as signs of sensation, I do not see how we can deny such sensation to the brainless animal which will also cease to cry, and will suck the delusive finger.

22. One of the earliest advocates of the Reflex Theory sums up his observations in these words: "It is clear that brainless animals, although without sensation, because not endowed with mind, nevertheless, by means of external impressions which operate incessantly on them, perform all the acts and manifest all the activity of the sentient animal; everything that is effected sensationally and volitionally, they effect by means of the organic forces of the impressions."† Call Sensibility one of the organic forces, if you please, but so long as the acts performed are not only the same as those of a sentient animal, but are performed by the same me-

* VOLKMANN, quoted by PFLÜGER.

† UNZER: *The Principles of Physiology* (translated for the Sydenham Society), p. 235.

chanism, they have every claim to the character of sensational acts which can be urged in the case of these animals when the brain is present. And the only reason on which this claim is disputed is the assumed loss of all sensation with the loss of the brain. Here, therefore, lies the central point to be determined.

CHAPTER II.

DEDUCTION FROM GENERAL LAWS.

23. The evidence is of two kinds: deductions from the general laws of nervous action, and inductions from particular manifestations. The former furnish a presumption, the latter a proof.

The central process which initiates a reflex action may be excited by the external stimulation of a peripheral nerve, by the internal stimulation of a peripheral nerve, or by the irradiation from some other part of the central tissue. The last-named stimulations are the least intelligible, because they are so varied and complex, and so remote from observation; among them may be placed, 1°, the organised impulses of Instinct and Habit, with their fixed modes of manifestation; 2°, the organised impulses of Emotion, which are more variable in their manifestations, because more fluctuating in their conditions; 3°, the organised impulses of Intellect, the most variable of all. Whether we shrink on the contact of a cold substance or on hearing a sudden sound,—at the sight of a terrible object,—at the imaginary vision of the object,—or because we feign the terror which is thus expressed,—the reflex mechanism of shrinking is in each case the same, and the neural process discharged on the muscles is the same; but the state of Feeling which originated the change,—or, in strictly physiological terms—the inciting neural process which preceded this reflex neural process—was in each case somewhat different, yet in each case was a mode of Sensibility.

24. The property of Sensibility belongs to the whole central tissue; and we have every reason to believe that unless it is excited no reflex takes place, whereas when it is exaggerated—as in epilepsy, or under strychnine—the reflex dis-

charges are convulsive. When anæsthetics are given, consciousness first disappears, and then reflexion. When the sensorium is powerfully excited by *other* stimuli, the normal stimulus fails to excite either consciousness or reflexion. Hence our conclusion is that for consciousness, on the one hand, and *normal* reflexion, on the other, the proximate condition is a change in the sensorium; or—to phrase it more familiarly—Feeling is necessary for reflex action.

The difficulty in apprehending this lies in the ambiguity of the term Feeling. Many readers who would find no difficulty in admitting Sensibility as a necessary element in reflex action, will resist the idea of identifying Sensibility with Feeling. But this repugnance must be overcome if we are to understand the various modes of Sensibility which represent Feeling in animals, and its varieties in ourselves. We understand how the general Sensibility manifests itself in markedly different sensations—how that of the optic centre differs from that of the auditory centre, and both from a spinal centre. The tones of a violin are not the same as the tones of a violoncello, both differ from the tones of a key-bugle: yet they all come under the same general laws of tonality. So, as I often insist, the tissues in brain and cord being the same, their properties must be the same, their laws of excitation, irradiation, and combination the same, through all the varieties in their manifestations due to varieties of innervation. Hence it is that there are reflex cerebral processes no less than reflex spinal processes: the motor impulse from the hemispheres on the *corpora striata*, or from posterior grey substance on anterior grey substance, is similar to that from the anterior grey substance on the motor nerves. The difference in reflexes arises from the terminal organs; as the difference in sensations arises from the surfaces stimulated. But not only are there reflex processes in the brain, of the same *order* as those in the cord, there are volitional processes in the cord of the same order as those in the brain. And in both the processes are sometimes conscious, sometimes unconscious. No evidence suggests that in the conscious action there is a sensorial process and a purely physical process in the unconscious action—only a different *relation* of one sensorial process to others.

25. Let us contrast a cerebral and a spinal process, in respect to the three stages of stimulation, irradiation, and discharge. A luminous impression stimulates my retina, this excites my sensorium, in which second stage I am conscious of the luminous sensation; the final discharge is a perception, or a mental articulation of the *name* of the luminous object. But the irradiation may perhaps not have been such as to cause a *conscious* sensation, because the requisite neural elements were already grouped in some other way; in this case there is an unconscious discharge on some motor group, and instead of perceiving and naming the luminous object, I move my head, or my hand, or my whole body, avoiding the object, or grasping at it. A third issue is possible: the irradiation instead of exciting a definite perception, or a definite movement, may be merged in the stream of simultaneous excitations, and thus form the component of a group, and the discharge of this group will be a perception or a movement.

It is the same with a spinal process. An impression on the skin is irradiated in the cord, and the response is a movement, of which we are conscious, or unconscious. Here also a third issue is possible: the irradiation may be merged in a stream of simultaneous excitations, modifying them and modified by them, thus forming a component in some ulterior discharge.

26. The obstacle in the way of recognising that cerebral processes and spinal processes are of the same order of sensorial phenomena, and have the same physiological significance when considered irrespective of the group of organs they call into activity, is similar to the obstacle which has prevented psychologists from recognising the identity of the logical process in the combinations of Feeling and the combinations of Thought, *i.e.*, the Logic of Feeling and the Logic of Signs. This obstacle is the fixing attention on the diversity of the effects when the same process operates with different elements. Because the spinal cord manifests the phenomena

of sensation and volition, we are not to conclude that it also manifests ideation and imagination; any more than we are to conclude that a mollusc is capable of musical feelings because it is affected by sounds.

27. The careless confusion of general properties with special applications of those properties, and of functions with properties, has been a serious hindrance to the right understanding of Sensibility and its operations. Instead of recognising that the nervous system has one general mode of reaction, which remains the same under every variety of combination with other systems, physiologists commonly lose sight of this general property, and fix on one mode of its manifestation as the sole characteristic of Sensibility. Sometimes the mode fixed on is Pain, at other times Attention. Thus, when an animal manifests no evidence of pain under stimulations which ordinarily excite severe pain, this is often interpreted as a proof that *all* sensation is absent; and if with this absence of pain there is—as there often is—clear evidence of the presence of some other mode of sensibility, the contradiction is evaded by the assumption that what here looks like evidence of sensation is merely mechanical reflexion. One would think that Physiology and Pathology had been silent on the facts of analgesia without anæsthesia, and of so much conscious sensation which is unaccompanied by pain.* Who does not know that a patient will lose one kind of sensibility while retaining others—cease to feel pain, yet feel temperature, or be insensible to touch, yet exquisitely alive to pain? † Inasmuch as Sensibility depends on the

* Even so eminent an investigator as GOLTZ has fallen into this confusion. He introduces an experiment to prove that the brainless frog is insensible to pain by the words "when an animal, placed under circumstances which would be very painful, makes no movement, although quite capable of moving, the least we can say is that it is improbable that the animal has sensation" (*Nervencentren des Frosches*, p. 127). I need not discuss the proof itself, having already done so in *Nature*, vol. ix. p. 84. The point to which I wish to call attention is the confusion of insensibility in general with insensibility to pain.

† See DUCHENNE: *De Électrisation localisée*, p. 398. GRIESINGER cites various examples of insane patients who have burned the flesh off their bones while manifesting a total indifference to these injuries:

condition of the centres, an abnormal condition will obviously transform the reaction of the centres into one very unlike the normal reaction. For example, Antoine Cros had a patient who was quite unable to feel the sensation of cold on her left side—every cold object touching her skin on that side was felt as a very hot one; whereas a hot object produced "the sort of sensation which followed the application of an intermittent voltaic current." * Thus also the experiments of Rose† and others have exhibited the effects of a dose of Santonine in causing all objects to be seen as yellow in one stage, and violet in another.

28. If, then, certain alterations in the organic conditions are accompanied by a suppression or perversion of some modes of Sensibility, without suppressing the rest, it is but rational to suppose that profound disturbances of the organic mechanism, such as must result from the removal of the brain, will also suppress or pervert several modes of Sensibility, and yet leave intact those modes which belong to the intact parts of the mechanism. Assuming that the spinal centres with the organs they innervate are capable of reacting under certain modes of sensation, these will not necessarily be suppressed by removal of the brain—all that will thereby be suppressed is their co-operation with the brain. I know it will be said that precisely this co-operation is necessary for sensation; and that the spinal reactions are simple reflexions in which sensation has no part. This, however, is the position I hope to turn. Meanwhile my assumption is that sensation necessarily plays a part in the reflex actions *of the organism*, and when that organism is truncated, its actions are proportionately limited, its sensations less complex. The spinal cord, separated from encephalic

Maladies Mentales, p. 94. FALRET says, "Nous avons vu plusieurs fois des aliénés s'inciser, s'amputer eux-mêmes diverses parties du corps sans paraître ressentir aucune souffrance:" *Leçons cliniques de Médicine Mentale*, 1854, i. 189. Patients incapable of feeling the contact of a hot iron with their skin, have felt subjective burnings in the skin thus objectively insensible.

* CROS: *Les Fonctions supérieures du Syst. nerveux*, 1875, p. 27.

† *Virchow's Archiv*, Bd. xxviii. p. 30.

connections, cannot react in the special forms of Sensation known as colour, scent, taste, sound, &c., because it does not innervate the organs of these special senses, nor co-operate with their centres. But it can, and does, react in other modes: it innervates skin and muscles; and the sensibilities, thus excited, it can also *combine* and *co-ordinate*. It has its Memory, and its Logic, just as the brain has: both no longer than they are integral parts of an active living organism: neither when the organism is inactive or dead. We do not expect the retina to respond in sounds, nor the ear to respond in colours: we expect each organ to have its special mode of reaction. What is common to both is Sensibility. What is common to brain and cord is Sensibility—and the laws of Grouping. Instead of marvelling at the disappearance of so many modes of Sensibility when the brain is removed, our surprise should be to find so many evidences of Sensibility remaining after so profound a mutilation of the mechanism.

29. The current hypothesis, which assumes that the brain is the sole organ of the mind, the sole seat of sensation, is a remnant of the ancient hypothesis respecting the Soul and its seat; and on the whole I think the ancient hypothesis is the more rational of the two. If the Soul inhabits the organism, using it as an instrument, playing on its organs as a musician plays on his instrument, we are not called upon to explain the mode of operation of this mysterious agent; but if the Soul be the subjective side of the Life, the spiritual aspect of the material organism, then since it is a synthesis of all the organic forces, the consensus of all the sentient phenomena, no one part can usurp the prerogatives of all, but all are requisite for each. And this indeed is what few physiologists would nowadays dispute. In spite of their localising sensation in the cerebral cells, they would not maintain that the cerebral cells, nor even the whole brain, could produce sensation—if *detached* from the organism; the cheek of the guillotined victim may have blushed when struck, but who believes that the brain felt the insult, or the blow? Obviously, therefore, when we read that thought is "a property of the grey substance of the brain, as gravitation

is of matter," or that the brain is the exclusive organ of Sensation, the writers cannot consistently carry out their hypothesis unless they silently reintroduce other organs as co-operating agents; for a neural process in the cerebrum is *in itself* no more a sensation than it is a muscular contraction, or a glandular secretion: the muscles must co-operate for the contraction, the gland for the secretion, the neural process being simply the exciting cause. In like manner the Sensorium is necessary for the sensation, the neural process—in cerebrum, or elsewhere—being simply the exciting cause.

30. And what is the Sensorium? A long chapter would be required to state the various opinions which have been held respecting its *seat*, although amid all the disputes as to the organ, there has been unanimity as to the function, which is that of converting stimulations into sensations. I cannot pause here to examine the contending arguments, but must content myself with expounding the opinion I hold, namely, that the Sensorium is the *whole* of the sensitive organism, and not any one isolated portion of it. When light falls on the optic organ, or air pulses on the auditory organ, the reaction of each organ determines the *specific* character of the sensation, *but no such sensation is possible unless there be a reaction of the organism;* and the nature of the product will of course vary with the varying factors which co-operate—a simple organism, a truncated organism, an exhausted or otherwise occupied organism, will react differently from a complex, a normal, or an unoccupied organism. Detach the optic organ with its centre from the rest of the organism, and no normal sensation of Sight will result from its stimulation; and in a lesser degree this is equally true of a stimulation of the optic organ when the sensorium is exhausted, or powerfully affected by other stimuli. Because of the great importance of the cerebrum, and its predominance in the nervous system, it has been supposed to constitute the whole of the sensorium, in spite of the evidence of varied Sensibility after the cerebrum has been removed. I do not wish to underrate the cerebral importance (see p. 147), yet I must say that the modern phrase *cerebration*, when employed as

more than a shorthand expression of the complex processes which a cerebral process initiates, and when taken as the objective equivalent of Consciousness or of Thought, seems to me not more justifiable than to speak of Combustion as the equivalent of Railway Transport. The railway waggons will not move unless the fuel which supplies the boiler be ignited; the organism will not think unless the cerebrum excites this peculiar mode of Sensibility by its action on the organs. *It is the man, and not the brain, that thinks:* it is the organism as a whole, and not one organ, that feels and acts.

31. Consciousness, or Sensation, is a complex product not to be recognised in any *one* of its factors. Cerebral processes and spinal processes are the elements we analytically separate, as muscular contractions are the elements of limb-movements. The synthetic unity of these elements is a reflex; this we analytically decompose into a sensation and a movement; and then we speak of sensation as the reaction of the sensory organ, the movement as the reaction of the muscular organ. By a similar procedure we separate the stimulation of a sensory nerve from the reaction of the sensory organ, and that from the reaction of the sensorium; and in this way we may come to regard Cerebration as Thought. But those who employ this artifice should remember that the organism is not an assemblage of organs, made up of parts put together like a machine. The organs are differentiations of the organism, each evolved from those which preceded it, all sharing in a common activity, all *inter*-dependent.

32. That co-operation of the Personality which is conspicuous in conscious actions is also inductively to be inferred in sub-conscious and unconscious actions. We know that a man reacts on an impression according to his physical and mental state at the moment—that through his individuality he feels differently, and thinks differently from other men, and from himself at other epochs, and in other states. Because he resembles other men in many and essential points we conclude that he will resemble them in all; but observation proves this conclusion to be precipitate.

Other men see a blue colour in the sky, or feel awe at sight of the setting sun; but he has perhaps not learned to discriminate this sensation, is not conscious of the blue; nor has he learned to feel awe at the setting sun. Why—having normally-constructed eyes—does he not see the blue of the sky? For the same reason that a dog, or an infant, fails to see it. The colour has no *interest* for him (and all cognition is primarily emotion), nor has this want of personal interest been rectified from an impersonal source: he has never been taught to distinguish the colour of the sky; and his eye wanders over it with the indifferent gaze with which a savage would regard a Greek codex.

33. The point here insisted on, namely, that every reaction on an impression is indirectly the reaction of the whole organism, and that no organ detached from the organism has more significance than a word detached from a sentence, is of far-reaching importance, and peculiarly worthy of attention in considering the Reflex Theory, because almost all the evidence urged in support of that theory presupposes the legitimacy of concluding what takes place in the organism from what is observed in an organ detached from its normal connections. No experimental proof is necessary to show that many actions take place unconsciously; the fact is undisputed. But does unconsciously mean insentiently? It is certain that the unconscious actions take place in a sentient organism, and involve organic processes of the same *order* as the actions which are conscious. It is also certain that many sentient processes take place unconsciously. For thousands of years men used their eyes, and saw as their descendants see, yet were unconscious of the blue sky and green of the grass. Were their visual reactions not of the same *order* as our own? So far as the optic apparatus is concerned, there cannot be a doubt on the point; yet in them the sensorium having a somewhat different disposition—the neural elements being differently combined—their reactions correspondingly differed. They too had optical Sensibility, and visual sensations; but they did not feel precisely what we feel.

34. I have chosen these somewhat remote illustrations for the sake of their psychological interest; but I might have confined myself to more familiar examples. Thus the contents of the consciousness of a man born blind cannot be *the same* as the contents of one who has had visual experiences, which will enter into the complex of every conscious state, because the visual organs will have affected his sensorium; nevertheless in the organism of the blind man there are conditions so similar to those of other men, and his experiences will have been so similar, that in spite of the modifications due to the absence of visual experiences, his consciousness will in the main resemble theirs. But now let us in imagination pursue this kind of modification, let us take away hearing, taste, and smell, and we shall have proportionately simplified the contents of consciousness—the reactions of the sensorium—in thus simplifying the organism. There still will remain Touch, Temperature, Pain, and the Systemic Sensations. There will still remain an organism to react on impressions. So long as there is a living organism, however truncated, there is a sentient mechanism. When the brain has been removed, the removal causes both a *disturbance* of function and a *loss* of function; the mechanism has been seriously interfered with; yet all those parts of the mechanism which still co-operate manifest their physiological aptitudes. The animal can live without its brain, *ergo* it can feel without its brain. Observation proves this, for it discovers the brainless animal manifesting various sensibilities, and combining various movements. The vision of the brainless animal is greatly impaired, but it nevertheless persists. The intelligence is greatly impaired, the spontaneity is reduced to a minimum; but still both intelligence and spontaneity are manifested.

35. The physiologist has only two conclusions open to him. Either he holds Sensation to be a *property* of nerve-tissue—and in that case he must assign it to the spinal cord as to the brain; or else he holds Sensation to be a *function* of an organ—and in that case, although analytically he may decompose the organism into separate organs, assigning special sensations to the reactions of each, he must still admit

that in reality these organs only yield sensations as component parts of the organism. The notion of a separate organ, such as the brain, being the exclusive seat of sensation is thus seen to be untenable.

In popular phrase, "it is not the eye which sees, but the mind behind the eye." It is not the stimulus which is the *object* felt—it is the change in consciousness—the reaction of the sensorium. No one would propound the absurdity that the retinal cells *see*, or the auditory cells *hear* (although by a conventional ellipsis these cells are said to be "percipient" of colours and sounds), yet many writers have no hesitation in asserting that the cerebral cells are the seats of these and all other sensations. In a hundred treatises may be read the most precise description of the transformation of molecular changes in the retinal cells into molecular changes in the cerebral cells, where, it is said, "we know that the stimulations become sensations." Now who knows this? How can it be known? Nay, who, on reflection, fails to see that this cannot be so? If a sensation of sight were not much *more* than a molecular change in the cerebrum stimulated by a molecular change in the optic tract, three conclusions would follow, each of which is demonstrably erroneous:—

I. The cerebrum in a decapitated animal would respond by a sensation of sight to a retinal stimulation.

II. The animal deprived of its cerebrum could not respond by a sensation of sight to a retinal stimulation.

III. The same retinal stimulation would always produce the same cerebral process and the same sensation; whereas the sensation depends on the condition of the sensorium at the time.

36. The difference between the Reflex Theory and that here upheld is important in its general relations, and yet turns on a point which may easily appear insignificant. The Reflex Theory asserts that when a sensory nerve is stimulated, the excitation of the centre may either subdivide into two waves, one of which passes directly to the brain and there awakens sensation, the other passes over to the motor-roots and causes muscular contractions; or, instead of thus subdi-

viding, the wave may pass at once to the motor-nerves, and then there is movement without sensation. This is obviously a restatement in anatomical terms of the observed fact that some reflexes take place consciously and some unconsciously. But what evidence is there for this anatomical statement? We have seen that there is none. According to all we actually know, and reasonably infer, the continuity of tissue and the irradiation of excitation are such that the stimulus wave must always affect the whole system, so that brain and cord being structurally united, their reactions must co-operate with varying energy dependent on their statical conditions at the time.*

37. The physiological fact that the irradiation is *restricted* to certain paths, and therefore only certain portions of the whole system are excited to discharge—the fact that stimulation takes effect along the lines of least resistance—is that which gives the Reflex Theory its plausible aspect. But this fact of restriction is not dependent on an *anatomical* disposition of structure, it is, as we have already seen (PROBLEM II. § 166), dependent on a fluctuating physiological disposition—a temporary statical condition of the centres. And it enables us to understand why the reflex action which is at one moment a distinctly conscious or even a volitional action, is at another sub-conscious or unconscious. When an object is

* The idea of a *fixed anatomical mechanism* for reflexion, such as that of an excito-motory system, is completely refuted by the fact that the grey substance may anywhere be cut away, and yet so long as a small bridge of grey substance remains the stimulation will be propagated through it. The idea of a *fixed pathway* is also refuted by the fact of the variations in the reflex responses, and the necessary irradiation even for very simple reflexes. Take, for example, that of breathing. An irritation of the bronchial filaments is transmitted by the pneumogastric to its centre in the medulla oblongata; from this, however, it is immediately irradiated *downwards* to the cervical and dorsal regions, which innervate the muscles of chest and diaphragm, and *upwards* to the brain, whether the stimulation awaken consciousness or not. One may say, indeed, that inasmuch as under normal conditions the bronchial irritation always causes a movement of a particular group of muscles, there is to this extent a fixed pathway of discharge; but, as I have formerly explained, this is only an expression of the particular tension of particular centres, and is variable with that tension; the other centres are also affected, even when they are not excited to discharge.

placed in the hand of an infant the fingers close over it by a simple reflex. This having also been observed in the case of an infant born without a brain,* one might interpret it as normally taking place without brain co-operation, were there not good grounds for concluding that normally the brain must co-operate. Thus if the object be placed in the hand of a boy, or a man, the fingers will close, or not close—not according to an anatomical mechanism, but according to a physiological condition: if the attention preoccupy his sensorium elsewhere, his fingers will probably close, probably not; if his sensorium be directed towards the object, either by the urgency of the sensitive impression, or by some one's pointing to the object, the fingers will close or not close, just as he chooses—perhaps the hand will be suddenly drawn away. The centre of innervation for the fingers is in the cord, and from this comes the final discharge of the sensitive stimulation; but the neural processes which preceded this discharge, and were consequent on the stimulation, were in each case somewhat different. In each case the impression on the skin was carried to the cord, and thence irradiated throughout the continuous neural axis, restricted to certain paths by the resistance it met with, but blending with waves of simultaneous excitations from other sources, the final discharge being the resultant of these component forces. We may suppose the brain to be the seat of consciousness, and yet not conclude that the brain was unaffected because the fingers closed unconsciously; any more than we conclude that the retina of the unoccupied eye is unaffected by light when with the other we are looking through a microscope, and only *see* objects with this eye—though directly we attend to the impressions on the other eye we see the objects which before were unseen. We know that the muscles of the back are all involved in walking, standing, &c., but we are seldom conscious of their co-operation till rheumatism or lumbago makes us painfully alive to it.

38. The two main positions of the Reflex Theory are, 1°, that reflex actions take place without brain co-operation,—

* LALLEMAND: *Recherches sur l'Encéphale*, iii. 310.

as proved by observation of decapitated animals; 2°, that they take place without brain co-operation,—as proved by our being unconscious of them.

To these the answers are: 1°. The proof drawn from observation of decapitated animals is defective, because the conditions of the organism are then abnormal—there is a disturbance of the mechanism, and a loss of some of its components. The fact that a reflex occurs in the absence of the brain is no proof that reflexes when the brain is present occur without its participation. 2°. The absence of consciousness cannot be accepted as proof of the brain not being in action, because much brain-work is known to pass unconsciously, and there are cerebral reflexes which have the same characters as spinal reflexes.

39. A prick on the great toe traverses the whole length of the spinal axis with effects manifested in various organs—the muscles of the limb, the heart, the chest, the eyes, &c. The leg is withdrawn, the heart momently arrested, the eyes turned towards the source of irritation, the thoughts directed towards relief. These effects can be observed—there are others which lie beyond our observation, and can only be revealed by delicate experimental tests. But even the observable effects are very fluctuating, because they depend on fluctuating conditions. All we can say is, that so long as there is continuity of structure, there must be continuity of excitation; and the brain structurally connected with the centre of a sensory impression, must necessarily co-operate more or less in the reactions of that centre. In other words, the brain, although not the exclusive seat of sensation, plays a part in every particular sensation, so long as it forms a part of the stimulated organism.

40. This view being so widely opposed to the views current in physiological schools, I was gratified to find Dr. Crichton Browne led by his researches to a conclusion not unlike it in essential features. In his essay on the Functions of the Optic Thalami * (well worthy of attention on other grounds) he says: "Allowing the spinal cord a power of independent

* *West Riding Lunatic Asylum Reports*, 1875, vol. v. pp. 252, *sq.*

action, it may still be that it generally acts reflexly through, or in association with, a superior centre. The sensorial ganglia can undoubtedly act alone in a reflex manner, but they almost invariably consult the cerebrum before dealing with the impressions which they receive; so it may be that the spinal cord, though capable of spontaneous reaction, may yet commonly refer to some higher seat of compound co-ordination before sending forth an answer to any message brought to it." What is here stated as a possible and occasional process, I consider to be a necessary and universal process. Dr. Browne acutely remarks that if "what may be termed the encephalic loop were an integral part of every reflex act, then the influence of an intracranial lesion in checking reflex action would not be difficult to understand"—and we may add the notorious influence of the brain in arresting reflex actions, and modifying them by the will, which is only explicable on the supposition that the cerebral and spinal centres are functionally associated. Dr. Browne further remarks: "In experimenting upon myself I have sometimes thought that when the toe is pricked the sensation of pain actually precedes the movement of withdrawal; and in experimenting upon patients with sluggish nervous systems I have certainly noticed that after the pricking of the toe the little cry of pain has anticipated the muscular contractions of the leg. Now this cry of pain is a secondary reflex act through the sensorial centre; it is the result of a discharge from efferent nerves from the summit of what we have spoken of as the encephalic loop line; and we should certainly not expect that it would be developed earlier than the primary reflexion upon the motor apparatus, unless indeed what we have regarded as the primary reflexion really itself took place by way of the loop line."

41. The difference between a voluntary and involuntary act is not, I conceive, that in the one case the brain co-operates and in the other is inactive, but that while in both the brain co-operates, the state of the sensorium known as mental prevision or ideal stimulation, is present in the one, and absent or less conspicuous in the other. So likewise

the difference between a normal reflex action accompanied, and the same action unaccompanied by consciousness, is not that the brain co-operates in the one and is inactive in the other, but that the state of the sensorium is somewhat different in the two cases. Movements which originally were voluntary and difficult of execution—accompanied therefore by brain co-operation—become by frequent repetition automatic, easy of execution, and unconscious—they are then said to depend on the direct action of the established mechanism. Granted. But what are the components of this mechanism? Are they not just those centres and organs which at first effected the movements? In becoming easy and automatic, the movements do not *change their mechanism* —the moving organs and the motor conditions remain what they were; all that is changed is the degree of consciousness, *i.e.*, the *state* of the sensorium which precedes and succeeds the movement. It is this which constitutes the difficulty of the question. Some readers may consider that all is conceded when unconsciousness is admitted. But this is not so. My present argument is the physiological one that the brain co-operates in reflex actions whenever the brain is structurally united with the reflex centres; the psychological question as to whether consciousness is also involved in this brain-co-operation must be debated on other grounds; and we have already seen that consciousness operates in gradations of infinite delicacy.

Observe a man performing some automatic action, such as planing a deal board, or cutting out a pattern, which he has done so often that he is now able to do it "mechanically." It is certain that his brain co-operates, and that he could not act thus with an injured brain; yet he is said to act unconsciously, his brain occupied elsewhere as he whistles, talks to bystanders, or thinks of his wife and children. Yet the brain is acting as an overseer of his work, attentive to every stroke of the plane, every snip of the scissors; and this becomes evident directly his attention is otherwise absorbed by an interesting question addressed to him, or an interesting object meeting his eye: then the work pauses, his hands are arrested, and the automatic action will only be resumed when his attention is released—when he has answered your question, or satisfied himself about the object.

42. This is a step towards understanding the co-operation of the brain even in those connate reflexes which were not originally voluntary acts, but were from the first organised tendencies, and are capable of being realised in the absence of the brain. I admit that it is difficult to find proof of brain-co-operation here, though I think the anatomical and physiological evidence render it highly probable. But distinct proof to the contrary would not suffice for the Reflex Theory—would not prove that reflex actions were insentient—unless there had previously been proved that which seems to me contradicted by the clearest and most massive evidence, namely, that the brain is the sole seat of sentience. This contradictory evidence we will now furnish.

CHAPTER III.

INDUCTIONS FROM PARTICULAR OBSERVATIONS.

43. In the last chapter we surveyed the deductive evidence, from which the conclusion was that Reflexion necessarily involves Sensibility, but not necessarily any one particular *mode* of Sensibility, such as Consciousness, Pain, Discomfort, Attention, or the reaction of any one of the special Senses. Although each or all of these modes may be involved in the sensorial process which determines a reflex act, each or all may be absent. Such is the fact of observation. This fact is interpreted on the hypothesis that Reflexion is the exclusive property of the spinal cord, as Sensation is of the brain. When we come to examine the evidence for this hypothesis, we find it to move in a circle: the brain is said to be the exclusive seat of sensation, because reflex actions can be effected after its removal; and reflex actions are said to be insentient because they take place in the absence of the brain.

A gentleman was one day stoutly asserting that there were no gold-fields except in Mexico and Peru. A nugget, dug up in California, was presented to him, as evidence against his positive assertion. He was not in the least disconcerted. "This metal, sir, is, I own, extremely *like* gold; and you tell me that it passes as such in the market, having been declared by the assayers to be undistinguishable from the precious metal. All this I will not dispute. Nevertheless, the metal is not gold, but *auruminium;* it cannot be gold, *because* gold comes only from Mexico and Peru." In vain was he informed that the geological formation was similar in California and Peru, and the metals similar; he had fixed in his mind the conclusion that gold existed *only* in Mexico and Peru:

this was a law of nature; he had no reasons to give why it should be so; but such had been the admitted fact for many years, and from it he would not swerve. He was not fond of newfangled notions, which, after all, would only lead us back to the exploded errors of the past. To accept the statement that gold was to be found elsewhere than in Mexico and Peru, would be to return to the opinion of the ancients, who thought there was gold in the upper regions of Tartary!

Sensation is not tangible, assayable, like gold. We can understand, therefore, that the very men who would make merry with the *auruminium*, would accept easily such a phrase as "reflex action." The decapitated animal defends itself against injury, gets out of the way of annoyances, cleans itself, performs many of its ordinary actions, but is said to do these things without that Sensibility which, if its head were on, would guide them. Even before the Reflex Theory was invented this line of argument was used. Gall, referring to the experiments of Sue, previously noticed, says that "Sue confounds the effects of Irritability with those of Sensibility." * Not gold, dear sir, but *auruminium!*

44. On investigating the phenomena we soon come upon two classes which must cause hesitation. We find that the brain has its reflex processes, of the same order as those of the cord; we find that these processes may be conscious or unconscious, voluntary or involuntary; so that we can no longer separate brain from cord on the ground of Reflexion. In this respect, at least, the two are mechanisms with similar powers. Turning now to the other class of phenomena, we find that precisely as the brain is an organ of Reflexion, the cord is an organ of Sensation. All the evidence we can have, from which to infer the presence of sensation, is furnished by the sensorial processes in the cord. Remove the brain, and the animal still manifests Sensibility, and this in degrees of energy and complexity proportional to the mechanisms still intact: some of these manifestations have the character of volitional actions, some of automatic actions, some of Memory, Judgment, and selective Adaptation. These we observe not

* GALL *et* SPURZHEIM: *Anat. et Physiol. du Système Nerveux*, i. 83.

indeed with the energy and variety of such manifestations when the brain co-operates, since the disturbance of the organism which is the consequence of the brain's removal—or the meagreness of the organism which is the correlative of the brain never having been developed—must of course involve a corresponding difference in the observed phenomena; but the point here brought forward is that phenomena of the same *order* are manifested by organisms with or without a brain.

45. Let us go seriatim through the evidence of these two classes:—

CEREBRAL REFLEXES.

While Theory separated the actions of the cord from those of the brain on the ground of their being at times unconscious and involuntary, Observation disclosed that this distinction could not be maintained.

This step was taken by Dr. Laycock in 1840. In a striking paper * read by him at the British Association in 1844, he brought together the evidence on which his view was founded. The idea has been adopted and illustrated in the writings of Dr. Carpenter, who now calls the action "unconscious cerebration."

"I was led to this opinion," Dr. Laycock says in announcing his view, "by the general principle that the ganglia within the cranium being a continuation of the spinal cord, must necessarily be regulated as to their reaction on external agencies by laws identical with those governing the spinal ganglia and their analogues in the lower animals. If, therefore, the spinal cord is a centre of reflexion, the brain must also be one." It is a matter of regret that Dr. Laycock did not extend this principle, and declare that whatever was true of the *properties* of the cranial centres, must also be true of the spinal centres; if the brain have Sensibility, the spinal cord must also have it.

Dr. Laycock refers to the curious phenomena of Hydro-

* Printed in the *British and Foreign Medical Review*, Jan. 1845.

phobia in proof that reflex actions may be excited by the optic nerves, or by a mere idea of water. When a mirror was presented to a patient, the reflexion of the light acting on his retina, in the manner of a reflexion from the surface of water, produced a convulsive sobbing, as in the attempt to swallow water, and the patient turned aside his head with expressions of terror. Money was given him to induce him to look a second time, but before he had looked a minute, the same effect was produced.

The *idea* of water excited similar convulsions. No sooner was it suggested that the patient should swallow a little water than he seemed frightened, and began to cry out. By kindly encouragements, he was brought to express his willingness to drink, but the *sound* of the water, as it was poured out again, brought on convulsions. In another case, "on our proposing to him to drink, he started up, and recovered his breath by a deep convulsive inspiration. On being urged to try, he took a cup of water in one hand, and a spoon in the other. With an expression of terror, yet with great resolution, he filled the spoon, and proceeded to carry it to his lips; but before it reached his mouth, his courage forsook him, and he was forced to desist. He repeatedly renewed the attempt, but with no more success. His arm became rigid and immovable whenever he tried to raise it to his mouth, and he struggled in vain against this spasmodic resistance."

In 1843 Griesinger—who appears to have known nothing of Dr. Laycock's paper—published his remarkably suggestive memoir on Psychical Reflexes,* in which he extends the principle of Reflexion to all the cerebro-spinal centres. The whole course of subsequent research has confirmed this view; so that we may say with Landry, "L'existence du pouvoir réflexe dans l'encéphale ou dans quelques unes de ses parties établit une nouvelle analogie entre le centre nerveux cranien et la moelle épinière." † Indeed we have only to consider

* GRIESINGER: *Abhandlungen*, 1872. The first volume contains a reprint of this memoir.

† LANDRY: *Traité des Paralysies*, i. 55. Conf. ZIEMSSEN: *Chorea* in

the Laughter which follows a ludicrous idea, or the Terror which follows a suggestion of danger,—the varying and involuntary expression of Emotion,—and the curious phenomena of Imitation and Contagion,—to see how large a place cerebral reflexion occupies.

46. The existence of cerebral reflexion having been thus made manifest, Dr. Carpenter classed all reflex actions under three heads: 1°, the excito-motor, determined by the spinal cord; 2°, the sensori-motor, determined by the ganglia at the base of the brain; 3°, ideo-motor, determined by the brain. From all these Consciousness is absent. From the first, he supposes Sensation to be absent. As an artifice, such a classification may have its value, but it is physiologically and psychologically misleading. It sustains the hypothesis of an imaginary excito-motor mechanism. It restricts Sensibility to one of its many modes. It fails altogether to connect Sensation with Thought, the Logic of Feeling with the Logic of Signs.

47. The view of Sensibility as common to the whole cerebro-spinal axis, is by no means new. Robert Whytt maintained it. Prochaska held that the spinal cord formed the greater part of the *sensorium commune;* and he adduced, in proof, the familiar facts of sensibility manifested by headless animals. The next writer whom I can discover to have held this opinion is J. J. Sue—the father of the celebrated French romance-writer—who, in 1803, conceived that his experiments proved the spinal cord to be capable of replacing, to a certain extent, the functions of the brain.* Next came Legallois,† who undertook to show, by a series of experiments, that the principle of sensation and movement, in the trunk and extremities, has its seat in the spinal

the *Handbuch der speciellen Pathologie*, Bd. xii. 2, p. 408. And LUYS: *Études de physiol. et pathol. cérébrales*, 1874, pp. 89–94.

* SUE: *Recherches Philosophiques sur la Vitalité et le Galvanisme*, p. 9. He was not consistent, however, but adopted Bichat's opinion respecting the sensibility of the viscera, p. 68.

† LEGALLOIS: *Expériences sur le principe de la vie.* Published, I conclude, in 1811; the edition I use is the one printed in the *Encyclopédie des Sciences Medicales*, iv.

cord. The mere division of the cord, he said, produces "the astonishing result of an animal, in which the head and the body enjoy separate vitality, the head living as if the body did not exist, and the body living as if the head did not exist. Guinea-pigs, after decapitation, seem very sensitive to the pain caused by the wound in the neck; they alternately carry first one hind-leg, and then the other, to the spot, as if to scratch it. Kittens also do the same."

A few years afterwards, 1817, Dr. Wilson Philip concluded that "the spinal marrow possesses sensorial power, as appears from very simple experiments;" but he held the brain to be the *chief* source of sensorial power.* The following year, Lallemand supported this opinion by the very curious phenomena exhibited by infants born without brains: these infants breathed, swallowed, sucked, squalled, and gave very unequivocal signs of sensibility. The value of such observations consists in disproving the objection frequently urged against the evidence of decapitated animals, namely, that in these animals the spinal cord preserves the remains of a sensibility endowed by the brain.

Longet here places an observation recorded by Beyer. A new-born infant, whose brain, during the birth, had been completely extirpated (to save the mother's life), was wrapped in a towel, and placed in the corner of the room, as a lifeless mass. While the surgeon was giving all his care to the mother, he heard with horror a kind of murmur proceeding from the spot where the body had been placed. In three minutes a distinct *cry* was heard. The towel was removed, and, to the surprise of all, this brainless infant was seen struggling with rapid movement of its arms and legs. It cried, and gave other signs of sensibility for several minutes.†

In 1828, Calmeil arrived at the same conclusion as that reached by Legallois, Wilson Philip, and Lallemand. Indeed when, in 1833, the Reflex Theory appeared, this opinion was so firmly rooted, that we find Mr. Grainger combating it as

* WILSON PHILIP: *Experimental Inquiry into the Laws of the Vital Functions*, pp. 209, 210.

† LONGET: *Traité de Physiologie*, ii. 105.

the established error of the day. He takes as much pains to show that physiologists are wrong in attributing sensation to the spinal cord, as I am here taking to show that they were right.* "It is, indeed, apparent," he says, "that the whole question concerning the truth or falsehood of the theory which attributes the reflex power to the spinal cord, hinges upon the correctness or incorrectness of the received doctrines respecting the seat of sensation and volition; so that until those doctrines are proved to be false, it is impossible to establish the hypothesis of Dr. Hall." †

The reader is requested to take note of this, because when we come to the evidence which proves the spinal cord to be a centre of sensation, we shall find that the *only* ground for rejecting that evidence is the assumed truth of the Reflex Theory, coupled with the assumption of the brain being the exclusive seat of sensation. Whereas if the evidence proves that the spinal cord *is* a sensational centre, then the Reflex Theory is destroyed, and cannot be urged against such evidence.

48. Thus many of the facts which prove the sensational function of the spinal cord were known, and even a vague conception of their real significance was general, until the Reflex Theory came to explain all such facts as the results of mechanical adjustment, and of a new nervous principle called "Reflexion." For many years this theory has reigned, and met with but little opposition. Yet the true doctrine has not wanted defenders in Germany. Nasse ‡ denied that decapitated animals showed no spontaneity; he asserted that they exhibited clear signs of mental activity. Carus sarcastically pointed out that the *word* "reflex" was replacing "irritability," as a key to unlock all puzzles; and he took up a position which is very similar to the one occupied in these pages, namely, that the spinal cord being formed of grey matter as well as of fibres, it must have sensibility and

* He cites Cuvier, Majendie, Desmoulins, and Mayo as maintaining this error.

† GRAINGER: *Structure and Functions of the Spinal Cord*, p. 66.

‡ NASSE: *Unters. zur Physiologie und Pathologie*, vol. ii. part 2.

power of reacting on nervous stimulus, no less than conductibility: that, in fact, it is a centre, and must act like all other nerve-centres.* J. W. Arnold opposed the Reflex Theory in a very remarkable little work, in which he vindicates the claim of the spinal cord as a sensory and motor centre, although denying to its actions any volitional character.† This was in 1844. Eleven years elapsed without any further opposition, when Edward Pflüger, in 1853, published his work on the Sensorial Functions of the spinal cord.‡ In this work he recurred to the old views of Prochaska and Legallois; but although he attacked Marshall Hall with merciless severity, he did not point out the fundamental error of the Reflex Theory, which theory he seems to accept. Nor did he give his views that philosophical and anatomical basis which could alone render his interpretations acceptable. Added to this, the tone of asperity in which his work was written, created some prejudice against him; and thus, while many admitted his facts, they rejected his conclusions.§

In 1858 Professor Owen read a paper of mine at the Leeds meeting of the British Association, on "The spinal cord as a centre of Sensation and Volition," in which a rapid indication of my point of view, and an account of some experiments to illustrate it, were given—*not*, I believe, conclusive to any of the audience. Indeed, the subject was too vast to be discussed in such a paper; and my object was rather to excite new inquiry, than to make converts to a view which could only be embraced after a thorough reinvestigation of the dominant theories.

In 1859 appeared Schiff's work;‖ and here we find a large space allotted to the discussion of Pflüger's doctrine. Schiff, whose immense experience as an experimentalist, and whose

* CARUS: *System der Physiologie*, iii. 101.

† J. W. ARNOLD: *Die Lehre von der Reflex-Function*, 86.

‡ PFLÜGER: *Die sensorischen Functionen des Rückenmarks der Wirbelthiere.*

§ Except AUERBACH, who repeated and varied the experiments; and FUNKE, who partially adopted the conclusions in his systematic treatise on Physiology.

‖ SCHIFF: *Lehrbuch der Physiologie*, 208.

acuteness and caution every one will highly estimate, frankly pronounces in favour of the sensational character of spinal actions; but he denies that they are volitional, and objects strongly to the introduction of any such idea as that of "psychical activity." He thinks it utterly untenable to suppose that impressions have reactions in the brain which they have not in the spinal cord:—if one has sensibility, the other must have it; and he thinks that, so far from the actions of the cord being distinguishable from those of the brain by the character of "reflexion," and depending on a mechanical arrangement—*all* actions, cerebral or spinal, are reflex; *all* depend on a mechanical arrangement.*

Since that time there has been the remarkable work of Goltz, so often cited in these pages,† and his subsequent experiments on dogs, which (although he does not decisively adopt the views of Pflüger) furnish ample evidence that sensation and volition cannot be exclusively localised in the brain.

49. Heubel's interesting experiments ‡ show that a frog may be thrown into a state of profound sleep by the withdrawal of all external stimulation, and in this state will remain lying on its back for hours. Now this position is one so very uncomfortable that, when awake, the frog will not retain it a moment, if free to turn round; and when asleep, a prick on the toe, a sudden noise, or a beam of light will awaken it, causing it to turn. That is to say, the withdrawal of the normal stimuli so lowers the sensibility of the frog's nerve-centres, that he does not feel the effects of the unusual position, but feels them directly the centres are

* LANDRY: *Traité des Paralysies*, 1859, maintains that the cord is a centre of sensation, and that there is in it a faculty *analogous* to the perception and judgment of the brain. Compare pp. 163 *et sq.* and 305. He also cites an essay by Dr. PATON of Edinburgh (*Edinburgh Medical Journal*, 1846), in which the sensational and volitional claims of the spinal cord are advanced.

† GOLTZ: *Beiträge zur Lehre von den Functionen der Nervencentren des Frosches*, 1869.

‡ *Pflüger's Archiv*, Bd. xiv. p. 158.

stimulated into activity. All this is intelligible enough on the supposition of the state of sleep being dependent on a lowering of the cerebral activity. But what shall we say on learning that precisely the same phenomena are manifested by a brainless frog? Every one knows that the brainless frog is intolerant of lying on its back, and immediately turns round, if placed on it. Yet the brainless frog may be thrown into deep sleep by the same exclusion of external stimuli; from which he also will be awakened by a prick, a noise, or a beam of light; and no sooner is he awakened than he at once turns round. Were the brainless frog incapable of sensation, a prick on his toe would cause a simple reflex withdrawal of the leg; but this is not the effect; on the contrary, the stimulus excites the whole spinal cord, and whatever sensation of discomfort may be caused by the abnormal position of the limbs in an uninjured awakened frog, is excited in the brainless frog.

50. I need not swell this chapter with examples of Sensibility in animals deprived of the brain; many have already been given, and any text-book of Physiology will supply more. No one disputes the observations, only the inference that these manifestations were sentient: they are said to have been merely mechanical reflexes. If, however, we can detect in them *some* evidence of what all recognise as peculiarly characteristic of Mind, the mechanical interpretation will be less plausible.

At the outset the reader must be warned against exaggerating and distorting the bearing of my remarks, and must not suppose that I disregard the vast differences between the Logic of Signs which belongs to Thought, and the Logic of Feeling which belongs to Sensation, nor suppose that I look upon the spinal cord as a mental organ having the *same* functions as the brain. All that I wish to establish is the common character of spinal and cerebal processes, modified as each is by the character of the actions initiated by the process.

51. This premised, let us begin with the evidence of

DISCRIMINATION.

Although this process is usually regarded as purely psychological, it must obviously have its physiological side; we find it in Sensation as in Ideation, and may expect to find it in unconscious as in conscious processes—in a word, in all sensorial processes whatever. Place a bit of marble on your tongue, and it will be touched, but not tasted: the sensations of contact and temperature will excite reflexes, but little or no reflexes from parotid and salivary glands. A difference in sensation has a corresponding difference in reflex action; which may be made evident by removing the tasteless marble, and replacing it by a pinch of carbonate of lime, *i.e.*, the marble in another state reduced to a powder: this will excite a sensation of taste, and a secretion from the glands. In both cases your sentient organism was affected, but it reacted differently because the difference of the stimulation was discriminated: consciously or unconsciously, you *felt* differently. Again: touch the back of your mouth with your finger, or a feather, and a convulsive contraction of the gullet responds, followed by vomiting, if the excitation be renewed. Yet these same nerves and muscles respond by the totally opposite action of swallowing, if instead of the stimulation coming from your finger, it come from the pressure of food or drink.

Analogous experiments on animals without their brains yield similar results.* The salivary secretion and the ordinary reactions of Taste are provoked by sapid substances. Still more conclusive are the observations made on a dog whose spinal cord has been divided, and who therefore according to the reigning ideas is incapable of feeling any impression made on parts below the section. A pencil inserted in the rectum causes a reaction of the muscles energetically resisting the entrance of this foreign body; yet this rectum so sensitive in its reaction on the stimulus of the pencil, responds by the totally different reaction—the relaxation of the muscles—on the stimulus of fæcal matters.

* See Prob. II. § 183.

52. "This is all mechanical," you say? Mechanical, no doubt, as all actions are; but the question here is whether among the conditions of the mechanical action Sensibility has a place? The answer can only be grounded on induction. The actions of the dog are analogous to the actions which you know were sentient in yourself. There was in both a discrimination, in both a corresponding reaction. I admit that what is here called "discrimination" is the application of a logical term to a mechanical process; I admit that if the spinal mechanism is insentient, the fact of discrimination may still be manifested; but I conceive that the many and coercive grounds for admitting that the mechanism is sentient gain further support in the evidence of discrimination. Every particular sensation has its corresponding reaction; and although this has been acquired during ancestral or individual experiences, so that in the majority of cases there is no consciousness accompanying the operation, this, as we have seen, is not a valid argument against the existence of a sensorial process. We have only to lower the Sensibility of the cord by anæsthetics, or to *preoccupy* its energies by some other excitation, and the reaction fails.

MEMORY.

53. "But discrimination, if not a purely physical process, implies Memory?" No doubt. And what is Memory—on its physiological side—but an organised tendency to react on lines previously traversed? As Griesinger truly says: "There is Memory in all the functions of the central organs, including the spinal cord. There is one for reflex actions, no less than for sense-images, words, and ideas." Gratiolet makes a similar assertion.* Indeed if, as we have seen, reflex actions are partly connate, and partly acquired, it is obvious that the second class must involve that very reproduction of

* "Il y a donc une mémoire par le cerveau et une mémoire par l'automate. Tous les organes ont une mémoire propre, c'est à dire *une tendance à* reproduire les séries d'actes qu'ils ont plusieurs fois executés."—GRATIOLET: *Anat. du Système Nerveux*, 1857, p. 464.

experiences, which in the sphere of Intellect is called Memory.

There is assuredly something paradoxical at first in this application of the terms of the Logic of Signs, yet the psychologist will find it of great service. But if the terms discrimination and memory be objected to, they may be replaced by some such phrase as the "adaptation of the mechanism to varying impulses." On its objective side, Discrimination is Neural Grouping; on its subjective side, it is Association of experiences.

INSTINCT.

54. If we can detect evidences of Volition and Instinct in the absence of the brain, our thesis may be considered less questionable. And such evidence there is. Goltz decapitated a male frog (in the pairing season), and observed that it not only sought, grasped, and energetically embraced a female, but could always discriminate a female from a male. Thus when a male frog closely resembling a female in size and shape was presented to this decapitated animal, he clasped it, but rapidly let it go again, whereas even the dead body of a female was held as in a vice. Goltz tried to *delude* this brainless animal in various ways, always in vain. Only a female would be held in his embrace. Goltz then presented a female in a reversed position, so that the head was grasped by the male. Now here, had there been simply a reflex machine, incapable of sentient discrimination, the clutched female would have been held in this position, just like any other object which excited the reflex; there would have been no "sense of incongruity," such as Goltz noticed in his frog, who at once began a series of movements by which he was enabled, without letting the female escape, to bring her into the proper position. To render this observation still more significant, I may add that Goltz did not find all male frogs act thus—many relinquished the female thus improperly presented to them. Such phenomena observed in frogs possessing brains, would be accepted as evidence of sexual instinct and volition.

Further: Goltz removed the brain from a frog, which he then held under water, gently pressing the body so as to drive the air out of its lungs; the body being then heavier than the water sank to the bottom, where it remained motionless. He repeated this procedure with another frog, not brainless but blinded. This one sank also, but in a few minutes rose to the surface to breathe. This difference naturally suggests that the brainless frog was insensible of the condition which in the other caused a movement of relief. The one felt impending suffocation, the other felt nothing. Such was the interpretation of a German friend in whose presence I repeated the experiment. But I had been instructed by Goltz, and bade my friend wait awhile. He did so, and saw the brainless frog slowly rise to the surface and breathe there like his blinded companion. So that the only difference observable was in the lessened sensibility of the brainless frog.

55. But Goltz records a still more conclusive case. In a large vessel of water he inverted a glass jar also containing water, which could then only be retained in the jar by atmospheric pressure. Through the neck of this inverted jar he thrust a blinded frog, not having pressed the air out of its lungs. It rose at once in the jar, touching the inverted bottom with its nose, and when the necessity of fresh air was felt, the frog began restlessly feeling about the surface of its prison till an issue was found in the neck of the jar, through which it dashed into the vessel, and at once rose to the surface of the water to breathe. In this observation are plainly manifested the stimulation of uneasy sensation, the volition of seeking relief, and the discrimination of it when found. If this frog was a sentient mechanism, what shall we say to the fact that a brainless frog was observed to go through precisely the same series of actions? Goltz pertinently remarks: "So long as physiologists satisfied themselves that the brain was the sole organ of sensation, it was easy to declare all the actions of the brainless animal to be merely reflex. But now we must ask, whether the greater part of these actions are not due to the *power of adaptation* in the central organs, and

are therefore to be struck out of the class of simple reflexes? If I bind one leg of a brainless frog and observe that he not only sees an obstacle, but crawls aside from it, I must regard these movements as regulated by his central power of adaptation; but now suppose I unbind the leg and remove the obstacle, then if I prick the frog he hops forward. Must I now declare this hop to have been a simple reflex? Not at all. In both cases the physiological processes have been similar."

56. There are no doubt readers who will dismiss all evidence drawn from experiments on frogs, as irrelevant to mammals and man. Let us therefore see how the evidence stands with respect to animals higher in the scale, endowed with less questionable mental faculties. In a former chapter (PROBLEM II. § 29) we recorded the marked results of removing the cerebral hemispheres; and at the same time suggested that these by no means justified the conclusion usually drawn respecting the hemispheres as the exclusive seat of sensation. And this on two grounds: First, because the absence of some sensitive phenomena does not prevent the presence of others: the mutilated organism is still capable of manifesting Sensibility in those organs which remain intact. Secondly, because were the mutilation followed by total destruction of Sensibility, this would not prove Sensibility in the normal organism to have its seat in the part injured. If the removal of a pin will destroy the chronometric action of a watch, we do not thence infer that the chronometric action was the function of this pin. And this objection has the greater force when we remember that one hemisphere may be removed without the consequent loss of a single function, and both may be removed without the loss of several functions usually ascribed to cerebral influence.*

* To obviate misunderstanding let me say that, unless the contrary is specified, I use the term Brain throughout this argument as equivalent to the cerebral hemispheres, because it is in these that sensation, volition, and consciousness are localised by the generality of writers, many of whom, indeed, regard the cells of the grey matter of the con-

57. Consider the analogous effects of injuries to or removal of the Cerebellum, in causing disturbance of locomotion, whence the conclusion has been drawn that the Cerebellum is the exclusive organ of muscular co-ordination, in spite of the unquestionable evidence that very many muscular co-ordinations still persist after this organ is removed. What is the part played by the Cerebellum I do not pause here to examine.* I only say that the movements of swimming, sucking, swallowing, breathing, crying, micturition, defecation, &c., are co-ordinated as well after removal of the Cerebellum as they were before, and that consequently *their* co-ordination has not its seat in the Cerebellum. The parallelism is obvious. Removal of the Cerebrum causes a disturbance in the combination of sensations, and the execution of certain sense-guided actions, but causes little appreciable disturbance in others. Removal of the Cerebellum causes a disturbance in the combination of certain muscular sensations, and the execution of certain co-ordinated actions, with little appreciable disturbance in others.

58. So little have the facts been surveyed and estimated in their entirety that there is perhaps no subject on which physiologists are more agreed than on the function of the Cerebellum being that of co-ordination. Yet consider this decisive experiment. I etherised three healthy frogs; from one I removed the entire cranial centres; from another I removed only the cerebellum; and, leaving the third in possession of an intact encephalon, I made two sections of the posterior columns of the spinal cord. The two first hopped,

volutions as the exclusive seat of these phenomena, dividing these cells into sensational, emotional, and intellectual. There are physiologists who extend sensation to the cerebral ganglia and grey masses of the medulla oblongata; but the medulla spinalis is so clearly continuous with the medulla oblongata that there is a glaring inconsistency in excluding sensation from the one if it is accorded to the other; and the grounds on which sensitive phenomena are admitted in the absence of the hemispheres, force us to admit analogous phenomena in the absence of the ganglia and medulla oblongata: in each case the phenomena are less complex and varied as the mechanisms become less complex.

* Compare Lussana e Lemoigne: *Fisiologia dei centri encefalici*, 1871, ii. 239, 240, 330.

swam, used their legs in defence, and exhibited a variety of muscular co-ordinations, although in both the supposed organ of co-ordination was absent. Whereas the third, which had this organ intact, and was capable of moving each limb separately, and each pair of limbs separately, was utterly incapable of moving all four simultaneously. Why was this? Obviously because in the first two frogs the motor mechanism remained intact, and only the cerebral and cerebellar influence was removed; in the third frog the sensory part of the motor mechanism had been divided, and no combination of the limbs was possible.

59. Physiological induction agrees with anatomical induction in assigning to the cerebrum and cerebellum the office of *incitation* and *regulation* rather than of *innervation*; for, as we have seen, no nerve issues directly from them (PROBLEM II. § 7). Consequently the effects of injuries to these centres are losses of spontaneity and of complexity in the manifestations. Inasmuch as in the intact organism all sensory impressions are propagated throughout the nervous centres, the reactions of these highest centres will enter into the complex of every adjusted movement; so the abolition of these centres will be the dropping of a link in the chain, the abolition of a special element in the complex group. The organs which are still intact will react, each in its own way, on being stimulated; but the reaction will be without the modifying influence of the absent centres. For instance, the retinal stimulation from a luminous impression normally calls up a cluster of associated feelings derived originally from other senses, and a perception of the object is associated with emotions of desire, terror, &c., according to the past history of the organism, and its organised reactions, due to hereditary or acquired experiences. It is these which form the complex feeling discharged in the particular movement of prehension, or flight. Remove the brain, and there can be no longer *this* cluster of associated neural groups excited; there will be therefore no emotion, simply the visual sensation, and such a movement as is directly associated with it. The brainless dog moans when hurt, it does not bark at the cat which it

nevertheless sees, and avoids as a mere obstacle in its path; the cat will cry, it will not mew. The present pain moves the vocal organs, but does not revive associated experiences. All those combinations by which a series of dependent actions result from a single stimulation are frustrated when the mechanism is disturbed, so that the mutilated animal can no longer recognise its prey or its enemy, to feed on the one and fly from the other; no longer builds its habitation, or rears its offspring. It can still live, feed, sleep, move, and defend itself against present discomfort; it cannot find its food, or protect itself against prospective discomfort. We must supply the place of its Intelligence. We must give it the food, and protect it from injuries.

There is therefore ample evidence to show that what is specially known as Intelligence is very imperfect after the cerebral influence has been abolished; but this does not prove the Cerebrum to be the exclusive seat of Intelligence, it only proves it to be an indispensable factor in a complex of factors. Still less does it prove the Cerebrum to be the exclusive seat of Sensation, Instinct, Volition; for these may be manifested after its removal, although of course even these will be impaired by the loss of one factor.

60. And here an objection must be anticipated. In spite of the familiar experience that one mode of Sensibility may be destroyed without involving the destruction of other modes, there is a general belief—derived from a mistaken conception of what is really represented by the unity of Consciousness—that Consciousness disappears altogether when it disappears at all; and hence, since Sensation is supposed to imply Consciousness, it also cannot be divisible, but must vanish altogether if it vanish at all. The first answer is that Sensation as an abstraction is neither divisible nor indivisible; but as a generalised expression of concrete sensorial processes it is reducible to these processes, and divisible as they are. No one doubts that we may lose a whole class of special sensations—sight, hearing, pain, temperature, &c.—yet retain all the others. No one doubts that we may lose a whole class of registered experiences—forget a language, or lose memory

of places so familiar as the streets of the small town we inhabit, or of faces so familiar as those of friends and relatives, while the names of these streets and friends are still remembered when the sounds are heard. Yet sensation and intelligence are not wholly lost. The mind is still erect amid these ruins.*

61. This premised, let us consider the experimental evidence. Flourens declares that when he removed the whole of the Cerebrum from pigeons and fowls, they lost *all* sensation, *all* perception, *all* instinct, and *all* volition. They lived perfectly well for months after the operation, if the food were placed in their mouths; but they never *sought* their food; they never *took* it, even when their beaks were plunged into it: they could swallow, and digest the grains; but they had no instinct to make them seek, no volition to make them pick up the grains. They *saw* nothing, although the iris remained irritable; they heard nothing; they could not smell. A state of stupor came on, resembling that of deep sleep. All voluntary action ceased. If they were thrown into the air, they flew; if irritated, they moved away; but if left to themselves, they remained motionless, with the head under the wing, as in sleep. Now, inasmuch as these effects always ensue when the Cerebrum is removed, and *never* when only the Cerebellum is removed, he concludes that all instincts, volitions, and sensations "belong exclusively to the cerebral lobes."

But all experimenters do not agree in other points named by Flourens; nor in the conclusions he has drawn. On the contrary, it is very certain, and we find evidence even in Flourens himself, that all instincts and all sensations are *not* destroyed by the removal of the cerebral lobes.

62. Let us hear Bouillaud on this subject.† He repeated the experiment of Flourens, removing the whole of the Cere-

* See a very interesting case of this special loss of memory in a priest who still occupied himself reading classic authors and performing his official duties many months after an injury to the brain. LUSSANA e LEMOIGNE: *Fisiologia dei centri encefalici*, i. 201.

† BOUILLAUD: *Recherches Expérimentales sur les Fonctions du Cerveau en général*, 1830, p. 5, *sq*.

brum from the Brain of a fowl; and he thus records his observations: "This fowl passes the greater part of her time asleep, but she awakes at intervals, and *spontaneously*. When she goes to sleep, she turns her head on one side and buries it in the feathers of the wing; when she awakes, she shakes herself, flaps her wings, and opens her eyes. In this respect there is no difference observable between the mutilated and the perfect bird. She does not seem to be moved at all by the noise made round about her, but a very slight irritation of the skin suffices to awaken her instantaneously. When the irritation ceases, she relapses into sleep. When awake, she is often seen to cast stupid glances here and there, *to change her place, and walk spontaneously*. If put into a cage, *she tries to escape;* but she comes and goes without any purpose, or rational design. When either foot, wing, or head is pinched, she withdraws it; when she is laid hold of, she *struggles to escape, and screams;* but no sooner is she liberated than she rests motionless. If severely irritated, she screams loudly; but it is not only to express pain that she uses her voice, for it is by no means rare to *hear her cackle and cluck a little spontaneously;* that is to say, when no external irritation affects her. Her stupidity is profound; she knows neither objects nor places, nor persons, and is completely divested of memory in this respect: not only does she not know how to seek or take food, she does not even know how to swallow it when placed in her beak—it must be pushed to the throat. Nevertheless her indocility, her movements, her agitation, attest that she *feels* the presence of a strange body. Inasmuch as external objects excite in her no idea, no desire, she pays no attention to them; but she is not absolutely deprived of the power of attention, for if much irritated her attention is awakened. She knows not how to escape an enemy, nor how to defend herself. All her actions, in a word, are blind, without reflexion, without knowledge."

In this recital, the evidence both of *sensation* and *instinct* is incontestable, to any unprejudiced mind. Bouillaud, in commenting on his observations, remarks, that assuredly *all* sensation was not destroyed, since the sensibilities of touch and pain were very manifest. Nor is it certain, he says, that the fowl heard nothing, saw nothing. It is true that she stumbled against objects, and knew not how to avoid them. She opened her eyes on awaking, looked about, and showed a sensibility in the pupil to light; which, he thinks, is incompatible with the absence of all sensation of sight.

63. The experiments of Longet * seem decisive on this latter point. Having removed the whole of the Cerebrum from a pigeon, he observed that whenever he approached a light brusquely to its eyes, there was contraction of the pupil, and even winking; but, what was still more remarkable, "when I gave a rotatory motion to the candle, and at such a distance that there could be no sensation of heat, the pigeon made a similar movement with its head. These observations, renewed several times in the presence of persons who were at my lectures, left no doubt of the persistence of sensibility to light after removal of the cerebral lobes." We have only to think of the baby following with its eyes the light moved before it, to understand the kind of impression produced by the candle on the pigeon. Longet also declares that his experiments prove the existence of sensations of sound, after removal of the whole cerebrum.

64. Dr. Dalton, giving the results of numerous experiments he performed, says that removal of the Cerebrum plunges the animal in "a profound stupor, in which he is *almost* entirely inattentive to surrounding objects. . . . Occasionally the bird opens its eyes with a vacant stare, stretches his neck, perhaps shakes his bill once or twice, or smoothes down the feathers upon his shoulders, and then relapses into his former apathetic condition. This state of immobility, however, is *not* accompanied by the loss of sight, of hearing, or of ordinary sensibility. *All these functions remain, as well as that of voluntary motion.* If a pistol be discharged behind the back of the animal, he at once opens his eyes, moves his head half round, and gives evident signs of having heard the report; but he immediately becomes quiet again, and pays no further attention to it. Sight is

* LONGET : *Traité de Physiologie*, ii. 240.

also retained, since the bird will sometimes fix its eye on a particular object, and watch it for several seconds together." *

While, therefore, Flourens concludes from his experiments that the Cerebrum is the seat of *all* sensation and all volition; and Bouillaud concludes that it is most probably the seat of *none;* Dr. Dalton concludes that the functions of the Cerebrum are restricted to those usually classed as intellectual. "The animal," he says, "is still capable, after removal of the hemispheres, of receiving sensations from external objects. But these sensations appear to make upon him no lasting impression. He is incapable of connecting with his perceptions any distinct succession of ideas. He hears, for example, the report of a pistol, but he is not alarmed by it; for the sound, although distinctly perceived, does not suggest any idea of danger or injury. The memory is altogether destroyed, and the recollection of sensations is not retained from one moment to another. The limbs and muscles are still under the control of the will; but the will itself is inactive, because apparently it lacks its usual mental stimulus and direction." †

Dr. Dalton reminds us how disturbance of the cerebral functions in human beings recalls these observations on animals. "In cases of impending apoplexy, or of softening of the cerebral substance, among the earliest and most common phenomena is a loss or impairment of the memory. The patient forgets the names of particular objects, or particular persons; or he is unable to calculate numbers with his usual facility. His mental derangement is often shown in the undue estimate which he forms of passing events. He is no longer able to appreciate the true relation between different objects and different phenomena. Thus he will show an exaggerated degree of solicitude about a trivial occurrence, and will pay no attention to other matters of importance. As the difficulty increases, he becomes careless of the directions and advice of his attendants, and must be watched and

* DALTON: *Human Physiology*, Philadelphia, 1859, p. 362.

† Ibid.

managed like a child or an imbecile. After a certain period he no longer appreciates the lapse of time, and even loses the distinction between day and night. Finally, when the injury to the hemispheres is complete, the senses may still remain active and impressible, while the patient is completely deprived of intelligence and judgment." *

65. Having seen how far other experimenters are from confirming the conclusions of Flourens, let us glance at his record of observations, and we shall find there evidence that *all* sensation and *all* volition cannot be localised in the Cerebrum. Speaking of a fowl whose Cerebrum was removed the day before, he says: "She shakes her head and feathers, sometimes even she cleans and sharpens them with her beak; sometimes she changes the leg on which she sleeps, for, like other birds, she sleeps habitually resting upon one leg. In all these cases she seems like a man asleep, who, without quite waking, changes his place, and reposes in another, from the *fatigue* occasioned by the previous posture: he selects one more *comfortable*, stretches himself, yawns, shakes himself a little, and falls asleep again. . . . On the third day the fowl is no longer so calm; she comes and goes, but without motive and without an aim; and if she encounters an obstacle on her path, she knows not how to avoid it." † In his second work he remarks of a Duck operated on in the same way: "As I mentioned last year *à propos* of fowls, the duck walks about oftener, and for a longer time together, when it is fasting, than when it is fed."

Here he observes the unmistakable evidence of feelings of Hunger, Fatigue, and Discomfort in animals which, according to him, have lost *all* sensation. He also observes the operation of instinct (cleaning the feathers), and of spontaneous activity (walking about), in animals said to have lost *all* instinct and *all* volition.

66. Still more decisive are the observations recorded by other experimenters. Leyden removed the hemispheres *and* the ganglia at their base from a hen; yet this hen moved about

* DALTON, p. 363. † FLOURENS, p. 89.

and clucked. Meissner noticed that a pigeon whose hemispheres had been removed always uttered its *coo*, and showed restlessness at the usual feeding-time.* Voit carefully extirpated the cerebrum from some pigeons, and kept them for many months in health. For the first few weeks they exhibited the well-known stupor. Then they began to shake this off, open their eyes, walk, and fly about *spontaneously*. They gave unmistakable signs of seeing and hearing. But the chief defect was in the inability to feed themselves, and the complete insensibility to danger. They also manifested signs of sexual feeling with lively cooings; though quite unable to gratify their desires.† Vulpian having removed the cerebrum, optic thalami, and corpora striata from a young rabbit, found that on pinching its tail it cried out and struggled to escape; and a rat thus mutilated not only struggled and cried when pinched, but manifested strong emotion. "Il est très craintif, très impressionable; il bondit pour peu qu'on le touche; le moindre bruit le fait tressaillir. Un certain bruit d'appel fait avec les lèvres, ou un soufflet brusque imitant celui qu'emettent les chats en colère excitent chez le rat une vive émotion." ‡

67. There are several well-authenticated cases on record of children born without a vestige of brain, and others with only a vestige, who nevertheless manifested the ordinary signs of sensation. I will cite but one, and it shall be one for which an illustrious physiologist, Panizza, is the guarantee. A male infant, one of twins, who lived but eighteen hours, during that period manifested such unquestionable signs of Sensibility as the following: the pupils contracted under light, sharp sounds caused flutterings, and a bitter solution when placed in the mouth was instantly rejected. This infant had not a vestige of cerebrum, cerebellum, or cerebral ganglia. The medulla oblongata was normal. There were no olfactory

* LEYDEN in the *Berliner klinische Wochenschrift*, 1867, No. 7. MEISSNER: *Jahresbericht über Physiol.*, 1867, p. 410.

† VOIT in the *Sitzungsberichte der Münchener Academie*, 1868, p. 105. Comp. also GOLTZ in *Pflüger's Archiv*, Bd. xiv. 435.

‡ VULPIAN: *Système Nerveux*, 542–48.

nerves, and the optic nerves terminated in a little mass of membrane.*

68. The observations of Lussana and Lemoigne are both extensive and precise, and the conclusion at which they arrive is that the removal of the Cerebrum is the abolition of Intelligence and Instinct, but is not the abolition of Sensation. Whereas Rolando, and after him Renzi, consider that only the Intelligence is abolished, the supposed loss of Instinct being really nothing more than the loss of the directive influence which makes the Instinct to be executed.

69. Here it becomes needful to understand

THE MECHANISM OF INSTINCT.

Were we dealing with an ordinary mechanism, and the disturbances produced in its actions by the removal of any part, we should attribute all observed effects to *interference with the conditions of dependent sequence:* we should infer that the actions were imperfectly performed, or wholly abolished, because their requisite mechanical conditions were disturbed. Let us be equally precise in dealing with the physiological mechanism. If we have deprived it of an organ in which certain combinations are effected, we must expect to find all actions which were dependent on such combinations to be now impossible; but all the actions which are not directly dependent on these combinations may still be possible. The actions of feeding, for example, are determined by certain sensations, when these are present in a particular sequence, but not otherwise; the sensation of sight does not suffice, because the animal must not only *see* the food, he must *perceive* it. The action of defence and flight are also determined by certain sensations, but only when these are connected in a certain sequence: the brainless animal will defend itself, or move out of the way, under the stimulus of unpleasant sensation; but will not be moved by a *prospective* injury, because he fails to associate it with the sight of the threatening object. In the same way a blind man shrinks at the actual

* For other examples see GINTRAC: *Pathologie Interne*, 1868, vi. 51-57.

contact of the heated poker, but does not shrink at the approach of that poker which he does not see. We do not deny him the possession of the so-called instinct of Self-preservation on this ground; why deny it to the brainless animal? The brainless fish or frog swims when placed in the water, because the sensation from the *moving* water * sets going the swimming mechanism. To call this a "swimming instinct" may seem extravagant; yet it is as fully entitled to the name as Self-defence is, or the Alimentary Instinct. In all three cases there is a connate mechanism set going by appropriate feelings.

70. Since all admit that there is an Alimentary Instinct, let us see what kind of mechanism it implies. There must be a state of feeling called Hunger, which—combined with other feelings—determines certain muscular adjustments in the search, recognition, capture, and finally the swallowing of the food:—a very complex series of actions, which lead to and sustain one another until the desire is gratified. On the mental side there are three constituents, all indispensable: the hunger must be felt, the food must be discriminated, the desire must be gratified; on the physical side there are also the indispensable arrangements of the motor mechanism. Now it is obvious that the *entire* mechanism of this instinct cannot be localised in the brain, even if its mental elements are localised there; and there is reason to believe that even the mental elements—the feelings of hunger, discrimination, and gratification—are not exclusively localised there. The brainless animal manifests if not the feeling of Hunger, at any rate that feeling of discomfort which is the basis of Hunger. The restlessness is that of a hungry animal. Now we know that some of the Systemic Sensibility is preserved, for we see the animal breathing, swallowing, urinating, sleeping, preening its feathers, changing its attitude, resting on one leg after the fatigue of the other, &c. We may therefore

* If the water is perfectly still the fish sinks to the bottom and remains motionless until the water be stirred. Mere *contact* does not suffice; there must be intermittent pulses from the moving water.

infer that other systemic sensations, such as Hunger and Thirst, arise under the usual conditions.

71. We have noted an indication of Hunger; but on further observation we discover that although the food is eaten, if brought within reach of that portion of the feeding mechanism which is still intact, yet the second step—the feeling of recognition—is wanting. The animal fails to perceive the food brought under his eyes, or even placed in his mouth; unless the back part of the mouth be touched no swallowing takes place. Hence the animal can no longer feed himself, and is therefore said to have lost his instinct. But although the mechanism of the instinct has been *disturbed*, its action is not wholly abolished. The brain is necessary for that combination of adjustments which normally accompany the perception of food through sight and scent; and its absence of course frustrates such combination; but we shall presently see that although certain sensible marks by which a perception is guided are absent, others may still be present, and suffice.

72. Before adducing examples let me say that we cannot legitimately attribute the abeyance of an instinct solely to the absence of the brain, 1°, because we observe a similar abeyance of the instinct and frustration of perception, even when the brain is present, and the animal is in its normal state. 2°. On the other hand, some instincts are unmistakably manifested, and some perceptions excited, after the brain has been removed. In fact, all that is needful is that some of the mental elements of such perception and such instinct be preserved; and this is the case so long as the leading element is present.

73. On the first point consider this unequivocal example. A healthy, hungry frog may be placed in a vessel in which lie a quantity of dead flies. He sees these flies, but sight is not enough; to him they are only so many black spots, in which he does not recognise his food, because the flies do not move, and the *leading element* in his perception of food is not a *coloured* form, but a *moving* form. Hence this frog, in spite of brain and an intact organism, will starve amidst appropriate food. Whereas the frog that will not snap at

motionless flies, snaps at any other small moving object, though it be not his food. Goltz observed one incessantly snapping at the moving tentacles of a slug which was in the vessel—as if that were possible food! Not only the stupid frog, but the more intelligent carnivora will starve in the presence of appropriate food which is unrecognised, because the leading element in the recognition is absent. The cat will not eat a dead mouse, unless she has killed it herself. Predatory animals must capture their food—unless the scent of blood excites their alimentary instinct. So intimately is this sensation of a moving object connected with the predatory impulse, that the cat which is unexcited by the dead mouse cannot resist springing on a moving ball. We need not suppose the cat to mistake this ball for food; but we must suppose that, accustomed to pounce upon moving food, it is unable to resist the impulse of this leading sensation.

74. The *presence* of the brain not sufficing, in the absence of the leading sensation, we shall now see that the *absence* of the brain will not prevent the execution of the instinctive action, if the leading sensation be present. The brainless bird sees a heap of grain, or a pan of water, but no more recognises them by sight alone than the frog recognises the dead flies; yet if the bird's feet be placed in the water, *this* sensation will suffice to make him drink; if placed amid the grain, this sensation will (sometimes) suffice to make him feed. Lussana and Lemoigne state that their brainless pigeons ate and drank with avidity when their feet were placed in grain and water.* M. Krishaber removed the hemispheres from a pigeon, and observed that when his beak was thrust into a heap of hempseed the head was quickly withdrawn, whereas when the beak was plunged into water the bird drank eagerly. Every day he was forced to feed the bird by pouring the seed into its throat, but every day it drank when the beak was thrust into the pan of water.† Brücke noticed that his brainless hen, which made no attempt to peck at the grain under her very eyes,

* LUSSANA e LEMOIGNE: *Op. cit.*, i. 15.

† *Archives de Physiologie*, 1869, p. 539.

began pecking if the grain were thrown on the ground with force, so as to produce a rattling sound. The sensation of hearing was here more perfect than that of vision, and sufficed to awaken the state of feeling necessary to initiate the pecking movement.*

75. Somewhat analogous phenomena are observed in Aphasia. The patient can see printed or written letters, and even copy them; but he cannot read, *i.e.*, interpret these symbols; as the birds see the grain, but cannot connect this sensation with others. These letters and words, which the patient cannot interpret when *seen*, he can interpret when *heard;* he can not only understand them when spoken, but write them if they are dictated to him. The birds recognise the grain and water (or act as if they did) when other sensations than those of sight are excited. Sound is the leading element in Language, both spoken and written. We hear the words even when we see them, but we do not see them when we hear them. The visible symbols are accessory and subordinate. But to the born deaf the visible symbols dominate. How one sensation will determine a particular group of movements which cannot be effected by any other stimulus is abundantly illustrated in disease no less than in experiment. Here is a very

* BRÜCKE: *Physiologie,* ii. p. 53. While these sheets are passing through the press, GOLTZ has published his second series of experiments on the brain. The following detail is a good illustration of what is said in the text. A dog deprived of a portion of both hemispheres displayed a marked imperfection in the execution of ordinary instincts. Although sight was impaired he could see, and recognise men and certain objects: the sight of a whip made him cower, but the sight of meat did not suffice to set the feeding mechanism in action. When meat was suspended above his head, the scent caused him to sniff about in search, but he failed to find it, and even when he was so placed that he could see the suspended meat, the *unusual* impression failed to guide him. If the meat were held towards him, or placed before him in a dish, he took it at once—this being the customary stimulation. So also, if the hand were held up, in the usual way when dogs are made to leap for food, this dog sprang vigorously up and caught the food; but he would spring up in the same way when the hand was held empty, and continue fruitlessly springing, whereas an uninjured dog ceases to spring when he sees the hand is empty.—*Pflüger's Archiv,* Bd. xiv. p. 419.

luminous example: Gratiolet had a patient for six months under his eye incapable of articulating a single word, owing to the incoherence of her incessant utterance—she babbled sounds, but could not group the syllables into a recognisable word. Yet she could sing the words of any song she knew, the musical sensations being sufficient to guide her vocal organs. "Ainsi la mémoire, infidèle dans le cas où les mots étaient des idées, devenait claire et précise quand les mots étaient des chansons."*

76. These illustrations plainly tell how the brainless animal may starve amid his food, failing to perceive it because the leading sensation is not excited; and how the same animal may manifest his feeding instinct if the mechanism be set going by a leading sensation. We are told, indeed, that in the absence of the brain the actions are mechanical reflexes from impressions, and not comparable with the complex processes determined by perception. I think, however, that the only difference is in degree of complexity: a combination of touch, temperature, and muscular movement will be simpler than one which also combines sight, smell, and the revived images of associated sensations. The sight of a sheep affects the instinctive mechanism of a wolf *only* when combined with the leading element of smell. Place a stuffed sheep in a field, and no wolf will approach and spring on it, whereas the blind wolf will find and capture the real sheep; and I believe that were it practicable to remove the brain without injury to the organ of scent and the powers of locomotion, the wolf would track and capture the living sheep.

77. The outcome of this discussion is that the mechanism of each instinct is the adjustment of the organs which effect the instinctive action; and this adjustment is not simply a cerebral process, but a complex of *many* sensorial processes; consequently the instinct cannot be exclusively localised in the brain, although the cerebral process may be a very important element in the adjustment. This is true even on the supposition that in speaking of Instinct we refer only to the state of feeling which originates the action—separating the

* GRATIOLET: *Anat. Comparée du Système Nerveux*, 1857, p. 459.

psychological from the physiological aspect of the phenomenon. For the brain *minus* the organism is obviously incapable of feelings; whereas the organism *minus* the brain is obviously capable of sensibilities adequate to determine the actions. Thus the feeling of hunger which prompts the alimentary actions does not arise if the animal is satiated, nor does the sexual feeling which prompts generative actions arise when the animal is castrated; but each arises when the organism is in a particular state. In vain will food be placed before the satiated animal, or a female before the castrated male; food and female are seen and recognised, but no desires are excited, in spite of the brain and its supposed instincts. On the contrary, when the brain is removed, the need of the organism for food is felt, and this need determines restless movements, which are directed by certain other sensations, and the instinctive action of feeding is finally effected; although, of course, the removal of the brain has so disturbed the normal mechanism of the instinct that the action is imperfect. Renzi says that an animal deprived of its brain has lost the intelligence which enables it to seek and seize its food, but not the instinct, since it still has the desire for food. The following experiment may illustrate this. Renzi wounded superficially one optic thalamus of a frog without injuring the external margin, or optic tract. The frog showed no appreciable loss of sight, but hopped timidly away whenever approached. Then both thalami were divided transversely, the optic tract still being spared. This frog remained motionless under every threat. It manifested no alarm, and even when directly irritated, only crawled or hopped away like a brainless frog. Sight still so far remained that obstacles were avoided.* Now since this animal's brain was intact, and its organs of movement were capable of responding to stimulation, how are we to explain the loss of its instinct of self-preservation? The frog perceived no danger in a threatening approach, yet perceived an obstacle and avoided it, getting under it if there were room enough, crawling beside it if that was the easier escape.

* LUSSANA e LEMOIGNE: *Op. cit.*, i. 363.

Why did one vision prompt the movements of escape, and another fail? Was it not that in the one case the normal pathway was still open, in the other closed? We know that one injury will destroy the perception of colour without destroying that of light and shadow; so one injury may destroy the combination of neural processes necessary for the perception of a *danger*, without destroying those necessary for the perception of a *hindrance*. If all actions depend on their mechanical conditions, they must be disturbed according to the disturbance of the conditions. Nothnagel found that after removing the *nucleus lentiformis* on both sides of a rabbit, leaving all the rest of the encephalon intact, the rabbit hopped when its tail was pinched; yet although starting at the sound when hands were loudly clapped, did not hop as a normal rabbit does; nor although closing his eyes when a light was brought near them, did he ever move aside. No feeling of danger was excited by sound or sight. In striking contrast are the phenomena manifested by a rabbit whose *corpora striata* have been removed: it is with difficulty made to hop by pinching its skin, whereas noises and sights cause it to make terrified bounds.*

78. No sooner do we analyse the conditions of an instinct than we see the error of regarding instincts as localised in the brain. The cerebral process is only one factor in the product—an important factor, no doubt, since the cerebrum is the supreme centre of incitation and regulation; but its absence does not wholly carry away the activity of the mechanism, sentient and motor, on which the instincts

* *Virchow's Archiv*, Bd. lx. pp. 130–33. Yet there are many physiologists who persist in placing the *motorium commune* in the *corpora striata!* And they place the *sensorium commune* in the optic thalami, although, not to mention the ambiguous evidence of Pathology, the experiments of NOTHNAGEL and VEYSSIÈRE show that destruction of the thalami does not destroy sensation. See VEYSSIÈRE, *Recherches sur l'hémianesthésie de cause cérébrale*, 1874, pp. 83, 84. I may observe, in passing, that the notion of the *corpora striata* being the necessary channel for volitional impulses, and the *optic thalami* for reflex actions, is utterly disproved by the experimental evidence recorded in the text, as well as in § 66.

depend, it only carries away one source of stimulation and regulation.

79. An instinct depends on a connate mechanism. Let us glance for a moment at a parallel case of an ordinary reflex action, also dependent on a connate mechanism, say that of sneezing. When the inner surface of the nose is stimulated by snuff, or other irritant, the nasal branch of the trigeminus is excited, and the effects are first a deep inspiration, then a closure of the respiratory orifices by the tongue, which in turn excites a spasmodic expiration. But the same effects are producible from quite different stimulations—namely, that of the ciliary nerves on sudden exposure to a glare of sunshine—or of the skin nerves on a sudden draught of cold air. Brücke remarks that there is perhaps no spot on the surface of the body from which this reflex may not be excited in very sensitive people. He knew a gentleman who always sneezed when in winter he laid hold of a cold door bell; and the fit of sneezing was only arrested by giving him a crust of bread or something hard to gnaw. Now just as the connate mechanism of sneezing may be set in action by a variety of stimulations, so may the connate mechanism of an instinct.

ACQUISITION.

80. Not only may Discrimination and Instinct be manifested in the absence of the brain, but even the acquisition of new modes of reaction, such as are classed under Learning through Experience. The objection is sometimes urged that animals without their brains only manifest single reactions on stimulation—the pinched foot is withdrawn, and then remains motionless until again pinched. But although the stimulation does not excite a consecutive series of movements, because there is no cerebrum to react in successive stimulation, this does not prove the absence of sensation in the one movement which is excited. If my hand be lying on the table, and something irritates it, my hand is withdrawn, and then remains as motionless as the limb of the brainless animal, *until* some fresh stimulation, external or internal, moves it. Although removal of the brain causes a manifest reduction in the variety and succession of the movements, all experimenters are agreed that animals acquire a certain dexterity in executing actions which they had previously failed to carry out after removal of their brains. "There is," says Freusberg, "a decided improvement acquired in the reactions of the motor centres after division of the spinal cord, not indeed in vigour, but in delicacy. Removed from the regulating influence of the brain, the legs acquired through practice a power of self-regulation." Nor is this wonderful: pathways are made easy by repetition of impulses, and new adaptations form new adjustments. It is thus all learning is effected—intelligent, and automatic. Nor is there any force in the objection that the power thus acquired speedily disappears, so that if the stimulations are effected at long intervals the reactions do not manifest their acquired dexterity. The spinal centres forget, as the cerebral centres forget; but they also remember, *i.e.*, they learn. Because an animal shows to-day none of the aptitude it acquired three days ago, we are not to deny that it had once acquired the aptitude it has now lost. Attempt to teach a child to read by giving it spelling lessons of two or three minutes at intervals of two or three months, and little will the acquisition be!

81. Hitherto we have been considering phenomena manifested in the absence of the cerebral hemispheres, because it is in these that the majority of writers place the sensorium. There are, indeed, many authoritative writers who regard the ganglionic masses at the base of the cerebrum, and even those of the medulla oblongata, as participating in this sensorial property, which they refuse to the lower ganglia in the spinal cord. I cannot follow their logic. The cerebrum is by its position as a centre of centres, and its detachment from all direct innervation of organs, so different from the rest of the neural axis, that we can understand how it should be assigned a special function; although being of the same tissue as the other ganglionic masses, it must have the same property.

And what that special function is I shall hereafter endeavour to set forth. But that the upper region of the spinal axis should differ so profoundly from the lower region as to be the seat of psychical processes, while the lower region is simply the seat of mechanical processes, is what I cannot understand, so long as the anatomical structure and physiological properties of the two regions are seen to be identical. The various centres innervate various organs, and have consequently various functions. As each centre is removed, we observe a corresponding loss of function—the organism is truncated, but continues to manifest such functions as have still their mechanisms intact. Let us suppose the brain or upper regions of the cord detached from the lower regions by a section of the cord; the animal will still live, and perform almost all its functions in the normal way, but there will be little or no consensus between the lower and the upper regions. Granting Sensibility to both, we must still see that the sensation excited in one will not be felt in the other. And this is the ground on which physiologists deny that the lower regions have Sensibility. Without pausing here to examine this point, which will occupy us in the next chapter, I assume that the positive evidence of Sensibility suffices to discredit that argument; and in furtherance of that assumption will cite an example of sensation and volition manifested by the lower portion of the cord when separated from the brain and upper portion.

82. The function of Urination is one which notoriously belongs to the voluntary class, in so far as it is initiated or arrested by a voluntary impulse, and it is one which, according to the classic teaching, has its centre in the brain. The grounds on which this cerebral centre is assigned are very similar to those on which other functions are assigned to cerebral centres, namely, observation of the suppression of the function when the pathway between certain organs and the brain is interrupted. But the careful experiments of Goltz * have demonstrated that the "centre" of Urination is not in the brain, but in the lower region of the cord. When

* *Pflüger's Archiv*, Bde. viii. and ix.

the cord is completely divided, Urination is performed in the *normal* way—not passively, not irregularly, but with all the characters of the active regular function. And, what is also noticeable, this function is so intimately dependent on Sensibility that it will be arrested—like any other function —by a sensation excited from the periphery—to be resumed when the irritation ceases. Now this arrest from a stimulation of sensory nerves takes place when the brain is cut off from the spinal centre, just as when the brain is in connection with it.

The same is true of Defecation, and the still more complex functions of Generation and Parturition. I can only refer the reader to the very remarkable case of Goltz's bitch with the spinal cord divided in the lumbar region, if evidence be wanted for the performance of complex functions so long as the spinal centres were intact. It is true that Goltz considers these functions to have been independent of *sensation;* but that is because he has not entirely emancipated himself from the traditional views; for my purpose it is enough that he admits the functions to be dependent on sensorial processes.

83. To sum up the evidence, we may say that observation discloses a surprising resemblance in the manifestations of the cord and brain. In both there are reflex processes, and processes of arrest; in both there are actions referable to conscious and unconscious processes; in both depression and exaltation are produced by the same drugs; in both there are manifestations interpretable, as those of Discrimination, Logic, Instinct, Volition, Acquisition, Memory; in both there is manifestation of Sensibility—how then can we deny Sensation to the one if we accord it to the other?

CHAPTER IV.

NEGATIVE INDUCTIONS.

84. I FANCY some reader exclaiming: "All your reasoning, and all your marshalled facts, are swept away by the irresistible evidence of human patients with injured spinal cords, whose legs have manifested reflex actions, and who nevertheless declared they had *no sensation whatever* in them. We can never be sure of what passes in an animal; but man can tell us whether he feels an impression, or does not feel it; and since he tells us that he does not feel it, *cannot*, however he may *try*, we conclude that reflex action may take place without sensation."

As this is the one solitary fact which is held to negative the mass of evidence, anatomical and physiological, in favour of the Sensibility of the spinal cord, it is necessary that we should candidly examine it. No reader will suppose that during the twenty years in which I have advocated the doctrine expounded in this volume I have not been fully alive to the one fact which prevented the general acceptance of the doctrine. From the first it has seemed to me that the fact has been misinterpreted.

85. Certain injuries to the spinal cord destroy the connection of the parts below the injury with the parts above it; consequently no impression made on the limbs below the injured spot is transmitted to the brain, nor can any cerebral incitation reach those limbs. The patient has lost all conciousness of these limbs, and all control over them. Hunter's patient on being asked if he felt any pain when the prick caused his leg to kick, answered, "No: but you see my leg

does." This answer has been regarded as a drollery; I think it expressed a physiological truth. For on the assumption that the whole of the cerebro-spinal axis had one uniform *property*, corresponding with its uniform structure, and various *functions*, corresponding with the variety of organs it innervates, a division of this axis would necessarily create two independent seats of Sensibility, and interrupt the consensus of their functions. In such a case it would be absurd to expect that the cerebral segment could be affected by, or co-operate with, what affected the spinal segment.

Now, when a man has a diseased spinal cord, the seat of injury causes, for the time at least, a division of the whole group of centres into two independent groups. For all purposes of sensation and volition it is the same as if he were cut in half; his nervous mechanism *is* cut in half. How then can any cerebral control be obeyed by his legs; how can any impression on his legs be felt by his cerebrum? As well might we expect the man whose arm has been amputated, to feel the incisions of the scalpel, when that limb is conveyed to the dissecting-table, as to feel by his brain impressions made upon parts wholly divorced from organic connection with the brain.

86. But, it may be objected, this is the very point urged. The man himself does not feel the impressions on his legs when his spine has been injured; he is as insensible to them as to the dissection of his amputated arm. Very true. *He* does not feel it. But if the amputated arm were to strike the anatomist who began its dissection, if its fingers were to grasp the scalpel, and push it away, or with the thumb to rub off the acid irritating one of the fingers, I do not see how we could refuse to admit that the *arm* felt although the *man* did not. And this is the case with the extremities of a man whose spine is injured. *They* manifest every indication of sensibility. In the frog and pigeon the legs manifest the unmistakable control which we ascribe to volition. It is true that the man himself, when interrogated, declares that he feels nothing; the cerebral segment has attached to it organs of speech and expressive features, by which *its* sensations can be communicated to others; whereas the spinal segment has *no* such means of communicating *its* sensations; but those which it *has*, it *employs*. You can ask the cerebral segment a question, which can be heard, understood, and answered; this is not the case with the spinal segment; yet if you *test* its sensibility, the result is unequivocal. You cannot ask an animal whether it feels, but you can test its sensibility, and that test suffices.

87. The question we have to decide, therefore, is not whether a patient, with an injured spine, can feel impressions on, or convey voluntary impulses to, limbs below the seat of injury—for as respects the nervous mechanism these limbs are separated from him, no less than if actual amputation had taken place—the question is, whether these separated limbs have any sensibility? And the answer seems to me unequivocally affirmative. I assert, therefore, that if there is ample evidence to show that the spinal centres have sensibility, when separated from the cerebral centres, such evidence can in no respect be weakened by the fact that a man with an injured spine is unconscious of impressions made below the seat of injury; since such a fact necessarily follows from the establishment of two centres: the parts above are then not sensitive to impressions on the parts below; nor are the parts below sensitive to impressions on the parts above; but each segment is sensitive to its own affections.

88. Every one knows that there are animals, low down in the scale, which may be cut in two, each half continuing to live, and each capable of reproducing its lost segments. Would any one, seeing these separated halves move and manifest ordinary signs of Sensibility, venture to say that the one half was a living, the other an insentient, mechanism? And since the one half had eyes, mouth, tentacles, &c., while the other half had none of these, would the observer be surprised that the functions of the one differed from those of the other in these respects? Why, then, should he not conclude the same of the two halves of the human mechanism, when disease had divided them?

89. The man, you urge, does not feel the prick on his leg. This is true, because "the man" here designates the seeing, hearing, tasting, smelling, talking, thinking group of organs —to the exclusion of the limb or limbs which are no longer in sensitive connection with this group. When a leg is amputated "the man" remains—a truncated man, indeed, yet still one having all the distinguishing human characters. Yet obviously in strict language we can no longer say that the man is the *same* as he was. "Man" or "animal" means the complex whole; and each anatomically separable part forms one constituent of that whole. The medulla oblongata and spinal cord innervate certain parts; the mesencephalon innervates others; the cerebrum rises above the whole. If after removing one limb, then another, we continued truncating the organism till we left only the head, should we call *that* the man? Clearly not. Should we even suppose that the intact brain—the supposed seat of sensation and volition—still felt, and willed? Clearly not. There is absolutely no evidence, however faint, of the isolated head manifesting any sensational and volitional phenomena; whereas there is ample evidence of the truncated spinal cord manifesting some of these phenomena. And this is intelligible when we understand that the nerve-centres stimulate into action the organs they innervate, but do not by themselves play any other part.

90. "The man" then does not feel the prick on his leg, but his leg feels it. The man has no consciousness of what takes place outside the sphere of his sensitive mechanism; and the leg is now outside that sphere. Consciousness —as distinguished from Sentience in general—we have seen to be a resultant of the composition of forces co-operating at the moment; the Sensibility of the spinal cord in the regions below the injury cannot *now* enter into that composition. It is detached from the upper organs. But inasmuch as the organs it innervates are still living and active, the functions of this detached portion are still displayed. We have seen the dog with divided cord capable of Urination,

Defecation, Generation, &c.; its hinder legs, though not moving in a consensus with the forelegs, yet moved independently; and all the normal reflexes of the parts followed on stimulations. To say that "the dog" showed no signs of Sensibility when its hinder limbs were irritated, is identifying "the dog" with the anterior half of the organism which was not in connection with the posterior half. It is equally true that the posterior half showed no signs of Sensibility when the anterior was irritated. The two halves were united by the circulation, nutrition, &c., but disunited as to sensation and volition.

91. Do I then suppose the separated half of an animal to feel pain and pleasure, hope and terror? The reader who has attentively followed the exposition will be at no loss to answer. Pain, pleasure, hope, and terror, are special modes of Sensibility, dependent on particular neural combinations. The organs comprised in the anterior half of the animal furnish the main conditions for these special modes, whereas the organs comprised in the posterior half furnish few or none of those—they contain none of the special Senses, and they are without the chief combining centre, the brain. But since we know that a large amount of normal Sensation is wholly without the special characters of pain, pleasure, hope, or terror, we need not hesitate to assign Sensation to the spinal cord because these characters are absent.

92. All I contend for is that the spinal centres have Sensibility of the same *order* as the cerebral centres; and that in the normal organism this Sensibility enters as a factor into the general Consciousness—no one portion of the nervous system being really independent of all the others, all co-operating in every result. Over and over again I have had to insist that the property of Sensibility is only the general condition of Sensation; and that each particular sensation receives its *character* from the organs innervated, *plus* the reaction of the whole organism. Obviously, therefore, the peculiar character of a sensation, or "state of consciousness," must vary with the variations in either of these factors. To say that every

segment of the spinal cord has Sensibility, is not saying that an excitation of that segment will produce a particular sensation of definite character; because for this definite character there is needed the co-operation of all those parts of the mechanism which enter into the complex product.

93. And here attention must be called to a double fallacy pervading the arguments on the other side. It is always assumed that the reactions of an organ, or part of the organism, when separated from the rest, are typical of their reactions when forming constituents of the normal organism. Nothing of the kind. The movement of a muscle or a limb separated from the body may resemble that movement when normally effected—but only as the movements of a mechanical bird resemble those of a living bird: the modes of production are different. So that were we to grant the postulate of the brain being the exclusive seat of sensation, we should still deny that an action which was effected after removal of the brain was typical of the action effected when the brain was present. The leg of Hunter's patient jerked when the skin was irritated; but this action could not be altogether the same as the similar action in a leg united with the rest of the sensitive mechanism. Nor is this all. The leg may have been insensible, the spinal segment which innervated it may have been wholly without Sensibility, and still we should have to question the logic which extended such an inference to the very different and far more complex actions of decapitated animals. On this ground:—The leg is, by the hypothesis, insensible because cut off from all connection with the sensitive mechanism. But this is not the case with the decapitated animal: there still remain the essential parts of a sensitive mechanism—all the chief organs are still in activity, still manifesting their functions. Decapitation has produced a great disturbance in the mechanism, and has removed an important centre; but nevertheless every impression excites a connected group of centres, and this group responds.

94. In conclusion, unless we adopt the opinion that Sensation—Consciousness—Sensibility, is something not belonging to the physiological properties of the nervous system in a vital organism (the opinion held by spiritualists), there seems no alternative but to adopt the opinion advocated in this volume, namely, that the physiological properties of the nervous system are inseparable from every segment of that system; and the functions are the manifestation of those properties as determined by the special organs with the co-operation of all.

THE END.

PRINTED BY BALLANTYNE, HANSON AND CO.
EDINBURGH AND LONDON.

Printed in Dunstable, United Kingdom

91220861R00288